Stroke Nursing

Second Edition

Stroke Nursing

Second Edition

Edited by

JANE WILLIAMS
Southern Health Foundation Trust
Southampton, UK

LIN PERRY
University of Technology Sydney
Northern Hospitals Network
South Eastern
Sydney Local Health District
Sydney, NSW, Australia

CAROLINE WATKINS
University of Central Lancashire
Preston, UK

WILEY Blackwell

Registered Office(s)
John Wiley & Sons, Inc., 111 River Street, Hoboken, NJ 07030, USA
John Wiley & Sons Ltd, The Atrium, Southern Gate, Chichester, West Sussex, PO19 8SQ, UK

Editorial Office
9600 Garsington Road, Oxford, OX4 2DQ, UK

For details of our global editorial offices, customer services, and more information about Wiley products visit us at www.wiley.com.

Wiley also publishes its books in a variety of electronic formats and by print-on-demand. Some content that appears in standard print versions of this book may not be available in other formats.

Library of Congress Cataloging-in-Publication Data

Names: Williams, Jane (Jane E.), editor. | Perry, Lin, editor. | Watkins, Caroline, editor.
Title: Stroke nursing / edited by Jane Williams, Lin Perry, Caroline Watkins.
Other titles: Acute stroke nursing
Description: Second edition. | Hoboken, NJ : Wiley-Blackwell, 2019. | Preceded by: Acute stroke nursing / edited by Jane Williams, Lin Perry, Caroline Watkins. 2010. | Includes bibliographical references and index. | Identifiers: LCCN 2018054706 (print) | LCCN 2018057605 (ebook) | ISBN 9781119111467 (AdobePDF) | ISBN 9781119111474 (ePub) | ISBN 9781119111450 (pbk.)
Subjects: | MESH: Stroke–nursing | Evidence-Based Nursing
Classification: LCC RC388.5 (ebook) | LCC RC388.5 (print) | NLM WY 152.5 | DDC 616.8/10231–dc23
LC record available at https://lccn.loc.gov/2018054706

Cover Design: Wiley
Cover Image: © KTSDESIGN/SCIENCE PHOTO LIBRARY/Getty Images

Set in 10/12pt Stix by SPi Global, Pondicherry, India
Printed in Singapore by C.O.S. Printers Pte Ltd

10 9 8 7 6 5 4 3 2 1

Contents

Editors and Contributors

Editors

Dr. Jane Williams

Jane Williams is Director for Transformation, Director of Transformation for physical health services based in Southern Health NHS Foundation Trust, Southampton, UK. She spent 20 years, until 2014, developing the stroke service in Portsmouth. During this time, Jane was involved in many national working parties, including the National Stroke Strategy, UK Forum for Stroke Training, and UK Stroke Forum. Jane has been a member of The Stroke Association research awards committee. A founder member of the National Stroke Nursing Forum, Jane undertook a term of office as chair.

Jane's current role is based in a large community health organisation which provides services across physical, mental health, and learning disabilities both in people's own homes and in bed-based services. The current foci of her work include development of new models for community health services, integration of intermediate care services, and how clinicians can use activation to support their own practice whilst supporting patients with health behaviour change techniques.

Professor Lin Perry

Lin Perry is Professor of Nursing Research and Practice Development, University of Technology Sydney and the Northern Hospitals Network, South Eastern Sydney Local Health District, Sydney, NSW, Australia. She has a specialist interest in chronic conditions, practice, and service development, particularly in relation to knowledge translation and change management for frontline staff. A past member of the Intercollegiate Stroke Working Party in the UK and current member of the Stroke Foundation Guidelines Working Party and Stroke Network, New South Wales Agency for Clinical Innovation in Australia, she has extensive experience with national guideline development, benchmarking, service review, and evaluation.

Professor Dame Caroline Watkins

Dame Caroline Watkins is Professor of Stroke and Older People's Care, Director of Research and Innovation, Faculty of Health & Wellbeing, University of Central Lancashire, Director of Lancashire Clinical Trials Unit, and Director of Lancashire research Institute For global health and wellbeing (LIFE), Preston, UK. She is Chair of the UK Stroke Forum. Her multidisciplinary team of researchers have a large portfolio of clinically relevant stroke research and contribute to stroke service development locally, nationally and internationally. Caroline's Services to Nursing and Older People's Care were recognised with the award of the DBE in the New Year Honours 2017.

Contributors

Professor Anne W. Alexandrov, Professor and Program Director for NET SMART at the Health Outcomes Institute, Fountain Hills, AZ, USA; a Professor of Nursing and a Professor of Neurology at the University of Tennessee Health Science Center at Memphis, Memphis, TN, USA; and the Chief Nurse Practitioner of the University of Tennessee – Memphis Mobile Stroke Unit, Memphis, TN, USA

Dr. Munirah Bangee, Research Associate, Faculty of Health & Wellbeing, University of Central Lancashire, Preston, UK

Dr. Elizabeth Boaden, Senior Research Fellow, School of Nursing, University of Central Lancashire, Preston, UK

Professor Dominique Cadilhac, Head of Translational Public Health and Evaluation Division in Stroke and Ageing Research, School of Clinical Sciences, Monash University, Clayton, VIC, Australia and Head of Public Health, Stroke Division, Florey Institute of Neuroscience and Mental Health, Parkville, VIC, Australia

Dr. Madeline Cruice, Reader/Associate Professor, School of Health Sciences, City, University of London, London, UK

Professor Kathryn Getliffe, Previously Professor of Nursing, School of Nursing and Midwifery, University of Southampton, Southampton, UK (now retired)

Dr. Josephine Gibson, Reader in Health Services Research, School of Nursing, University of Central Lancashire, Preston, UK

Clare Gordon, Consultant Nurse, Stroke Services, Royal Bournemouth and Christchurch Hospitals NHS Foundation Trust, Bournemouth, UK

Kirsty Harrison, Senior Lecturer, School of Health Sciences, City, University of London, London, UK

Professor Katerina Hilari, Professor of Acquired Communication Disorders, School of Health Sciences, City, University of London, London, UK

Dr. Stephanie Jones, Senior Research Fellow, School of Nursing, University of Central Lancashire, Preston, UK

Vicky Kean, Advanced Nurse Practitioner, George Eliot Hospital NHS Trust, Nuneaton, UK

Dr. Cherry Kilbride, Senior Lecturer in Physiotherapy, Brunel University London, London, UK and Lead Therapist, Research and Practice Development, Royal Free London NHS Foundation Trust, London, UK

Dr. Peter Knapp, Senior Lecturer in Evidence-based Decision Making, Department of Health Sciences & the Hull York Medical School, University of York, York, UK

Dr. Rosie Kneafsey, Head of School for Nursing, Midwifery and Health, Coventry University, Coventry, UK

Professor Diana Lee, Professor of Nursing, The Nethersole School of Nursing; Director of the Y.K. Pao Foundation Centre for Nursing Excellence in Chronic Illness Care; and Deputy Director of the CUHK Jockey Club Institute of Ageing at the The Chinese University of Hong Kong

Dr. Elizabeth Lightbody, Reader in Health Services Research, Faculty of Health & Wellbeing, University of Central Lancashire, Preston, UK

Mary Lyons, Senior Lecturer in Public Health, Liverpool School of Tropical Medicine, Liverpool, UK; and Senior Research Fellow, University of Central Lancashire, Preston, UK

Professor Jane Marshall, Professor, Division of Language and Communication Science, School of Health Sciences, City, University of London, London, UK

Professor Sandy Middleton, Professor of Nursing and Director of the Nursing Research Institute, a joint collaboration between St Vincent's Health Australia (Sydney) and Australian Catholic University, Syndey, NSW, Australia

Dr. Elaine Pierce, Independent Lecturer and Researcher

Associate Professor Julie Pryor, Nursing Research & Development Leader, Royal Rehab, Sydney, NSW, Australia and Clinical Associate Professor, University of Sydney, Sydney, NSW, Australia

Dr. Judith Redfern[†], Senior Research Fellow, School of Nursing, University of Central Lancashire, Preston, UK

Dr. Clare Thetford, Senior Research Fellow, Faculty of Health & Wellbeing, University of Central Lancashire, Preston, UK

Dr. Lois Thomas, Reader in Health Services Research, School of Health Sciences, University of Central Lancashire, Preston, UK

[†]Judith Redfern sadly lost her battle with cancer in February 2018, prior to the publication of this book. Judith started her research career in 1993 as a student working at the Home Office on the British Crime Survey. After graduating in Mathematics and Psychology, she moved into health services research. Her first research post was at University College London, working with Ann Bowling on a study into the appropriateness of outpatient care in the North Thames region. Judith has made an important contribution to the field of stroke since 1999, including a national study into the longer-term needs of stroke survivors. Jude joined the University of Central Lancashire in 2013 and was a Senior Research Fellow until her death in February 2018. During this time, she contributed to various research outputs, including the development of the Stroke Patient Concerns Inventory.

Foreword: Stroke Nursing

Stroke has become a recognised nursing specialty worldwide, supported by practice standards that blend nursing knowledge and clinical skills in both neurovascular and cardiovascular physiology [1]. The challenge and responsibility that we accept when caring for stroke patients requires acknowledgment of their highly vulnerable physiological and psychological states, for we provide care at a most fearful time in patients' lives. The disruption to family dynamics and their social, economic and spiritual needs are substantial.

There is much we can offer patients for primary prevention, rapid diagnosis, treatment, complication avoidance, rehabilitation, and secondary prevention. However, many factors limit provision of 'state of the science' stroke care. System and economic factors limit availability of stroke resources in some centres, including: lack of access to sophisticated imaging techniques to diagnose stroke and determine pathogenic mechanism, or inability to provide timely reperfusion treatment. Workforce factors may mean nursing, physician, and therapy specialists best equipped to diagnose, treat and prevent stroke are not available. Political and geospatial factors may result in stroke patients being taken to the nearest, rather than best, comprehensive facility. Finally, human factors may limit patients' and families' understanding and acceptance of risk factors, preventative medicine, and early notification of emergency personnel.

As nurses, we try to understand how these factors affect our ability to offer patients high-quality evidence-based care. Discomfort with our programs' limitations motivates us to generate powerful advocacy strategies to increase awareness and build consensus in support of program improvement. As exciting advancements in nursing and healthcare emerge, we must use our dissatisfaction when particular evidence-supported methods are unavailable in our workplaces, cities, or countries, and ask, 'Why not?'

This text will prepare nurses new to stroke practice and further the knowledge and skills of current stroke nurses. Readers will learn evidence-based nursing and medical care supported by research generated across the world. As you read, I encourage you to perform a self-inventory of content that you have yet to master, and consider the gaps in the stroke systems of care (diagnosis, treatment, prevention, and rehabilitation) at your facility. Consider what you can do to improve your own care and that of your interdisciplinary peers, and actively work towards achievement of best practice.

To accept the role of 'stroke nurse' is an honour and a privilege. We are the most trusted health professions by patients and families [2, 3], the most numerous of all healthcare providers, and well-positioned as key drivers of healthcare quality. I hope that you will accept this responsibility and use this text to support your stroke nursing journey.

Professor Anne W. Alexandrov
PhD, RN, AGACNP-BC, ANVP-BC, NVRN-BC, CCRN, FAAN
University of Tennessee Health Science Center at Memphis, Memphis, TN, USA

References

1. The Association of Neurovascular Clinicians. Scope and standards for neurovascular nursing 2018. Available from: www.anvc.org. [30 November 2018]
2. Gallup. Honesty/ethics in professions 2017. Available from: http://news.gallup.com/poll/1654/honesty-ethics-professions.aspx. [30 November 2018]
3. American Nurses Association. Nurses rank as most honest, ethical profession for 14th straight year 2015. Available from: https://www.prnewswire.com/news-releases/nurses-rank-as-most-honest-ethical-profession-for-14th-straight-year-300195781.html [30 November 2018]

Foreword: Stroke Services in Australia

In Australia, as elsewhere globally, stroke is a leading cause of death and disability [1] and optimal management is imperative. Provision of care for stroke patients in dedicated units by a coordinated multidisciplinary team is a pivotal strategy for improving patient outcomes [2]. This evidence has underpinned health reforms for hospitalised stroke patients worldwide. Data from the 2017 Stroke Foundation national audit showed 89% of Australian hospitals (with ≥75 people with acute stroke admitted annually) have a stroke unit (Kevin Hill, pers. comm., 18 April 2018) [3]. However, access to stroke unit care is not guaranteed; only 69% of stroke patients admitted to audited hospitals with a stroke unit received treatment on that unit [3]. The national thrombolysis rate is low (13%), but some hospitals achieve thrombolysis rates of up to 23% [3]. This demonstrates a major challenge for Australia – provision of equitable access to care. Australian stroke units are primarily (92%) in urban locations rather than rural settings, potentially disadvantaging non-metropolitan inhabitants [4]. However, 'hub and spoke' models, where larger stroke services provide coordinated care across a defined geographic region [5], are promising as support strategies for smaller rural hospitals.

Nationally, initiatives are informing and supporting improvements in the quality and planning of Australia's acute stroke services. The Stroke Foundation has developed a National Acute Stroke Services Framework [5], providing recommendations and definitions for general hospital and stroke specialist services. This is informed and supported by Australian Clinical Guidelines for Stroke Management [6]. In 2015, the Australian Commission on Safety and Quality in Health Care launched the Acute Stroke Clinical Care Standard [7]. Developed in consultation with consumers, clinicians, researchers, and health organisations, and consisting of seven quality statements and measurable indicators, the standard aims to improve early assessment and management of stroke, including initiation of an individualised rehabilitation plan. Collection of data for the stroke standard is not currently mandatory, but data for these key stroke processes of care could drive practice change.

Collection of reliable, nationally comparable data is imperative to drive clinical practice change. The Stroke Foundation organises alternate-year clinical audits which enable benchmarking across states for key stroke processes of care. In 2015, the Australian Stroke Coalition launched the Australian Stroke Data Tool (AuSDAT), underpinned by a national stroke data dictionary. AuSDaT is an online data collection tool for stroke clinical performance monitoring and improvement and is the method of data collection for the Australian Stroke Clinical Registry (AuSCR). Established in 2009, AuSCR is a collaborative national stroke registry collecting prospective stroke data, using a minimum data set of four key stroke indicators (eight in Queensland), to monitor, promote, and improve the quality of acute stroke care nationally. Importantly, AuSCR collects follow-up data at 90–180 days post-stroke and is linked with the National Death Index, providing mortality data and patient outcomes [8]. Data from the Stroke Foundation audit and AuSCR have been used to improve the quality of Australian stroke care [9].

Australian nurses play a pivotal role in the delivery of high-quality acute stroke care [10]. Education and research are two important factors in the delivery of evidence-based care. The Acute Stroke Nursing Education Network (established in 2013) facilitates the delivery of evidence-based acute stroke care by providing educational networking opportunities for stroke clinicians. This network runs regular webinars on clinically relevant topics for acute stroke nurses [11]. Australia has a thriving multidisciplinary stroke research community. Many stroke units throughout the country are involved in multi-centre, national and international clinical trials and research projects aimed at improving stroke services. Importantly for nurses, since publication of the first edition of this book, results from the Quality in Acute Stroke Care (QASC) Trial have been published. This landmark trial demonstrated the key role of nurse-led management of fever, hyperglycaemia, and swallowing difficulties and the consequent significant reduction of death and dependency when nurses do these 'simple' things well [12–14].

Excitingly for stroke nursing, in recent years several stroke nurse practitioners have graduated in Australia. 'Nurse practitioner' is a protected title in Australia and only available to those with an approved nurse practitioner qualification at Masters degree level who demonstrate advanced nursing practice in a clinical leadership role in a particular area of practice. These senior clinical nurses will have a pivotal role in shaping future stroke services, including new models of nurse-led care.

Australia has well-developed support for stroke survivors in the form of local state-based organisations and networks and the Stroke Foundation, working together to improve stroke care. This book sets out in detail what excellence in stroke nursing looks like. It makes a unique and essential contribution to dissemination of evidence-based practice and promotes improvements to stroke nursing care internationally.

Professor Sandy Middleton RN PhD
Professor of Nursing and Director, Nursing Research Institute
St Vincent's Health Australia (Sydney) and
Australian Catholic University, Sydney, NSW, Australia

References

1. Australian Institute of Health and Welfare (2013). Stroke and its Management in Australia: An Update. Canberra: Australian Institute of Health and Welfare.
2. Trialists'Collaboration SU (2013). Organised inpatient (stroke unit) care for stroke. Cochrane Database Systematic Review. (9): (Art. No. CD000197).
3. Stroke Foundation (2017). National Stroke Audit Acute Services Report. Melbourne: National Stroke Foundation.
4. National Stroke Foundation (2013). National Stroke Audit Acute Services – Organisational Survey. Melbourne: National Stroke Foundation.
5. National Stroke Foundation (2015). National Acute Stroke Services- Framework. Melbourne: National Stroke Foundation.

6. Stroke Foundation (2017). Clinical Guidelines for Stroke Management. Melbourne: Melbourne Stroke Foundation.

7. Australian Commission on Safety and Quality in Health Care (2015). Acute Stroke Clinical Care Standard. Sydney: Australian Commission on Safety and Quality in Health Care.

8. Cadhilac, D.A., Lannin, N.A., Anderson, C.S. et al. (2014). The Australian Stroke Clinical Registry Annual Report 2013. Victoria: The Florey Institute of Neuroscience and Mental Health.

9. Cadilhac, D.A., Andrew, N.E., Salama, E. et al. (2015). Improving discharge from hospital after stroke: a focus on prevention medication and discharge planning. International Journal of Stroke 10 (S3): 10.

10. Middleton, S., Grimley, R., and Alexandrov, A.W. (2015). Triage, treatment, and transfer. Evidence-based clinical practice recommendations and models of nursing care for the first 72 hours of admission to hospital for acute stroke. Stroke 46 (2): e18–e25.

11. Acute Stroke Nurses Education Network. ASNEN: Acute Stroke Nurses Education Network. Available from: www.asnen.org. [30 November 2018]

12. Middleton, S., McElduff, P., Ward, J. et al. (2011). Implementation of evidence-based treatment protocols to manage fever, hyperglycaemia, and swallowing dysfunction in acute stroke (QASC): a cluster randomised controlled trial. The Lancet 378 (9804): 1699–1706.

13. Middleton, S. (2012). Doing the simple things well. Collegian 19 (2): 65–66.

14. Middleton, S., Coughlan, K., Mnatzaganian, G. et al. (2017). Mortality reduction for fever, hyperglycemia, and swallowing nurse-initiated stroke intervention: QASC Trial (Quality in Acute Stroke Care) Follow-Up. Stroke 48 (5): 1331–1336.

Foreword: Stroke Care in Hong Kong

In Hong Kong, stroke is the fourth commonest cause of death [1], with at least 20,000 people becoming paralysed or losing their functional abilities as a result each year [2]. Death and disability from stroke will increase as the population rapidly ages in the coming decades.

Over 90% of Hong Kong stroke patients are managed in public hospitals. As elsewhere, acute stroke management depends largely on effective intervention within hospitals where organised care is provided by stroke units, using standardised stroke orders and integrated stroke pathways managed by multidisciplinary professionals. Stroke units are effective in reducing stroke mortality, increasing the proportion of patients returning home at six weeks, and reducing the need for institutional care [3]. Since 2016, 15 acute stroke units (260 beds) have been set up in acute public hospitals, which enhance acute stroke management so that patients benefit from early intervention [4]. However, access to these units is not always assured, as these 260 beds are serving over 90% of Hong Kong's 7.3 million population. Three acute stroke units have been provided with upgraded facilities to become referral centres for acute stroke patients from across Hong Kong.

The use of thrombolytic treatment in managing acute ischaemic stroke was conservative until the early 2010s [5]. This was due to a reported higher rate of intracranial haemorrhage from thrombolysis because of racial differences [6] and a lack of resources in our public health system. To facilitate neurologists' remote thrombolysis assessment during non-working hours, a Security-Enhanced Mobile Imaging Distribution System (SEMIDS) was introduced in 2012. Based on this telestroke system, 24-hour thrombolytic services have been implemented in most hospitals, resulting in a threefold increase in stroke patients receiving thrombolysis. SEMIDS thrombolytic service relieves the local shortage of neurologists and has greatly improved healthcare for acute stroke patients [7]. Prompt recognition of stroke and rapid access to appropriate treatment are critical in improving stroke outcomes. Fast-track Transient Ischaemic Attack (TIA) Priority Clinics have also been set up to provide timely treatment for mild stroke patients and reduce the risk of neurological events through multidisciplinary collaboration.

Reliable, comparable, and up-to-date data are imperative to improving practice and the quality of stroke care. While a Hong Kong city-wide stroke data bank is not yet available, the Hospital Authority (HA), which manages all of Hong Kong's public hospitals, has maintained a computerised 'Clinical Management System' (CMS) for clinical management since 1999. As over 90% of all hospital stroke admissions are to hospitals run by the HA, the clinical data for these patients are captured in the CMS database. A territory-wide 'Electronic Health Record' (eHR) has also been developed (2009) by the HA to enhance access to and sharing of participating patients' health data by authorised healthcare providers in the public and private sectors. This has enhanced our endeavours to continuously improve service quality and safety for stroke care.

Nurses in Hong Kong play a critical role in all phases of stroke care. Nurse-led TIA clinics, stroke clinics, and transition care programmes for discharged stroke survivors provide stroke care and management from initial evaluation and diagnostic workup through to rehabilitation. When nurse consultants were established in the HA (2009), stroke nurse consultants were also appointed. Whilst these consultants have a clinical leadership role to promote nurse-led stroke care, the development is in its infancy, as only a few have been appointed since 2009.

In Hong Kong, and other Asian regions (e.g. China, Korea, and Japan), improvement in stroke care has paradoxically increased the number of stroke survivors. Most stroke survivors need long-term preventive medicine, intense rehabilitation, and caregiver support. In Hong Kong, there is active participation of public institutions, charity funds, non-government organisations, and professional organisations in promoting public awareness and improving local stroke services and rehabilitation. The Hong Kong Neurological Society and the Hong Kong Stroke Society, for example, have developed guidelines and protocols on many aspects of the general management of stroke patients from admission to rehabilitation. These guidelines are used by professionals in both public and private hospitals. A wide range of innovative rehabilitation services (i.e. use of video games, music therapy, and robots) have been piloted by different professional stroke organisations and non-government organisations.

One salient feature of Hong Kong's stroke care is the integration of Chinese and Western medicine in stroke treatment and rehabilitation. Local research has found that the use of integrative medicine, which includes the basic treatment of Western medicine and routine rehabilitation in conjunction with acupuncture and Chinese medicine, improves stroke patient outcomes [8]. Since 2014, the HA has developed the Integrated Chinese-Western Medicine (ICWM) programme for three disease areas, including stroke rehabilitation. With this programme, Chinese medicinal treatment options, including acupuncture, cupping therapy, tui na, and herbal medicine, have been introduced at an earlier stage for stroke patients in public hospitals.

As in other developed cities, one-third of the stroke sufferers in Hong Kong are less than 65 years old, and numbers are increasing in younger people [1]. Primary prevention by promoting healthy lifestyle changes and screening individuals for known risk factors will continue to be a key mechanism for reducing the burden of stroke in the wider Hong Kong community. However, Hong Kong is yet to develop a well-established policy or territory-wide primary care network or programme capable of effectively achieving these aims.

This book, a unique stroke nursing text, provides a stimulus for nurses to anchor stroke care in the reality of life in the acute stroke wards and in the community of the stroke survivors and caregivers. This work is significant, not only because it recognises the complexity and delicacy of stroke care, but also because it makes explicit the depth of knowledge and understanding necessary for such care provision. The precepts of this excellent book could both illuminate and ultimately change stroke care practice. It is essential reading for all nurses, not just for stroke care nurse specialists.

Professor Diana Lee PhD RN FAAN JP
Professor of Nursing, The Nethersole School of Nursing
Director, Y.K. Pao Foundation Centre for Nursing
Excellence in Chronic Illness Care
Deputy Director, CUHK Jockey Club Institute of Ageing
The Chinese University of Hong Kong

References

1. Department of Health (2015). Health Facts of Hong Kong. Hong Kong: Department of Health.
2. Yu, R., Chau, P.H., McGhee, S.M. et al. (2012). Trends of Disease Burden Consequent to Stroke in Older Persons in Hong Kong: Implications of Population Ageing. Hong Kong: The Hong Kong Jockey Club.
3. Ko Kwai, F. and Sheppard, L. (2006). The contribution of a comprehensive stroke unit to the outcome of Chinese stroke patients. Singapore Medical Journal 47 (3): 2008–2212.
4. Information Services Department (2016). Hong Kong: The Facts. Hong Kong: The Information Services Department.
5. Wong, G.K.C., Tam, Y.Y.W., Zhu, X.L.Z., and Poon, W.S. (2014). Incidence and mortality of spontaneous subarachnoid hemorrhage in Hong Kong from 2002 to 2010: a Hong Kong hospital authority clinical management system database analysis. World Neurosurgery 81 (3–4): 552–556.
6. Ueshima, S. and Matsuo, O. (2002). The differences in thrombolytic effects of administrated recombinant t-PA between Japanese and Caucasians. Thrombosis and Haemostasis 87 (3): 544–546.
7. Chan, E. (2012). Thrombolytic service of acute ischaemic stroke in Hong Kong. Hong Kong Medical Journal 18 (2): 170.
8. Fang, J., Chen, L., Chen, L. et al. (2014). Integrative medicine for subacute stroke rehabilitation: a study protocol for a multicentre, randomised controlled trial. British Medical Journal Open 4 (12): 1–7.

Acknowledgements

We would like to acknowledge the chapter authors of the previous edition, Michael Leathley, Chris Burton, Wendy Brooks, Aeron Ginnelly, Sheila Payne, Peter Humphrey, Louise Brereton, Jill Manthorpe, and Graham Williamson, who were no longer involved in this edition.

The editors would also like to acknowledge the editorial support team: Kerry Hanna, Alison Doherty, Naoimh McMahon, and Kateryna McDonald.

CHAPTER 1

Setting the Scene

Caroline Watkins[1] and Dominique Cadilhac[2,3]
[1] University of Central Lancashire, Preston, UK
[2] School of Clinical Sciences, Monash University, Clayton, VIC, Australia
[3] Stroke Division, Florey Institute of Neuroscience and Mental Health, Parkville, VIC, Australia

KEY POINTS

- Transforming stroke services is of paramount importance in the quest to save lives and reduce dependency.
- Translating research evidence into clinical practice is challenging but many examples show that this is both achievable and worthwhile.
- Continued development of stroke nursing through expansion of the stroke nursing knowledge base and demonstration of competence and skill is pivotal to the future of the specialism.
- Continued development of stroke nursing is essential for development of stroke services, locally, nationally, and internationally.

1.1 Introduction

Internationally, stroke – and its impact on people's lives – is finally gaining the recognition it deserves, not only as an acute event and a chronic disease, but also as a preventable condition. The profile of stroke has more recently increased because a greater number of effective treatments, including those for prevention, have become available, and mechanisms for implementation have been established. However, in order to make these treatments available for everyone who might benefit, it is imperative that the public knows about, and has a heightened awareness of, stroke risk factors and stroke symptoms.

Public awareness campaigns are planned to raise the profile of modifiable stroke risk factors: smoking, hypertension, and atrial fibrillation, amongst others. Public campaigns for recognising the signs of stroke have been graphically driving home the message that if a stroke is suspected, the emergency medical services should be contacted. Emergency services must respond rapidly and get patients to centres providing specialist acute-stage treatments, ongoing rehabilitation, and long-term support. Throughout this care pathway, best-available treatment can only be provided if staff have stroke-specific knowledge and skills commensurate with their roles, and if all agencies involved work collaboratively, providing a seamless journey for the person affected by stroke. Nurses are the largest section of the workforce, and are involved throughout the entire stroke care pathway. Consequently, nurses have the greatest opportunity to play a primary role in providing leadership and ensuring the delivery of evidence-based stroke care.

The focus of this chapter is to describe the importance of stroke nursing in the context of wider systems. The extent of the problem of stroke is illustrated, and the reason stroke has become a burning issue for healthcare and research is explored. Policy imperatives are discussed, as well as the present and future of stroke-specific infrastructure. Importantly, the need to support stroke service developments and put in place mechanisms to produce evidence for practice is outlined, and how evidence can be implemented into practice is clarified. Fundamental to delivery of this huge agenda is the development of a stroke-specialist workforce. Staff delivering care along the stroke pathway need the right knowledge, skills, and experience in stroke, and should achieve recognition for it. Suitable recognition for specialising in stroke care should ensure that the most able staff pursue rewarding careers in stroke care. This then should establish a virtuous circle, whereby able staff stay in the speciality and contribute further to advancing the field, including delivery of sustainable quality improvements into the future. Staff can then also participate in ongoing audits of care, reflection on performance, and instigation of further improvements, and thus constantly drive up the quality of care.

1.2 Stroke Epidemiology

Stroke is a major cause of mortality and morbidity in adults. Globally, it is the second leading cause of disease burden after ischaemic heart disease given the combined effects of premature death and long-term disability [1]. In addition, over 90% of this stroke burden is attributed to modifiable risk factors, with about 74% being associated with behavioural factors such as smoking, poor diet, and physical inactivity [2]. Therefore, much could be done to reduce the incidence and prevalence of stroke. Crude incidence varies greatly amongst countries, according to both the different risk factor profiles and the timing of different studies. The reported age-adjusted incidence rates range from 54 per 100 000 population per year in Lagos, Nigeria (2007–2008) to 146 per 100 000 per year in Iwate, Japan (based on World Health Organization World standard population) [3]. Stroke incidence rates are generally greater in men that in women, and women will generally experience their stroke event at an older age. Greater mortality in women is mostly explained by age, but also by stroke severity, atrial fibrillation, and pre-stroke functional limitations [4]. Case-fatality rates within 28–30 days also range widely amongst countries, from about 10% in Dijon, France to 37% in rural Trivandrum, India [3].

Many countries are experiencing increases in life expectancy. Since age is the strongest factor contributing to stroke incidence, there are concerns that the numbers will rise and this will impact on the ability of the health systems to manage stroke effectively. Currently, trends are unclear, and further research is needed to understand what the future holds. Whilst stroke incidence may not increase, and may even decrease [5], it is clear that more people are surviving stroke and living with the sequelae [6]. Surviving with moderate to severe disability can have profound effects in all domains of life [7], and poor quality of life has been associated with greater unmet needs over the longer term. Whilst we want acute stroke interventions to improve survival rates, we also want them to ensure independent survival.

Importantly, we also need prevention interventions to be a priority, given that the overall global burden of stroke is substantial. Summary measures of population health capture both morbidity and mortality and are used to describe the burden of disease. These summary measures include Health Adjusted Life Expectancy (HALE), Disability Adjusted Life Years (DALYs), and Quality Adjusted Life Years (QALYs). The HALE value represents the number of expected years of life equivalent to years lived in full health adjusted for time spent in poor health, based on current rates of ill health (e.g. chronic disease) and mortality in a community. The DALY is a health gap measure and captures the years of life lost (YLL) due to premature mortality and the years of life lived with disability (YLD), for example as a consequence of experiencing stroke. QALYs are based on a similar conceptual framework (life expectancy plus quality of life), but assumptions and methods differ. In recent work to determine the health gap experienced by stroke survivors compared to the normal population, it was determined that the QALYs lost per first-ever stroke were about 5.09 for ischaemic stroke and 6.17 for intracerebral haemorrhage [8]. In other words, if a stroke was prevented, this represents the health gain that could be achieved on average per person.

1.3 Cost Burden

The costs of stroke are substantial, due to the complexity and chronic nature of this condition. The greatest costs incurred in the first year are associated with hospital care and rehabilitation [9]. Comparing results of cost-of-illness studies between countries is complicated due to the different methodological approaches, such as the types of costs included and the time horizon [10]. Since the costs of stroke peak within the first year and decline over time, it is important to quantify long-term resource use in order to gain a greater understanding of the potential lifetime impact on society. Furthermore, the direct costs of informal care and indirect costs of productivity losses (inability to work or perform important home duties) after stroke are often omitted, despite these costs being substantial. Using 10 years of follow-up data, the authors of the North East Melbourne Stroke Incidence study (Australia) estimated the average lifetime costs at US$68,769 for ischaemic stroke and US$54,956 for intracerebral haemorrhage in 2010 [11]. In other recent work undertaken in a more remote geographic Australian location, the lifetime costs of stroke were substantially larger (US$207,218), and the greatest costs were associated with patients who had an Indigenous background, renal disease, heart disease, or hypertension [12].

In contrast, 5-year costs per stroke in the United Kingdom have been reported as £29,405 in 2001–2002, if informal care was included [13]. In the United States, the average costs within 1 year of hospitalisation per stroke averaged US$47,790 in 2008 [14], and the lifetime health costs were estimated to be US$140,000 per patient with ischaemic stroke in 2010 [15, 16]. To contain the growing total costs of stroke and associated health expenditure, it is essential that cost-effective prevention and treatment policies are put in place. That is, the investment of healthcare funding is strategically used to maximise the potential health benefits that can be achieved at an acceptable cost to society. These costs are based on those of high-income countries (HICs), and as yet there is a dearth of evidence, not only of the costs of stroke care in low- and middle-income countries (LMICs), but also of the incidence and prevalence of stroke. Costs are also difficult to determine because of the lack of stroke specialist services; there are fewer than 50 stroke units in India, for example, where approximately 3,500 are required to serve this large population.

1.4 Stroke Policy

1.4.1 Developing Stroke as a Healthcare Priority

Over the last 20 years, much has been achieved – at least in HICs – in providing guidance on best-practice care and establishing methods of monitoring adherence to clinical guideline recommendations. Unfortunately, this work has shown repeatedly that eligible patients may not always receive recommended therapies even in well-resourced settings [17]. Information about underperformance against expected standards of care can be used to guide policy and practice decisions and to make improvements to health services [18]. In a recent Australian simulation study whereby average performance was modelled to meet achievable benchmarks established from the top-performing hospitals, it was found that considerable gains in health could be achieved at relatively low additional costs to the health system [17].

The World Stroke Organization has recently released guidelines and a quality action plan framework to inform stroke policy and set strategic directions to elevate standards of stroke care [19]. However, even in HICs, delivering equitable access to stroke services remains a challenge. Some of the issues include the lack of specialist staff, the cost of experienced staff, and the lack of basic infrastructure to support diagnostic investigations and rehabilitation in hospital [19]. To address this problem, in the United Kingdom, the National Stroke Strategy (NSS) [20] encouraged the introduction of acute stroke units in all hospitals (2007), and centralised Hyperacute Stroke Units have also been developed in at least eight hospitals. Further centralisation of services will follow the forthcoming National Stroke Plan (NSP) (due for publication in 2019), which will be driven by the need for thrombectomy services. In Australia, the Stroke Foundation developed an Acute Stroke Services Framework as part of a strategy to improve the quality of acute stroke services [21]. This framework describes the main features and minimum criteria for acute stroke units and recommends that all hospitals admitting more than 100 acute strokes per year have a stroke unit. There is evidence that adverse outcomes are more frequent where patients are treated in hospitals treating <50 strokes per year (low volume) compared to than in those treated in high-volume hospitals (100+ strokes per year) [22]. This recommendation was further strengthened using data from the Australian National Acute Services Audit, whereby hospitals treating 100 or more patients per year in a stroke unit were found to provide better care and to have fewer serious adverse patient outcomes than those managing similar numbers of patients without a stroke unit [23].

Within the United Kingdom, stroke has received increasing attention from professional healthcare providers and the government. A similar situation has been seen in Australia (see Foreword: Stroke Services in Australia). When the first National Sentinel Audit (NSA) was performed in 1998, it highlighted the poverty of stroke services. Amongst the biggest problems were the lack of stroke units and how few people were admitted to a stroke unit at some point during their hospital stay. This was particularly discouraging because the benefits of organised inpatient care had been known for over two decades [24, 25]. Not long after this first audit, the first edition of the National Clinical Guidelines for Stroke [26] was developed. From the start, guideline developers agreed that patients' views would be an important factor in determining how services should be run. Focus groups were used to elicit the experiences of those affected by stroke and their preferences and recommendations for service provision [27]. The guidelines give healthcare providers best-practice recommendations, underpinned by evidence from research or expert consensus, and incorporate the views of those affected by stroke. Both the NSA and the clinical guidelines have been important levers in the improvement of stroke care, demonstrating the influence that stroke metrics (data collection points) and clinician-led practice standards can achieve. The success of this model has led to its replication in Australia and other countries.

Key components of stroke care are assessment, management, and treatment, and evidence to underpin these has been used to produce and update the UK National Clinical Guidelines for Stroke [26, 28–31]. Concurrently, successive rounds of the NSA Intercollegiate Stroke Working Party, now the Sentinel Stroke National Audit Programme (SSNAP) [32], have revealed the relationship – and shortfalls – between evidence and practice. Overall, the judgement has been that response to suspected stroke has not been fast enough, either in terms of actions taken for an individual experiencing a stroke or in implementing into practice what scientific literature indicates should be done [33]. Despite some improvements, there remains much to be achieved [34]. Scientific advances are not consistently or rapidly translated into clinical practice, and it is estimated that implementation takes on average 17 years [35]. Some services have vastly improved, whilst others still lag behind. It is precisely this situation which has led to continued benchmarking of stroke services and the establishment of registries or audit programmes in many countries [36].

The SSNAP demonstrates these milestones still have not been fully met. Furthermore, it has taken time to ensure that all important milestones are recognised. Whilst the importance of reducing the time between symptom onset and arrival at hospital was raised in the addendum [37] to the Clinical Guidelines for Stroke (2004) [38], and Emergency Stroke Calls: Obtaining Rapid Telephone Triage (ESCORTT) results [39] have shown that recognition by call handlers can be improved, mechanisms to achieve national rollout have yet to be implemented. Whilst hospital trusts have been endeavouring to reduce door to needle times for intravenous (IV) thrombolysis, the ambulance service has yet to implement call-to-arrival time as a performance indicator [34]. Services should work together to identify opportunities to streamline the whole stroke pathway, and not just sections of it.

Between 2004 and 2005, the UK Stroke Association developed the Face, Arm, Speech Test (FAST) to raise public awareness of stroke [40]. The campaign was revised in 2009, with the 'T' now standing for time, emphasising the importance of rapid response. The campaign ran alongside a Department of Health public awareness campaign, also using FAST, through television and radio advertising. There were striking reductions in the time to both seeking and receiving medical attention after stroke in the United Kingdom coinciding with the start of the 2009 FAST TV campaign [41]. Similar impacts of public campaigns have also been reported in Australia, whereby awareness of stroke advertising increased 31–50% between 2004 and 2010, as did unprompted recall of two or more most common stroke warning signs (20–53%) [42]. Awareness of stroke advertising was independently associated with this recall, illustrating the value of public education efforts [42].

The potential value of such campaigns is great. Stroke has been calculated to cost the National Health Service (NHS) £2.8 billion annually in direct costs, as well as £1.8 billion due to lost productivity and disability and £2.4 billion in informal care costs [33]. The National Audit Office report states that response to stroke is not as fast and effective as it could be and that, with more efficient practice, there is scope for potential savings of £20 million annually, with 550 deaths avoided and over 1700 people recovering from their stroke each year who would not otherwise do so [33].

1.4.2 UK Stroke Policy

Throughout the world, countries have been developing documents and guidelines to mandate the provision of quality stroke care. In England, the NSS [20] and other service investments and reorganisations have achieved significant improvements in stroke care and a reduction in mortality [34]. The proportion of patients dying within 10 years of their stroke has reduced from 71 to 67% since 2006 [34]. The United Kingdom's forthcoming NSP (due for publication in 2019) aims to renew vigour in stroke service redesign and improvement.

Further successful implementation of such strategies should save lives and reduce disability, decrease health and social care costs, and limit the devastating effects on people's lives. Nevertheless, ensuring that 'the system provides patients with the precise interventions they need, delivered properly, precisely when they need them' [43] is challenging. Whilst the NSP can tell us what we need to achieve, we must determine how this can be delivered in local healthcare systems. The results of implementation research demonstrate that approaches to achieving delivery are not as obvious as they may seem. The North West's quality improvement collaborative is a case in point [44]. Despite a huge investment of public funds, researcher support, and stroke staff engagement over a protracted period of time, there has been a spectacular failure to achieve improvements in delivery of bundles of care. The research team even questioned the benefits of collaboration, revealing negative undertones of unhealthy competition and 'free riding', where hard-working innovative trusts were being exploited by their less proactive peers [45]. This is in stark contrast to the spectacular achievements of the Quality in Acute Stroke Care (QASC) study, where a simple implementation strategy negotiated with individual trusts, working through issues on a unit-by-unit basis, not only resulted in improvements in the monitoring of patients, but also delivered much better outcomes in patients at 90 days post-stroke [46]. This evidence for stroke unit care has now been rolled out as a service development initiative across New South Wales, with evidence of similar success [47]. The challenges in implementing the Fever, Sugar Swallowing intervention in the real world were informed by an understanding of the context (organisational, geographical, demographic, etc.) in which the intervention was originally tested [48] and of the use of protocols and external facilitation. In complementary work conducted within Victoria and NSW, the role of stroke clinical facilitators in increasing access to evidence-based stroke care has been found to be an effective model, regardless of whether this role is permanent or is time-limited to only a few years [49, 50].

Often, studies report the effectiveness of an intervention whilst only providing an outline of its content; methods of testing are detailed, but processes (barriers, facilitators, etc.) of introduction are rarely explained. Without detailed knowledge of how to implement research evidence into practice, implementation is hampered, and potential benefits to patients are not fully realised. Consequently, despite having effective treatments for stroke and transient ischaemic attack (TIA), unless we understand the healthcare delivery models that can ensure timely access to treatment and care, people with TIA will continue to go on to have completed stroke, and those with completed stroke will be more likely to die or to survive with severe disability.

In determining the service developments required and how to implement them, evidence of effectiveness and evidence-based approaches to implementation must be employed. Currently, one of the biggest challenges to the effectiveness of the NSP is the implementation of existing research evidence [51]. Implementation issues and potential tensions include consideration of:

- organisational context and culture (research-focused, specialist teaching centres, as compared with district general hospitals; teaching general practitioners (GPs) as compared with non-teaching GPs; level and type of leadership; communication strategies, etc.);
- geographical location (metropolitan, urban, suburban, rural, or remote);
- team structures (specialist, generalist, coordination, or professional/discipline-specific leadership);
- professional roles (traditional, new ways of working); and
- research culture (competences for participation and utilisation)

Participation in clinical trials is promoted via the UK Clinical Research Network (UKCRN: www.uksrn.ac.uk); there is a sub-specialty for stroke. Hospitals that are involved in clinical trials tend to deliver better care to their recruited patients, which might be partly explained by the closer monitoring associated with the experience of being in a study [52].

Whilst trials provide evidence of what can work, it is imperative that applied health research undertakes the translational work to demonstrate how this evidence can be applied within routine clinical services. This requires close collaborative working between clinicians, stroke care networks, research networks, and academics. For example, for people with suspected stroke, stroke care networks will facilitate the development of new pathways of care, including hub-and-spoke models of hyper-acute stroke care. This might mean that within a geographical region, one centre provides hyper-acute treatments (e.g. thrombolysis) whilst others offer specialist care in the form of stroke units. This process will need to be supported to enable accurate early identification of people with suspected stroke, optimal choice of destination, and effects on current local services, including ambulance services. This will require work to determine local feasibility, and later evaluation of cost-effectiveness.

1.5 Stroke Management Strategies

1.5.1 Stroke Unit Care

The mainstay of stroke services is dedicated stroke units, whereby beds for patients with stroke are co-located and skilled interdisciplinary care is provided. More than 24 years ago, a statistical overview provided the first strong evidence of the value of specialist stroke units [25]. Much has been written since, and further meta-analyses of outcomes of stroke unit care have been regularly published as Cochrane reviews [53–55]. Stroke unit care has been shown to reduce mortality and dependency, and there is no indication that organised stroke unit care increases hospital stay [53].

Outcomes from clinical trials may not directly reflect what can be achieved when trial interventions become routine clinical practice, but combined evidence from observational studies also demonstrates significant benefit from stroke unit care [56]. Given the range and strength of this evidence, admission of all stroke patients to stroke units is recommended in the guidelines of many countries, including Australia [57], the United Kingdom [31], and the United States [58]. As most stroke patients can potentially benefit by this model of care, it has been described as the most important treatment for stroke patients [59].

Organised inpatient care is, by definition, not a single intervention. This, together with the fact that stroke unit trials have not systematically measured component interventions, has meant that the contents of the 'black box' of stroke unit care have gone unknown [60]. Researchers have aimed to unpack this black box and identify the key components of organised inpatient care [61]. In a survey of 11 stroke unit trials, the following similar approaches were identified:

- assessment procedures (medical, nursing, and therapy assessment);
- management policies such as early mobilisation and treating suspected infection; and
- ongoing rehabilitation policies such as coordinated multidisciplinary team (MDT) care [61].

The value of these approaches has been demonstrated by recent studies showing the benefits of assessment [46] and preventing complications [62]. The benefits of early mobilisation [63] have been brought into question, with patients in the control arm (not mobilising until after 24 hours' post-stroke) doing better [64]. A blanket policy of trying to prevent infection with prophylactic antibiotics in acute stroke has not been found to be beneficial [65], although there is a lack of evidence for targeted antibiotics in those with suspected infection.

Nurses play a key role in identifying complications after an acute stroke through physiological monitoring. With their constant presence along the care continuum [61], particularly in the first 72 hours, nurses are best placed to be vigilant, and to detect and act on any physiological variations. However, simply connecting patients to monitoring equipment is only part of the process. Nurses must also respond to variations in physiological parameters, because up to one-third of stroke patients deteriorate neurologically during the first few days (mostly in the first 24 hours), and over 25% of patients suffer 'stroke progression' (significant, persisting neurological deterioration) after admission to hospital [66]. Stroke progression can dramatically worsen outcome; about half of those who die or are left with serious long-term disability have undergone stroke progression in the first 72 hours [67]. In some cases, progression is due to intracerebral processes such as the 'ischaemic cascade', the prevention of which has been the focus of much pharmacological research [68]. In many cases, progression is associated with systemic haemodynamic, biochemical, or physiological disturbances that are potentially treatable [69]. Organised acute stroke care should therefore include intensive acute-stage monitoring and responsive interventions.

The underlying pathology of 85% of strokes is cerebral infarction, which implies that treatment directed at this group has the potential to make the greatest impact. Therefore, a key component of effective treatment for ischaemic stroke entails optimal uptake of thrombolysis, and more recently thrombectomy, in locations where delivery is safe. Practical barriers to local introduction of thrombolysis (which will also likely apply to thrombectomy, although this is yet to be explored) in the United Kingdom [70] include:

- lack of knowledge about thrombolysis for stroke;
- lack of the necessary skill mix;
- nursing fears of the haemorrhagic side-effects; and
- consent issues.

Consequently, for safe delivery of thrombolysis, appropriate training is required, which must ensure capacity and competence within stroke services. Safe delivery of acute and intensive interventions requires specialist training. In the United Kingdom, currently only medical staff have a (recently introduced) formal route to becoming a stroke specialist, but in the United States, stroke specialist credentialing is not limited by discipline. In the United Kingdom, nurses and allied health professionals need to develop standardised stroke specialist qualifications and training, which need to be available and accessible to all (see Section 1.6.2).

1.5.2 Stroke as a Medical Emergency

Benefit can be gained by treating stroke as a medical emergency and ensuring that all patients receive effective treatment early. Effective short-term treatment brings long-term gain, including cost benefit. To achieve this, signs and symptoms of stroke need to be recognised and acted on as a medical emergency by the public and healthcare providers. The call handler needs to recognise and react quickly to a potential stroke identified in a phone call [71], the paramedics need to react quickly to suspected stroke, and the patient should be triaged to a Category 1 response (currently, within 7 minutes), with rapid arrival at the scene. Rapid action at the onset of stroke symptoms is a key issue within the NSS [20] because stroke outcomes can be improved by timely care [72].

Once at the scene, ambulance personnel need to be able to recognise the symptoms of suspected stroke, triage, and transport patients rapidly to the most appropriate hospital. Early presentation to an appropriate hospital provides greater opportunity for time-dependent stroke treatment, such as thrombolysis [72] and thrombectomy [73]. Over time, advances in brain imaging technology and development of new interventions will increase the proportion of acute stroke patients eligible for treatments. More immediate access to organised stroke care will also positively impact survival and dependency rates [74]. Therefore, rapid access has the potential to reduce severity of stroke, health service usage, and length of stay, with overall reduction of the burden of stroke for individuals, carers, and society as a whole.

In the United Kingdom, a rapid ambulance protocol was established in 1997 to facilitate rapid transport of patients to an acute stroke unit [75]. A FAST assessment forms part of the process (see Chapter 4 for discussion of stroke identification tools). Paramedics using the FAST showed good agreement with physicians' ratings of stroke patients [76]. Development of valid scales is only the first part of the process; local staff education and training is also required. Training is important for first-line paramedic staff, as well as for call handlers and ambulance dispatchers [71]. A multilevel educational programme has been shown to improve rapid hospitalisation and paramedic diagnostic accuracy, and to increase the number of patients presenting for evaluation within a 3-hour time window for thrombolysis [72].

1.5.3 Innovative Use of Technology to Reduce Inequity of Access to Acute Treatment

Telemedicine used for the purpose of delivering expert advice for stroke care exploits the growing technology capability of telecommunication that can be applied to healthcare. The application in stroke is not new, but has advanced significantly as technology has evolved. It was significantly leveraged with the era of stroke thrombolysis in the late 1990s [77], and more recently with the advances in urgent care related to endovascular clot retrieval [78]. A major driver for its use has been the need to ensure better equity for patients in accessing this time-critical therapy in urban, suburban, and rural regions [77], particularly where there are limited numbers of stroke specialist physicians [79].

Important considerations in establishing a telestroke service include understanding the workforce cultural issues surrounding changes in working practices and the complex relationships that use of this service may entail. In addition, it is important to sort out the governance prior to implementation of a service, and any credentialing, licensing, or liability for physicians providing remote consultations [80].

Such matters require adequate time to be resolved, and establishment of any new services must take this set-up period into account.

Other important practical considerations include the need for practice in the use of new software or equipment; building relationships with clinicians in remote hospitals; and having a well-coordinated rota. Strategies to increase confidence and working relationships may include a pilot phase with mock telestroke consultations and the provision of joint education and training to fill knowledge gaps and foster greater mutual understanding and familiarity amongst the service providers at both ends of the telestroke interchange [81, 82]. Whilst the focus is often on the role of physicians, nurses with stroke specialist training have also been highlighted as playing an important role in facilitating telemedicine consultations, including neurological examination [79]. Regardless of the types of clinical staff involved in telemedicine consultations, it is clear that to ensure high-quality care and high quality governance, all staff must have the right knowledge and skills for their role in the stroke care pathway (see http://www.stroke-education.org.uk). This can allow the accommodation of different workforce models, such as the utilisation of highly skilled stroke specialist nurses (e.g. those having participated in the Neurovascular Education and Training in Stroke Management and Acute Reperfusion Therapies (NET SMART) programme, where nurses have a major role in differential diagnosis of stroke and patient selection eligibility assessment for thrombolysis) [83].

It has also been suggested based on work in this area from the United States that pre-existing local connections should be leveraged in establishing a new network [80]. However, increased personal work, and it's appropriate recompense, have previously been indicated as barriers to the implementation of telestroke [84]. This is essential to ensuring a successful and coordinated system whereby there is strong clinician commitment.

Importantly, building familiarity amongst the service providers and achieving stakeholder acceptance of telestroke as a viable alternative option for clinical decision-making support has been found to increase access to thrombolysis [80]. Another important advantage of telestroke services is that they support rapid access to new evidence. Effective use of telemedicine to identify patients for endovascular thrombectomy in regional areas and facilitate patient transfers to hospitals that are capable of performing this complex procedure has been achieved in Australia as part of the Victorian Stroke Telemedicine programme. The sharing and pooling of knowledge and experience from across different countries helps to promote and ensure further successes in supporting effective telestroke models.

1.6   Research and Education

Research plays an important part in service development; support and facilitation of research are national priorities around the world. Various strategies are employed to support research capacity development and to maximise engagement at the stroke unit level and recruitment of individual stroke patients. In the United Kingdom, this has included establishment of the UKCRN.

1.6.1 UK Clinical Research Network

The UKCRN aims to facilitate clinical stroke research by enhancing NHS research infrastructure and exploring ways to remove barriers to conducting world-class studies. This has entailed facilitation of collaborative working between academics, stroke clinicians, stroke service users, and research funders. The UKCRN comprises a UK Coordinating Centre, Local (regional) Research Networks (CRNs), Research Networks in Scotland, Northern Ireland, and Wales, and a UK Steering Group. A number of local clinical leads have been tasked with promoting research portfolio development and advising on the suitability of studies for the portfolio. The role of local CRNs is to increase participation in stroke research studies and involve people with stroke and their carers in network activities. They support the set-up and running of research studies within the UKCRN portfolio on local sites, development of the local research workforce, and establishment of service user groups.

1.6.2 Specialist Training

High-quality care and services for people with stroke require staff with appropriate knowledge and skills; in the United Kingdom, there are presently no coordinated mechanisms to achieve this. The UK Forum for Stroke Training was established in the wake of the NSS; it has now been encompassed within the UK Stroke Forum, which is working towards the achievement of recognised, quality-assured, and transferable education programmes in stroke. This UK Stroke Forum is responsible for linking training and education, workforce competences, professional development, and career pathways. The UK Stroke Forum Steering Group has representation from stroke-specific and stroke-relevant professional bodies, health and social care, voluntary organisations, and service users. The Stroke-Specific Education Framework (SSEF), based around the 16 elements of care, covers the whole stroke care pathway. The SSEF's symbols (see Appendix A) have been utilised throughout this book to give an indication to the reader of the aspects of care that are covered wholly, or partially, within each chapter. The UK Stroke Forum supports the infrastructure for further development, sustainability, accreditation, and embedding of the SSEF for the delivery of a stroke-skilled workforce.

The overall purpose of the SSEF is to add stroke-specific knowledge and skills to the generic skills that health, social, voluntary, and independent care staff already possess. To achieve this, it will be fundamental to consider how to:

- build on existing skills, knowledge, and experience – *generic competences*;
- develop stroke-specific knowledge and skills – *stroke-specific competences*; and
- develop the ability to implement knowledge and skills gained through education and training in practice – *work-based learning*.

The relationship between these three aspects is essential to the provision of a stroke-skilled workforce. In order to reinforce learning from participation in education and training opportunities, individuals reflect upon how practice relates to new knowledge, and theoretical knowledge to practice. Ideally, this utilises work-based practice opportunities, where clinical mentors facilitate such reflection.

Through engagement with the UK Stroke Forum, the NHS, Social Services, and voluntary and independent sector organisations can contribute to the development of a stroke-specialist workforce. Staff delivering care along the stroke pathway must have the right knowledge, skills, and experience in stroke and the opportunity to participate in clearly defined career pathways. Improving recognition of stroke as a prestigious specialism will ensure future quality improvement through investment in stroke-specific and stroke-relevant services and the workforce required to deliver them.

1.7   Conclusion

This chapter describes the recent stroke service context, setting out how stroke has developed to become recognised as a policy priority, with national strategies, service and management developments, and networks to support education and research. Similar processes are underway in the United Kingdom and other HICs, but LMICs have a long way to go. If implementation is possible, these developments will ensure that stroke services achieve the best possible outcomes for patients and families affected by stroke. Stroke services can now provide staff with stimulating work environments, and with educational and professional development within clear career pathways. From a hard-to-recruit-to clinical backwater, stroke is maturing into an exciting, challenging, and progressive specialism; the following chapters, which include anonymised case examples, set out in detail what this entails for stroke nurses, and the wider team.

Stroke nursing is now a rewarding specialism, and provides opportunities for nurses to become active in exciting cutting-edge clinical practice, research, and education. This book aims to inspire and enthuse nurses to become involved and drive the specialism forward.

Acknowledgement

We gratefully acknowledge Dr Michael Leathley, who contributed to the first edition of this chapter.

References

1. Murray, C.J., Barber, R.M., Foreman, K.J. et al. (2015). Global, regional, and national disability-adjusted life years (DALYs) for 306 diseases and injuries and healthy life expectancy (HALE) for 188 countries, 1990-2013: quantifying the epidemiological transition. The Lancet 386 (10009): 2145–2191.
2. Feigin, V.L., Roth, G.A., Naghavi, M. et al. (2016). Global burden of stroke and risk factors in 188 countries, during 1990-2013: a systematic analysis for the Global Burden of Disease Study 2013. The Lancet Neurology 15 (9): 913–924.

3. Thrift, A.G., Thayabaranathan, T., Howard, G. et al. (2017). Global stroke statistics. International Journal of Stroke 12 (1): 13–32.

4. Phan, H.T., Blizzard, C.L., Reeves, M.J. et al. (2017). Sex differences in long-term mortality after stroke in the INSTRUCT (INternational STRoke oUtComes sTudy): a meta-analysis of individual participant data. Circulation Cardiovascular Quality and Outcomes 10 (2): https://doi.org/10.1161/CIRCOUTCOMES.116.003436.

5. Dey, P., Sutton, C., Marsden, J. et al. (2007). Medium Term Stroke Projections for England 2006 to 2015. London: Department of Health.

6. Patel, A., Berdunov, V., King, D. et al. (2017). Executive Summary Part 2: Burden of Stroke in the Next 20 Years and Potential Returns from Increased Spending on Research. London: Stroke Association.

7. Jagger, C., Matthews, R., Spiers, N. et al. (2006). Compression or Expansion of Disability?: Forecasting Future Disability Levels under Changing Patterns of Diseases. Leicester: University of Leicester.

8. Cadilhac, D.A., Dewey, H.M., Vos, T. et al. (2010). The health loss from ischemic stroke and intracerebral hemorrhage: evidence from the North East Melbourne Stroke Incidence Study (NEMESIS). Health and Quality of Life Outcomes 8: 49.

9. Cadilhac, D.A., Carter, R., Thrift, A.G., and Dewey, H.M. (2009). Estimating the long-term costs of ischemic and hemorrhagic stroke for Australia: new evidence derived from the North East Melbourne Stroke Incidence Study (NEMESIS). Stroke 40 (3): 915–921.

10. Wilson, A., Bath, P.M.W., Berge, E. et al. (2017). Understanding the relationship between costs and the modified Rankin scale: a systematic review, multidisciplinary consensus and recommendations for future studies. European Stroke Journal 2 (1): 3–12.

11. Gloede, T.D., Halbach, S.M., Thrift, A.G. et al. (2014). Long-term costs of stroke using 10-year longitudinal data from the North East Melbourne Stroke Incidence Study. Stroke 45 (11): 3389–3394.

12. Zhao, Y., Condon, J., Lawton, P. et al. (2016). Lifetime direct costs of stroke for indigenous patients adjusted for comorbidities. Neurology 87 (5): 458–465.

13. Youman, P., Wilson, K., Harraf, F., and Kalra, L. (2003). The economic burden of stroke in the United Kingdom. Pharmacoeconomics 21 (1): 43–50.

14. Husaini, B., Levine, R., Sharp, L. et al. (2013). Depression increases stroke hospitalization cost: an analysis of 17,010 stroke patients in 2008 by race and gender. Stroke Research and Treatment 2013: 846732.

15. Lloyd-Jones, D., Adams, R.J., Brown, T.M. et al. (2010). Heart disease and stroke statistics—2010 update a report from the American Heart Association. Circulation 121 (7): e46–e215.

16. Heidenreich, P.A., Trogdon, J.G., Khavjou, O.A. et al. (2011). Forecasting the future of cardiovascular disease in the United States a policy statement from the American Heart Association. Circulation 123 (8): 933–944.

17. Kim, J., Andrew, N.E., Thrift, A.G. et al. (2017). The potential health and economic impact of improving stroke care standards for Australia. International Journal of Stroke 12 (8): 875–885.

18. Asplund, K., Hulter Asberg, K., Appelros, P. et al. (2011). The Riks-Stroke story: building a sustainable national register for quality assessment of stroke care. International Journal of Stroke 6 (2): 99–108.

19. Lindsay, P., Furie, K.L., Davis, S.M. et al. (2014). World Stroke Organization global stroke services guidelines and action plan. International Journal of Stroke 9 (Suppl. A100): 4–13.

20. Department of Health (2007). National Stroke Strategy. London: Department of Health.

21. National Stroke Foundation (2011). Acute Stroke Services Framework 2011. Melbourne: National Stroke Foundation.
22. Saposnik, G., Baibergenova, A., O'Donnell, M. et al. (2007). Hospital volume and stroke outcome: does it matter? Neurology 69 (11): 1142–1151.
23. Cadilhac, D.A., Kilkenny, M.F., Andrew, N.E. et al. (2017). Hospitals admitting at least 100 patients with stroke a year should have a stroke unit: a case study from Australia. BMC Health Services Research 17 (1): 212.
24. Indredavik, B., Bakke, F., Solberg, R. et al. (1991). Benefit of a stroke unit: a randomized controlled trial. Stroke 22 (8): 1026–1031.
25. Langhorne, P., Williams, B.O., Gilchrist, W., and Howie, K. (1993). Do stroke units save lives? The Lancet 342 (8868): 395–398.
26. Intercollegiate Stroke Working Party (2000). National Clinical Guidelines for Stroke. London: Royal College of Physicians.
27. Kelson, M., Ford, C., and Rigge, M. (1998). Stroke Rehabilitation: Patient and Carer Views. A Report by the College of Health for the Intercollegiate Working Party for Stroke. London: Royal College of Physicians.
28. Intercollegiate Stroke Working Party (2004). National Sentinel Stroke Audit. London: Royal College of Physicians.
29. Intercollegiate Stroke Working Party (2008). National Sentinel Audit for Stroke. London: Royal College of Physicians.
30. Intercollegiate Stroke Working Party (2012). National Clinical Guidelines for Stroke. London: Royal College of Physicians.
31. Intercollegiate Stroke Working Party (2016). National Clinical Guidelines for Stroke. London: Royal College of Physicians.
32. Royal College of Physicians (2015). Sentinel Stroke National Audit Programme (SSNAP). London: Royal College of Physicians.
33. National Audit Office (2005). Reducing Brain Damage – Faster Access to Better Stroke Care. London: The Stationery Office [updated 12th March 2018]. Available from: www.nao.org.uk/report/department-of-health-reducing-brain-damage-faster-access-to-better-stroke-care. [30 November 2018].
34. National Audit Office (2010). Progress in Improving Stroke Care. London: National Audit Office.
35. Morris, Z.S., Wooding, S., and Grant, J. (2011). The answer is 17 years, what is the question: understanding time lags in translational research. Journal of the Royal Society of Medicine 104 (12): 510–520.
36. Cadilhac, D.A., Kim, J., Lannin, N.A. et al. (2016). National stroke registries for monitoring and improving the quality of hospital care: a systematic review. International Journal of Stroke 11 (1): 28–40.
37. Jones, S.P., Jenkinson, M.J., Leathley, M.J. et al. (2007). The recognition and emergency management of suspected stroke and transient ischaemic attack. Clinical Medicine 7 (5): 467–471.
38. Intercollegiate Stroke Working Party (2004). National Clinical Guidelines for Stroke. London: Royal College of Physicians.
39. Watkins, C.L., Leathley, M.J., Jones, S.P. et al. (2013). Training emergency services' dispatchers to recognise stroke: an interrupted time-series analysis. British Medical Council Health Services Research 13 (1): 318.
40. Harbison, J., Hossain, O., Jenkinson, D. et al. (2003). Diagnostic accuracy of stroke referrals from primary care, emergency room physicians, and ambulance staff using the face arm speech test. Stroke 34 (1): 71–76.
41. Wolters, F.J., Paul, N.L., Li, L., and Rothwell, P.M. (2015). Sustained impact of UK FAST-test public education on response to stroke: a population-based time-series study. International Journal of Stroke 10 (7): 1108–1114.

42. Bray, J.E., Johnson, R., Trobbiani, K. et al. (2013). Australian public's awareness of stroke warning signs improves after national multimedia campaigns. Stroke 44 (12): 3540–3543.
43. Woolf, S.H. and Johnson, R.E. (2005). The break-even point: when medical advances are less important than improving the fidelity with which they are delivered. The Annals of Family Medicine 3 (6): 545–552.
44. Carter, P., Ozieranski, P., McNicol, S. et al. (2014). How collaborative are quality improvement collaboratives: a qualitative study in stroke care. Implementation Science 9 (1): 32–43.
45. Power, M., Tyrrell, P.J., Rudd, A.G. et al. (2014). Did a quality improvement collaborative make stroke care better? A cluster randomized trial. Implementation Science 9 (1): 40.
46. Middleton, S., McElduff, P., Ward, J. et al. (2011). Implementation of evidence-based treatment protocols to manage fever, hyperglycaemia, and swallowing dysfunction in acute stroke (QASC): a cluster randomised controlled trial. The Lancet 378 (9804): 1699–1706.
47. Middleton, S., Lydtin, A., Comerford, D. et al. (2016). From QASC to QASCIP: successful Australian translational scale-up and spread of a proven intervention in acute stroke using a prospective pre-test/post-test study design. BMJ Open 6 (5): e011568.
48. Craig, L.E., Churilov, L., Olenko, L. et al. (2017). Testing a systematic approach to identify and prioritise barriers to successful implementation of a complex healthcare intervention. BMC Medical Research Methodology 17 (1): 24.
49. Cadilhac, D.A., Purvis, T., Kilkenny, M.F. et al. (2013). Evaluation of rural stroke services: does implementation of coordinators and pathways improve care in rural hospitals? Stroke 44 (10): 2848–2853.
50. Purvis, T., Moss, K., Francis, L. et al. (2017). The benefits of clinical facilitators on improving stroke care in acute hospitals: a new program for Australia. Internal Medicine Journal 47 (7): 775–784.
51. Tooke, J. (2008). Aspiring to Excellence. Findings and Final Recommendations of the Independent Inquiry into Modernising Medical Careers. London: Aldridge Press.
52. Purvis, T., Hill, K., Kilkenny, M. et al. (2016). Improved in-hospital outcomes and care for patients in stroke research: an observational study. Neurology 87 (2): 206–213.
53. Stroke Unit Trialists Collaboration (2013). Organised inpatient (stroke unit) care for stroke. Cochrane Database of Systematic Reviews 9 (Art. No.: CD000197). https://doi.org/10.1002/14651858.CD000197.pub3.
54. Stroke Unit Trialists' Collaboration (1997). Collaborative systematic review of the randomised trials of organised inpatient (stroke unit) care after stroke. British Medical Journal 314 (7088): 1151–1159.
55. Stroke Unit Trialists' Collaboration (2007). Organised inpatient(stroke unit) care for stroke. Cochrane Database of Systematic Reviews 4 (Art. No.: CD000197). https://doi.org/10.1002/14651858.CD000197.pub2.
56. Seenan, P., Long, M., and Langhorne, P. (2007). Stroke units in their natural habitat: systematic review of observational studies. Stroke 38 (6): 1886–1892.
57. National Stroke Foundation (2017). Clinical Guidelines for Stroke Management. Melbourne: National Health and Medical Research Council.
58. Adams, H.P. Jr., del Zoppo, G., Alberts, M.J. et al. (2007). Guidelines for the early management of adults with ischemic stroke: a guideline from the American Heart Association/American Stroke Association Stroke Council, Clinical Cardiology Council, Cardiovascular Radiology and Intervention Council, and the Atherosclerotic Peripheral Vascular Disease and Quality of Care Outcomes in Research Interdisciplinary Working Groups: the American Academy of Neurology affirms the value of this guideline as an educational tool for neurologists. Stroke 38 (5): 1655–1711.
59. Indredavik, B. (2009). Stroke unit care is beneficial both for the patient and for the health service and should be widely implemented. Stroke 40 (1): 1–2.

60. Gladman, J., Barer, D., and Langhorne, P. (1996). Specialist rehabilitation after stroke. British Medical Journal 312 (7047): 1623–1624.
61. Langhorne, P. and Pollock, A. (2002). What are the components of effective stroke unit care? Age and Ageing 31 (5): 365–371.
62. Govan, L., Langhorne, P., and Weir, C.J. (2007). Does the prevention of complications explain the survival benefit of organized inpatient (stroke unit) care? Further analysis of a systematic review. Stroke 38 (9): 2536–2540.
63. Bernhardt, J., Chitravas, N., Meslo, I.L. et al. (2008). Not all stroke units are the same: a comparison of physical activity patterns in Melbourne, Australia, and Trondheim, Norway. Stroke 39 (7): 2059–2065.
64. Bernhardt, J., Collier, J., Dewey, H. et al. (2015). Efficacy and safety of very early mobilisation within 24 h of stroke onset (AVERT): a randomised controlled trial. The Lancet 386 (9988): 46–55.
65. Westendorp, W.F., Vermeij, J.-D., Zock, E. et al. (2015). The Preventive Antibiotics in Stroke Study (PASS): a pragmatic randomised open-label masked endpoint clinical trial. The Lancet 385 (9977): 1519–1526.
66. Jorgensen, H., Nakayama, H., Reith, J. et al. (1996). Factors delaying hospital admission in acute stroke: the Copenhagen Stroke Study. Neurology 47 (2): 383–387.
67. Birschel, P., Ellul, J., and Barer, D. (2004). Progressing stroke: towards an internationally agreed definition. Cerebrovascular Diseases 17 (2–3): 242–252.
68. Davis, S.M. and Donnan, G.A. (2002). Neuroprotection: establishing proof of concept in human stroke. Stroke 33 (1): 309–310.
69. Davis, M. and Barer, D. (1999). Neuroprotection in acute ischaemic stroke. II: Clinical potential. Vascular Medicine 4 (3): 149–163.
70. Innes, K. (2003). Thrombolysis for acute ischaemic stroke: core nursing requirements. British Journal of Nursing 12 (7): 416–424.
71. Watkins, C.L., Jones, S.P., Leathley, M.J. et al. (2014). Emergency Stroke Calls: Obtaining Rapid Telephone Triage (ESCORTT) – a programme of research to facilitate recognition of stroke by emergency medical dispatchers. Southampton: NIHR Journals Library.
72. Wojner-Alexandrov, A.W., Alexandrov, A.V., Rodriguez, D. et al. (2005). Houston paramedic and emergency stroke treatment and outcomes study (HoPSTO). Stroke 36 (7): 1512–1518.
73. Berkhemer, O.A., Fransen, P.S.S., Beumer, D. et al. (2015). A randomized trial of intraarterial treatment for acute ischemic stroke. New England Journal of Medicine 372 (1): 11–20.
74. Stroke Unit Trialists' Collaboration (1997). Collaborative systematic review of the randomised trials of organised inpatient (stroke unit) care after stroke. British Medical Journal 314 (7088): 1151.
75. Harbison, J., Massey, A., Barnett, L. et al. (1999). Rapid ambulance protocol for acute stroke. The Lancet 353 (9168): 1935.
76. Nor, A.M., McAllister, C., Louw, S.J. et al. (2004). Agreement between ambulance paramedic- and physician-recorded neurological signs with Face Arm Speech Test (FAST) in acute stroke patients. Stroke 35 (6): 1355–1359.
77. Bladin, C.F. and Cadilhac, D.A. (2014). Effect of telestroke on emergent stroke care and stroke outcomes. Stroke 45 (6): 1876–1880.
78. Akbik, F., Hirsch, J.A., Chandra, R.V. et al. (2016). Telestroke – the promise and the challenge. Part one: growth and current practice. Journal of Neurointerventional Surgery https://doi.org/10.1136/neurintsurg-2016-012291.
79. French, B., Day, E., Watkins, C. et al. (2013). The challenges of implementing a telestroke network: a systematic review and case study. BMC Medical Informatics and Decision Making 13: 125.
80. Akbik, F., Hirsch, J.A., Chandra, R.V. et al. (2016). Telestroke – the promise and the challenge. Part two: expansion and horizons. Journal of Neurointerventional Surgery https://doi.org/10.1136/neurintsurg-2016-012340.

81. Bagot, K.L., Bladin, C.F., Vu, M. et al. (2016). Exploring the benefits of a stroke telemedicine programme: an organisational and societal perspective. Journal of Telemedicine and Telecare 22 (8): 489–494.

82. Cadilhac, D.A., Vu, M., and Bladin, C. (2014). Experience with scaling up the Victorian Stroke Telemedicine programme. Journal of Telemedicine and Telecare 20 (7): 413–418.

83. Alexandrov, A.W., Brethour, M., Cudlip, F. et al. (2009). Postgraduate fellowship education and training for nurses: the NET SMART experience. Critical Care Nursing Clinics of North America 21 (4): 435–449.

84. Moskowitz, A., Chan, Y.F., Bruns, J., and Levine, S.R. (2010). Emergency physician and stroke specialist beliefs and expectations regarding telestroke. Stroke 41 (4): 805–809.

CHAPTER 2

What Is a Stroke?

Anne W. Alexandrov

Health Outcomes Institute, Fountain Hills, AZ, USA

University of Tennessee Health Science Center at Memphis, Memphis, TN, USA

University of Tennessee – Memphis Mobile Stroke Unit, Memphis, TN, USA

KEY POINTS

- Stroke is a common and complex neurovascular disease, an important public health issue, and a healthcare professional priority topic.
- Given stroke's complexity, the variety of presentations, and the differences between optimum treatment regimes for different stroke types, it is essential that all clinical staff involved with stroke have a thorough understanding of its underpinning anatomy, physiology, and disease processes.
- This chapter details neurological examinations and tools to support stroke assessment.

This chapter maps to criteria within the following sections of the Stroke-Specific Education Framework (SSEF):

2.1 Introduction

As the third most common cause of death and a leading cause of adult disability in most countries, stroke is an important neurovascular disease. This chapter provides an overview of processes in the development of stroke, the normal neurological anatomy and physiology, and the neurovascular clinical examination used to identify stroke.

2.2 Stroke Classification

Stroke is broadly divided into two main categories: ischaemic infarction and haemorrhagic. Ischaemic stroke is the most common, accounting for 70% or more of stroke events [2]. Stroke is defined as a rapidly evolving syndrome of sudden onset, presenting with non-epileptic neurological deficit that follows a discreet vascular territory in the brain, retina, or spinal cord. Transient ischaemic attack (TIA) cannot be differentiated from ischaemic stroke without brain magnetic resonance imaging (MRI) to determine if infarction has occurred. Infarction may be clinically silent, lacking any signs or symptoms, and in these circumstances, only an MRI can image brain tissue to allow differentiation of stroke from TIA [2]. Throughout mainly the English-speaking world, MRI has become standard of care, mostly performed pre-discharge in patients admitted for stroke or TIA.

When blood flow to an area is disrupted through occlusion of blood vessels, an infarcted core rapidly develops. The core is surrounded by an ischaemic halo, or 'penumbra', that is vulnerable to permanent infarction, but this tissue may survive if the area is reperfused rapidly. Collateral blood flow within the penumbra is generally limited, and in some cases may not exist; therefore, practitioners are under tremendous pressure to rapidly diagnose and treat patients with therapies capable of breaking down clots or removing them, limiting infarction growth.

Ischaemic stroke develops through a number of mechanisms. Probably the most common categorisation is TOAST, developed for the **T**rial of **O**rg 10172 (Danaparoid) in **A**cute **S**troke **T**reatment [3].

2.2.1 Large Artery Atherosclerosis (LAA)

Large artery atherosclerosis (LAA) involves significant (>50%) stenosis (narrowing) of a major brain artery or cortical branch artery, presumably due to atherosclerosis, with infarct size generally >1.5 cm. Within this category, mechanisms resulting in stroke include intracranial thrombosis and intra- and extracranial artery-to-artery embolisation, such as that occurring with rupture of a carotid plaque. Clinical findings of LAA include impairments indicating damage to the cortical, brainstem, or cerebellar locations. Patients with LAA may demonstrate evidence of widespread atherosclerotic disease, such as intermittent claudication, coronary artery disease, extracranial carotid stenosis, or TIA occurring in the same vascular territory. For this classification, there should not be any indication of a cardioembolic mechanism [3]. In the Stroke Data Bank of the US National Institute of Neurological Disorders and Stroke (NINDS), LAA is responsible for about 6% of strokes, with another 4% categorised as tandem artery occlusions [4].

2.2.2 Cardioembolism

Cardioembolism produces a stroke from emboli arising within the heart. At least one cardiac source must be identified to use this classification, and LAA must be ruled out. The categories of LAA and cardioembolism are mutually exclusive [3]. Conditions associated with cardioembolism are listed in Table 2.1. Patients with

TABLE 2.1 Conditions associated with cardioembolic stroke

High-risk sources	Medium-risk sources
Mechanical prosthetic valves	Mitral valve prolapse
Mitral stenosis with atrial fibrillation	Mitral annulus calcification
Atrial fibrillation	Mitral stenosis without atrial fibrillation
Left atrial/atrial appendage thrombus	Left atrial turbulence
Sick sinus syndrome	Atrial septal aneurysm
Recent myocardial infarction (<4 wk)	Patent foramen ovale
Left ventricular thrombus	Atrial flutter
Dilated cardiomyopathy	Lone atrial fibrillation
Akinetic left ventricular segment	Bioprosthetic cardiac valve
Atrial myxoma	Non-bacterial thrombotic endocarditis
Infective endocarditis	Congestive heart failure
	Hypokinetic left ventricular segment
	Myocardial infarction (>4 wk, <6 mo)

cardioembolic stroke may have evidence of multiple brain emboli over a period of time. About 14% of NINDS Stroke Data Bank patients are classified as having cardioembolic stroke [4].

2.2.3 Small Vessel Occlusion (SVO)

Small vessel occlusion (SVO) is commonly referred to as 'lacunar stroke'. Originally thought to be caused exclusively by lipohyalinosis (small vessel disease, with deposits of eosinophilic cells within the vessel walls), SVO secondary to atherosclerosis is now considered to be a common mechanism. Patients with lacunar stroke present with symptoms that include pure sensory or motor dysfunction, or combined sensory and motor findings. SVOs usually occur in the subcortex and brainstem, and these patients often have longstanding hypertension, diabetes, and hyperlipidaemia, and are frequently smokers [3]. Vascular imaging of the large intracranial arteries using magnetic resonance angiography (MRA) or computed tomographic angiography (CTA) should show that there are no occlusions, because the small perforating arteries producing lacunar stroke are too tiny to show up on current forms of vascular imaging. In the NINDS Stroke Data Bank, 19% of stroke patients are classified as having SVOs [4].

2.2.4 Stroke of Other Determined Aetiology

This category includes unusual stroke mechanisms such as non-atherosclerotic vasculopathies, hypercoagulable states, haematological disorders, arterial dissections, venous thrombosis, cocaine or other illegal drug-associated causes, and unusual embolic sources (iatrogenic gas or small particles, neoplasms, parasites, fat). Stroke location and size vary depending on the associated cause, and cardiac embolism, SVO, and LAA lesions must be ruled out [3].

2.2.5 Stroke of Undetermined Aetiology

This classification of stroke mechanism, which is also called 'cryptogenic stroke', is reserved for patients: where no aetiological factor can be identified, with incomplete aetiological work-up; or where there is more than one contributing aetiological factor [3]. As determination of stroke mechanism can be challenging, in the NINDS Stroke Data Bank, 28% of patients fall into this category [4]. Patients with occult right-to-left intrathoracic vascular shunts may mistakenly be placed into this category in the absence of a thorough work-up. For example, patent foramen ovale (PFO) was identified in 50–56% of young stroke patients previously diagnosed with cryptogenic stroke [5–7], resulting in recategorisation as cardioembolism. When cryptogenic classification is the result of incomplete work-up, patients are vulnerable, because without knowing the cause of their stroke, secondary stroke prevention strategies may be inadequate. With paroxysmal atrial fibrillation (AF) now capable of detection using implanted loop recorders over extended periods of time [8], patients previously classified with cryptogenic stroke can now be correctly identified as cardioembolic and receive anticoagulation prophylaxis for secondary prevention [9, 10].

2.2.6 Stroke Due to Haemorrhage

Haemorrhage causes less than 30% of stroke events [4, 11]. Intraparenchymal haemorrhage (IPH; also referred to as intracerebral haemorrhage, ICH) associated with hypertensive emergency is the most frequently encountered form of haemorrhagic stroke. Less commonly, IPH may result from amyloid angiopathy (most common in older persons) or rupture of an arteriovenous malformation or aneurysm. Subarachnoid haemorrhage (SAH), from rupture of an intracranial aneurysm, is a less common but still important cause of haemorrhagic stroke, particularly in the Asian population [12].

2.3 Risk Factors for Stroke

The risk factors for stroke are similar to those for cardiovascular disease, and can be either non-modifiable or modifiable [13]. Non-modifiable risk factors are characteristics that patients cannot change, including age, low birth weight, race/ethnicity, and genetic factors. Modifiable risk factors are further subdivided into first- and second-tier factors. The first-tier risk factors, in order of importance, are hypertension, diabetes mellitus, cigarette smoking, AF, and left ventricular dysfunction. The first three contribute to about 50% of the total risk for stroke compared to other factors, and are the most important areas for stroke prevention [2]. Second-tier risk factors include hyperlipidaemia, asymptomatic carotid stenosis, sickle cell disease, oestrogen replacement therapy, diet, obesity and body fat distribution, alcohol and/or drug abuse, sleep-disordered breathing, migraine, and hypercoagulable states [2]. Many second-tier risk factors are associated with development of first-tier risk factors; for example, obesity is a risk factor for both hypertension and diabetes. Vigilant management of all contributing risk factors is needed to prevent first-ever or secondary stroke. There is more on risk factor management in Chapter 3.

2.4 Anatomy, Physiology, and Related Stroke Clinical Findings

The brain and spinal cord make up the central nervous system (CNS) and are amongst the most delicate, and yet important, organs of the body. Protection is provided to these structures by the skull, which forms a rigid bony vault around the brain, with one large opening at its base – the foramen magnum – through which the brainstem projects and connects to the spinal cord [14]. As the skull cannot expand in adults, an increase in brain size (e.g. in oedema), cerebrospinal fluid (CSF) (e.g. hydrocephalus), or blood collection (e.g. haematoma) will result in brain compression and increased intracranial pressure if treatment is not administered quickly [15].

The meninges lie just beneath the skull and vertebral column, and consist of three layers: the dura mater, the arachnoid mater, and the pia mater. The dura mater makes up the outermost layer of the meninges; the term 'dura' in Latin means 'tough'. This layer supports the brain and spinal cord, holding nerves and blood vessels in place [14]. Within the double layer of the dura mater are venous sinuses that collect blood drained from intracranial and meningeal veins for return to the systemic venous circuit via the internal jugular veins [14]. Within the cranium, four extensions of the dura mater provide direct support for brain structures and separate specific areas of the brain:

- The falx cerebri vertically divides the right and left hemispheres of the brain from the frontal to the occipital lobe.
- The tentorium cerebelli forms a tent-like extension between the occipital lobes and the cerebellum, separating the cerebrum from the brainstem and cerebellum. Brain structures located above the tentorium cerebelli are commonly called 'supratentorial', whilst those below the tentorium are referred to as 'infratentorial', making up a region of the brain often called the posterior fossa.
- The falx cerebelli divides the two lobes of the cerebellum.
- The diaphragma sellae creates a roof-like covering for the sella turcica, which houses the pituitary gland [14].

The arachnoid mater lies directly under the dura mater, with the area between the two considered a 'potential space', containing a large number of unsupported small veins. These can tear during traumatic impact, resulting in development of a subdural haematoma [14]. The arachnoid is a delicate membrane, with fine threads of elastic tissue called trabeculae connecting it to the pia mater, creating a web-like structure called the subarachnoid space. Large arteries are carefully bound by trabeculae to the surface of the brain from the point at which they enter the skull [14]. Within the subarachnoid space, CSF freely circulates; rupture of an intracranial artery within the subarachnoid space (SAH) causes blood and CSF to mix. CSF is absorbed into arachnoid villi: membranous tufts that project into the superior sagittal and transverse venous sinuses and provide conduits into the venous system. Normally, adults produce approximately 20 ml of CSF per hour, so arachnoid villi reabsorption is largely driven by increased hydrostatic pressure within the subarachnoid space as CSF volume continuously builds. Should these delicate structures become obstructed with blood, as in SAH, reabsorption may be significantly impacted, resulting in increased CSF, commonly referred to as 'communicating hydrocephalus' [14].

The pia mater adheres directly to brain and spinal cord tissue, following all the folds and convolutions of the CNS surface. The pia is rich in small blood vessels, which supply a large volume of arterial blood to the CNS. Within the lateral third and fourth ventricles, tufts of pia mater form a portion of the choroid plexus, which is responsible for CSF production [14].

Four CSF-filled canals lined with ependymal cells make up the ventricular system (Figure 2.1). At the uppermost part of the system, two lateral ventricles extend from the frontal to the occipital lobes [14]. The right lateral ventricle is commonly the site for cannulation when CSF drainage by ventriculostomy/shunt or intracranial pressure monitoring is required. The two lateral ventricles are connected by the foramen of Monro to the third ventricle, which lies directly above the midbrain of the brainstem. The aqueduct of Sylvius – the cerebral aqueduct – connects the third and fourth ventricles, and is located between the brainstem and cerebellum. Two openings at the base of the fourth ventricle, the foramina of Luschka and Magendie, open into the subarachnoid space [14]. Blockage of CSF flow within the ventricular system, which may develop from a cerebellar infarct with oedema formation, produces a non-communicating hydrocephalus as CSF continues to

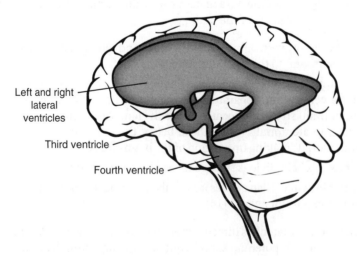

Left and right
lateral
ventricles

Third ventricle

Fourth ventricle

FIGURE 2.1 The ventricular system. *Source: Reproduced with permission of Stephen DiBiase Designs.*

TABLE 2.2   Composition of cerebrospinal fluid (CSF)

CSF characteristics and components	Normal values
pH	7.35–7.45
Appearance	Clear and colourless
Specific gravity	1.007
Total volume	135–150 ml
Pressure:	
• Lumbar	70–200 cmH$_2$O
• Intraventricular	0–15 mmHg
Cell content:	
• White blood cells	0
• Red blood cells	0
• Lymphocytes	0–10
Glucose	50–75 mg dl^{-1}; typically 66% of blood glucose
Protein	5–25 mg dl^{-1}

be formed but can neither circulate nor be reabsorbed. This causes dilation of the ventricles from trapped CSF, and may produce increased intracranial pressure [15]. The ventricular system and subarachnoid space are filled with CSF, which protects the CNS through 'shock absorption' during traumatic injury. Whilst not well understood, it probably also plays a role in providing glucose to nourish neurons. CSF flows from the lateral ventricles through the foramen of Monro into the third ventricle, through the cerebral aqueduct into the fourth ventricle, and out of the foramen of Magendie and the foramina of Luschka into the subarachnoid space of the brain and spinal cord (Table 2.2) [14].

2.4.1   Arterial Circulation

The brain makes up only 2% of body weight but uses approximately 20% of resting cardiac output to maintain its vital functions. It requires approximately 750 ml blood flow per minute, extracting up to 45% of the arterial oxygen to meet its normal metabolic needs [14–16]. There are no reserves of oxygen or glucose in the brain, so disruption of arterial blood flow dramatically affects normal cellular function. Two pairs of arteries, the internal carotid and vertebral arteries (VAs), provide blood to the brain; these pairs comprise the anterior and posterior circulations, and are connected at the brain's base to form the circle of Willis (see Figure 2.2) [14, 16]. The brain's arterial distribution is illustrated in Figure 2.3.

The anterior circulation derives from the right and left internal carotid arteries (ICAs) and their branches. Originating as the common carotids, the left common

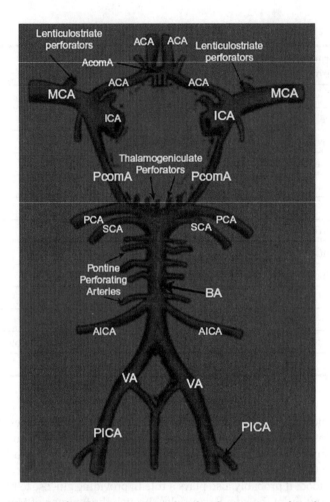

FIGURE 2.2   The circle of Willis. *Source: Reproduced with permission of Stephen DiBiase Designs.* MCA, middle cerebral artery; ACA, anterior cerebral artery; AComA, anterior communicating artery; PComA, posterior communicating artery; PICA, posterior inferior cerebellar artery; VA, vertebral artery; BA, basilar artery; AICA, anterior inferior cerebellar artery; SCA, superior cerebellar artery; PCA, posterior cerebral artery.

carotid takes off from the arch of the aorta and the right common carotid from the innominate artery. They then split at the level of the cricothyroid junction to form the external carotid artery (ECA) and ICA, with the face, scalp, and skull fed by branches of the former. The ICA enters the skull's base through an opening in the petrous bone. It gives off the right and left middle cerebral arteries (MCAs), the right and left anterior cerebral arteries (ACAs) (connected by the anterior communicating artery, AcomA), and the two posterior communicating arteries (PcomAs) [16, 17]. The anterior circulation provides 80% of blood flow to the cerebral hemispheres, including the frontal lobes, most of the parietal and temporal lobes, and subcortical structures located above the brainstem [14, 16]. The ophthalmic artery (OA) is also derived from the ICA, just before it divides into the ACA and MCA. The OA supplies blood to the retina and optic nerve; if the ICA is occluded, the

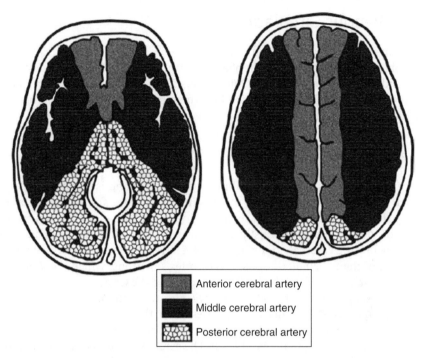

FIGURE 2.3   Arterial distribution for the brain. *Source: Reproduced with permission of Stephen DiBiase Designs.*

OA may reverse its course to supplement the anterior circulation's arterial blood volume [16].

The posterior circulation is derived from the two VAs, which originate from the subclavian arteries and travel posteriorly through small openings in the lateral spinous processes of the cervical spine. The VAs enter the skull through the foramen magnum; at the level of the pons, they fuse to form the basilar artery (BA). Two important arterial branches are derived from the terminal portion of the VAs prior to their fusion into the BA – the posterior inferior cerebellar arteries (PICAs). The BA gives rise to two major infratentorial branches – the anterior inferior cerebellar arteries (AICAs) and superior cerebellar arteries (SCAs); along with the PICAs, these arteries and their branches supply blood to the cerebellum and brainstem. The distal BA gives off the two posterior cerebral arteries (PCAs) that supply the posterior regions of the cerebral cortex [14, 16].

The circle of Willis (Figure 2.2) is a unique vascular supply system made up of the major branches of the anterior and posterior circulation. Each side of the anterior circulation is connected by the AcomA, which lies between the two ACAs; the posterior circulation is connected to the anterior circulation by the two PcomAs [14]. Approximately 50% of the population has a complete circle of Willis; atretic (small, non-functional or hypoplastic) segments are common, however, and are often found in the A1 branch of the ACAs, the P1 branch of the PCAs, and the PComAs [16]. When the circle of Willis is complete, it can support some collateral blood flow if an artery is occluded, although sufficient blood supply is not guaranteed.

2.4.2 Venous Circulation

The brain's venous drainage occurs through venous sinuses, many housed in the dura mater. Brain capillaries drain blood into venules, which connect to cerebral veins and ultimately empty blood into venous sinuses. The sinuses empty blood into the internal jugular veins, which in turn empty into the superior vena cava. The brain's veins have valves [14].

2.4.3 Cerebrum

The cerebrum makes up 80% of the brain's weight [14] and is composed of right and left hemispheres separated by the longitudinal fissure and connected at the base by the corpus callosum. The cerebral cortex makes up the outer aspect, consisting of grey matter that constitutes neuronal cell bodies. White matter lies directly below the cerebral cortex in what is referred to as the subcortical region, consisting of the myelinated axons of the cortex's neurons, which communicate impulses from neuronal cell bodies to other areas of the CNS.

The cerebrum has four anatomical divisions: the frontal, parietal, temporal, and occipital lobes. A fifth lobe is sometimes listed, the rhinencephalon or limbic lobe, although many see this structure deep within the cerebrum as anatomically associated with the temporal lobe [14, 18]. The cerebral cortex's primary functions include intellect, language, sensory, and motor functions [14]. Cerebral cortical cell architecture was classified in 1909 by Brodmann, who identified more than 100 unique areas of specialised cortical function (Figure 2.4). The functions within Brodmann's classification that are commonly assessed by nurses are as follows.

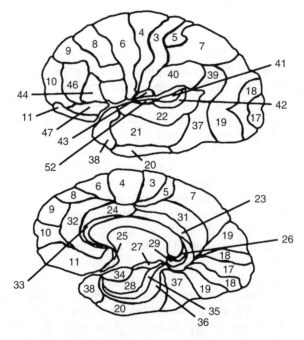

FIGURE 2.4 Brodmann areas of the cortex, numbered according to Brodmann's original plan; missing in this series are 13–16 and 48–51, which Brodmann's plan does not specify clearly. *Source: Reproduced with permission of Stephen DiBiase Designs.*

2.4.3.1 Frontal Lobes
These lie beneath the frontal bone, separated from the parietal lobe posteriorly by the central sulcus (fissure of Rolando) and from the temporal lobe inferiorly by the lateral fissure (Sylvian fissure). The frontal lobes' major functions include cognitive function (orientation, memory, insight, judgement, arithmetic, and abstraction), expressive language (verbal and written), and voluntary motor function.

- *Cognition* is controlled in Brodmann's areas 9–12 (ACA territory), in the prefrontal cortex, located just behind the forehead [14, 15]; this region focuses on intellectual appraisal and response to environmental stimuli. Intellectual capacity is blended with socially learned and accepted emotional responses and practices and with autonomic nervous system responses, such as tachycardia in relation to perceived threats. Injury here may dramatically alter intellectual capacity and social responses to environmental stimuli, profoundly affecting quality of life.

- *Expressive language* is housed in Brodmann's area 44 (MCA territory), also called Broca's area. This region is located in the inferior frontal gyrus, close to the motor strip's facial distribution. It is on the left side of the frontal lobe in most people, designating the left hemisphere as dominant in function, although occasionally it may be located in the right frontal hemisphere [14]. Broca's area is responsible for the formation of both verbal and written communication. Injury to this brain area results in disability ranging from word-finding difficulties to an expressive or non-fluent aphasia with significantly compromised verbal and written communication.

- *Voluntary (pyramidal) motor function* is controlled in Brodmann's area 4 (MCA territory) – the motor strip. Most voluntary motor tracts cross over to the opposite side as they descend through the brainstem (in the pyramids of the medulla – hence the name 'pyramidal motor function'), so the right motor strip represents voluntary motor function for the left side of the body and vice versa [14]. Figure 2.5 shows the motor homunculus, commonly used to depict the layout of motor function in area 4. The homunculus appears as an upside-down man; the foot is illustrated on the superior medial aspects of the frontal lobes, with the knees, hips, trunk, and shoulders extending along the lateral surfaces, and the hands, thumb, head, face, and tongue represented in a lateral inferior distribution extending to the Sylvian fissure. The larger the areas illustrated on the homunculus, the greater the amount of frontal cortex dedicated to the particular motor function [14]. For example, the hands require significantly more motor control than the trunk of the body and are therefore represented by a larger graphical distribution on the homunculus. When the motor strip is damaged by stroke or injury, motor function on the opposite side of the body is impaired. Table 2.3 summarises the clinical examination techniques used to assess frontal lobe function.

2.4.3.2 Parietal Lobes
The parietal lobes are situated posterior to the frontal lobe on the opposite side of the central sulcus. Posteriorly, the parieto-occipital fissure separates the parietal lobe from the occipital lobe. The primary function of the parietal lobes is integration of sensory stimuli, such as awareness of body parts and their positioning, recognition of the size, shape, and texture of objects, and interpretation of touch, pressure, and pain.

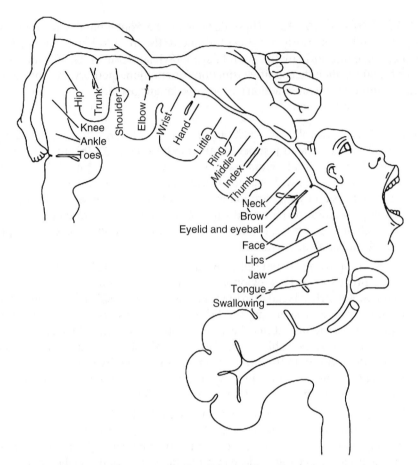

FIGURE 2.5   Motor homunculus. *Source: Reproduced from Patestas and Gartner [19], copyright 2007 with permission of Blackwell Publishing.*

Similar to the frontal lobe's motor strip, the parietal lobe contains a sensory strip (Brodmann's areas 1, 2, and 3; MCA territory) that is also organised as a sensory homunculus, or upside-down man (Figure 2.6), representing those areas that receive and analyse sensory information from different parts of the body. These areas are concerned with both deep and internal sensations, as well as cutaneous sensations such as touch, with sites of greater sensory need occupying larger areas on the sensory strip [14]. When injury occurs to a particular site, sensory loss or alteration on the opposite side of the body results.

Brodmann's areas 5 and 7 (MCA territory) are considered associative areas that further assess sensory stimuli to determine the precise purpose, relevance, and importance of sensory data. These areas are concerned with awareness of body parts, perceptual orientation in space, and recognition of environmental spatial relationships [14]. When injury occurs in these areas, perceptual neglect or inattention may occur [15, 17].

TABLE 2.3   **Frontal lobe function examination techniques**

Brodmann's area	Arterial territory	Related clinical examination
9–12	Anterior cerebral artery	Orientation to time, place, and person
		Short- and long-term memory
		Cognitive insight
		Judgement, decision-making
		Abstract processes (e.g. spelling a word backwards) and arithmetic (e.g. subtracting 7 from 100, 5 times)
4	MCA (arms), ACA (legs)	Grade motor function on a scale from 0 (absent) to 5 (normal):
		• 0/5 = No movement
		• 1/5 = Flicker of movement
		• 2/5 = Cannot overcome gravity
		• 3/5 = Cannot overcome resistance
		• 4/5 = Weak power
		• 5/5 = Normal power
		Arm pronator drift
	MCA (face)	Speech articulation
		Facial expression testing (CN VII – motor component)
		Clench teeth (CN V – motor component mandibular branch)
		Dysphagia testing
44	MCA	Expressive language
		Word-finding difficulties
		Language fluency

Brodmann's area 22 (MCA territory) is also called Wernicke's area. Most commonly located on the left side of the cerebral cortex, it is concerned with reception of both written and verbal language. It is intricately connected to other parts of the brain concerned with auditory and visual functions, as well as cognitive appraisal, emotion, and, ultimately, expressive language [14]. When this area is injured, disability ranging from minor receptive language dysfunction to receptive or fluent aphasia is likely. Those with receptive aphasia retain the ability to produce language, but its content is illogical, being described as 'word salad'. When brain injury includes areas responsible for both expression (Broca's) and reception (Wernicke's) of language, a global aphasia may result, significantly impacting quality of life through loss of most or all language ability. Table 2.4 summarises the clinical examination techniques used to assess parietal lobe function.

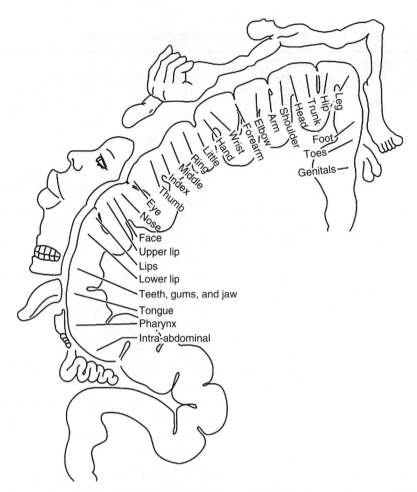

FIGURE 2.6 Sensory homunculus. *Source: Reproduced from Patestas and Gartner [19], copyright 2007 with permission of Blackwell Publishing.*

TABLE 2.4 Parietal lobe function examination techniques

Brodmann's area	Arterial territory	Related clinical examination
1–3	MCA (arms), ACA (legs)	Primary sensory testing: • Pin-prick • Touch • Vibration • Position-sense
5, 7	MCA (arms), ACA (legs)	Complex sensory testing: • Stereognosia • Double simultaneous stimulation (visual and tactile) • Graphaesthesia
22	MCA	Receptive language

2.4.3.3 Temporal Lobe
The temporal lobe lies in a lateral position beneath the temporal bone and separated from the frontal and parietal lobes by the lateral fissure. The primary functions of the temporal lobe include hearing, speech, behaviour, and memory [14].

Brodmann's areas 41 and 42 (MCA territory) are the primary auditory areas that receive sound impulses and assist in determining the source and meaning of sound. Auditory loss may be the outcome of injury to these areas. The portion of the temporal lobe where the frontal, parietal, and temporal lobes meet is an interpretive area for auditory, visual, and somatic association responsible for integrating input into complex thought and memory. Seizures originating from this region may produce auditory, visual, and sensory hallucinations. Clinical examination of temporal lobe function is primarily centred on auditory function; whilst loss of function may be associated with acute stroke, it is less common.

2.4.3.4 Occipital Lobe
The most posterior lobes in the cerebrum are the occipital lobes, which are concerned with interpretation of visual stimuli. Brodmann's area 17 (PCA territory) is the primary visual cortex, receiving impulses from the optic nerve (cranial nerve II). Impulses received here are referred to Brodmann's areas 18 and 19 (PCA territory), the visual associative areas responsible for interpretation and integration. Cortical blindness is likely following occipital lobe injury, where the ability to receive and interpret visual stimuli is lost, although the eye structures themselves remain intact [14, 17]. Clinical examination techniques pertinent to the occipital lobe are presented in Table 2.5.

2.4.4 Subcortical Region

Fibre tracts from the cerebrum converge in the area of the brain known as the *internal capsule* as they progress towards the brainstem and spinal cord. This area's arterial supply is from small perforating arterial branches of the MCA originating at the proximal portion of each hemisphere's main arterial trunk. Afferent (sensory) stimuli destined for the cortex travel from brainstem to thalamus to internal capsule to cerebral cortex. Efferent (motor) fibres leaving the cortex pass through the internal capsule en route to the brainstem and spinal cord [14]. With injuries to this area of the brain, pure sensory/motor or a combined sensory and motor loss on the opposite side of the body may occur, with preservation of cortical function [15, 17].

The *basal ganglia* comprise four pairs of nuclei (corpus striatum (caudate nucleus, putamen, and nucleus accumbens), globus pallidus, substantia nigra, and subthalamic nucleus) that regulate involuntary (extrapyramidal) motor function

TABLE 2.5 Occipital lobe function examination techniques

Brodmann's area	Arterial territory	Related clinical examination
17–19	Posterior cerebral artery	Visual field testing

and are located deep within the white matter of the cerebral hemispheres. They receive input from the cerebral cortex that stimulates their output, which is then sent to the brainstem and thalamus for relay back to the frontal cortex. The basal ganglia integrate associated movements and postural adjustments with voluntary motor movement; they suppress skeletal muscle tone as needed to provide fluid, smooth motor function. Damage to the basal ganglia typically results in tremor or other involuntary movements, rigid non-fluid muscle tone, and slowness of movement without paralysis.

The *thalamus* is made up of two ovoid masses of grey matter that form the lateral walls of the third ventricle. These serve as a relay station and gatekeeper for both motor and sensory stimuli, preventing or enhancing transmission of impulses based on situational need. Sensory and/or motor dysfunction may occur with thalamic injury, as normal impulse pathways are interrupted [15].

Located below the thalamus is the *hypothalamus*, connected to the pituitary gland by the hypothalamic or pituitary stalk. The hypothalamus coordinates many neural systems associated with emotion (including the limbic system) to control bodily behavioural responses. It is the primary control centre for internal homeostasis, stimulating autonomic nervous system responses and endocrine system functions in relation to body needs. Through these mechanisms, the hypothalamus plays a significant role in the regulation of temperature, food and water intake, pituitary hormone release, and overall autonomic nervous system function [14].

2.4.5 Cerebellum

The cerebellum (Figure 2.7), also called the 'hind brain', is separated from the cerebrum by the tentorium cerebelli. It accounts for one-fifth of the brain's overall size. The cerebellum consists of two lateral hemispheres connected by the vermis. Similar to the cerebrum, it is composed of an outer layer of grey matter, or cortex, with a core of white-matter tracts beneath [14].

The cerebellum transmits impulses to descending motor pathways to integrate spatial orientation and equilibrium with posture and muscle tone, ensuring synchronised adjustments in movement that maintain overall balance and motor coordination. The cerebellum monitors and adjusts motor activity simultaneously with movement, enabling control of fine motor function. Cerebellar injury results in ataxia, which clinically presents as preservation of motor strength without control or coordination of motor function. The AICA has very poor collateral blood supply, making this arterial territory highly susceptible to ischaemia. Typical presentation of an AICA territory stroke may include vertigo without hearing loss or tinnitus, and gaze-evoked nystagmus [15]. Cerebellar function examination techniques are presented in Table 2.6.

2.4.6 Brainstem

The brainstem is made up of three major divisions: the midbrain, pons, and medulla oblongata. This brain area is packed with sensory and motor pathways that travel between the spinal cord and the brain, as well as centres that regulate the body's vital mechanisms.

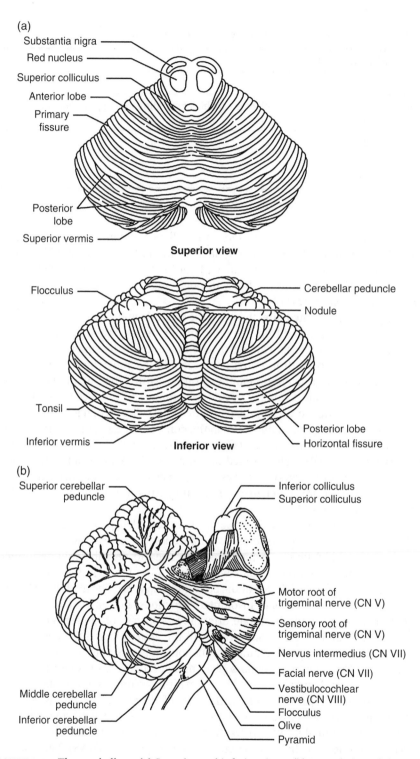

FIGURE 2.7   The cerebellum. (a) Superior and inferior views. (b) Lateral view of the cerebellum and medulla. *Source: Reproduced from Patestas and Gartner [19], copyright 2007 with permission of Blackwell Publishing.*

TABLE 2.6   **Cerebellar function examination techniques**

Clinical examination
Finger–nose–finger
Romberg's balance testing (if patient is capable of standing; not appropriate for hyperacute stroke assessment)
Speech articulation
Tandem gait testing
Heel–shin testing

Note: Cerebellar dysfunction commonly occurs alongside brainstem dysfunction.

The midbrain joins the brainstem to the diencephalon above and the pons below. Cranial nerves III and IV originate in the midbrain (Table 2.7), and the cerebral aqueduct is located in this area. Major functions of the midbrain include relay of stimuli to and from the brain through ascending sensory tracts and descending motor pathways [14].

The pons is positioned directly above the medulla and also participates in the relay of information to and from the brain through sensory and motor pathways. The upper surface of the fourth ventricle is made up of the superior part of the pons. Two respiratory control centres are located in the pons: the apneustic centre controls the length of inspiration and expiration, whilst the pneumotaxic centre controls respiratory rate. Cranial nerves V (trigeminal), VI (abducens), VII (facial), and VIII (acoustic) are located in the pons (Table 2.7). The medial longitudinal fasciculus (MLF), an important fibre tract in the pons, connects cranial nerves III, IV, and VI with the vestibular portion of the acoustic nerve and pontine paramedian reticular formation (RF), also located in the pons. The MLF fosters coordinated and appropriate movements of the eyes in response to noise, motion, position, and arousal; this is used by clinicians assessing the structural integrity of the brainstem by caloric testing [14, 17].

The medulla oblongata is situated between the pons and the spinal cord. Voluntary motor fibres cross over (decussate) in the pyramids of the medulla – pyramidal fibres – which are often used to describe voluntary motor function. This crossing over explains why stimuli from the right side of the brain control movement for the left side of the body and vice versa. The medulla oblongata houses the centres for control of involuntary functions such as swallowing, vomiting, hiccoughing, coughing, heart rate, arterial vasoconstriction, and respiration. The medullary respiratory centre works with both the apneustic and the pneumotaxic centres in the pons to control respiratory function, and is responsible for the rhythm of respiration. Cranial nerves IX (glossopharyngeal), X (vagus), XI (spinal accessory), and XII (hypoglossal) are also located in the medulla oblongata (see Table 2.7) [14].

The brainstem's RF is located at the core of the brainstem and is active in modulating sensation, movement, consciousness, reflexive behaviour, and the activities of the cranial nerves arising from the brainstem (III–XII) [14]. Ascending RF is commonly called the reticular activating system (RAS), because it is responsible for increasing wakefulness, vigilance, and responsiveness of cortical and thalamic neurons to sensory stimuli. Specifically, the RAS activates both the relay and the diffuse projection nuclei of the thalamus to increase distribution of

TABLE 2.7 Cranial nerve anatomy, physiology, and assessment

Cranial nerve	Anatomy	Physiology	Assessment
I. Olfactory (sensory)	Cell body located in the nasal mucosa. Axon passes through the ethmoid's cribriform plate to olfactory bulbs, with temporal lobe interpretation of smell	Smell; participates in the stimulation of additional systems triggered by smell interpretation, including peristalsis, salivation, and sexual stimulation	Rarely tested; with the eyes closed, the patient is presented with different familiar non-irritating odours. Commercial kits such as 'Sniffin' Sticks' may be used
II. Optic (sensory)	Retinal ganglionic cells converge in the optic disc, forming the optic nerve. Nerve fibres travel through the optic chiasm and the lateral geniculate body, terminating in the occipital lobe	Vision, including visual acuity and peripheral vision	• Ophthalmoscope inspection of the optic fundi • Visual acuity: Often deferred in critical care; pocket-size Snellen cards may be used, but are usually impractical • Visual fields: Four quadrants of vision are tested by confrontation in the cooperative patient, or by assessing blink to threat in the uncooperative patient • Visual neglect may be tested using double simultaneous stimulation (DSS) by having the patient identify simultaneous movement in the examiner's right and left fingers. Note: Neglect is *not* visual loss, but inability to discriminate between two simultaneous stimuli
III. Oculomotor (motor)	Cell body located in the midbrain. Supplies motor fibres to the superior, inferior, and medial recti, as well as the inferior oblique of the eye. Also supplies the levator muscle of the eyelid and gives off parasympathetic fibres to the ciliary muscles and iris	Extraocular movements; moves the eye in the following directions: superior rectus – elevation medial rectus – adduction (medially) inferior rectus – depression (downward) inferior oblique – extorsion (up and in) Raises eyelid and constricts the pupil	• Assess for unilateral eyelid drooping (III) • Assess pupil size (range 1–6 mm) and symmetry. Note: 20% of people have anisocoria – a difference in pupil size of 0.5 mm. Anisocoria is normal if pupil light response is normal (III) • Assess pupil response to light: Direct response – the pupil of the eye directly receiving the light stimulus contracts; consensual response – the pupil of the eye not receiving the light stimulus contracts. Pupillary response is noted to be brisk, sluggish, or non-reactive (III)

(continued)

TABLE 2.7 Cranial nerve anatomy, physiology, and assessment (*continued*)

Cranial nerve	Anatomy	Physiology	Assessment
IV. Trochlear (motor)	Cell body located in the midbrain. Supplies motor fibres to the superior oblique muscle of the eye	Extraocular movements; moves the eye down and in (intorsion)	• Eye movement is coordinated through the internuclear pathway of the medial longitudinal fasciculus (MLF), and involves the integrated responses of the III, IV, and VI cranial nerves, as well as input from the VIII nerve
V. Trigeminal (sensory and motor)	Cell body located in the pons. Gives off three branches: ophthalmic (sensory), maxillary (sensory), and mandibular (sensory and motor)	Ophthalmic branch: provides sensation to the cornea, ciliary body, iris, lacrimal gland, conjunctiva, nasal mucosa, forehead, and nose Maxillary branch: provides sensation to the skin of the cheek and nose, lower eyelid, upper jaw, teeth, mouth mucosa, and maxillary sinuses Mandibular branch: provides sensation to lower jaw and motor function to muscles of mastication	• The ophthalmic branch is tested by eliciting a corneal reflex; in the unconscious patient, a blink should normally occur in response to gentle contact with the cornea by a cotton wisp • The maxillary branch is tested with dull/sharp discrimination using a pin • The mandibular branch is a mixed motor and sensory branch and may be tested by palpating muscles of the jaw during clenching of the teeth
VI. Abducens (motor)	Cell body located in the pons. Supplies motor fibres to the lateral rectus muscle	Extraocular movements; moves the eye laterally (abduction)	• Ability of the eye to move in the six cardinal directions is assessed; the conscious patient is asked to follow the examiner's finger movements with his or her eyes; the examiner moves his or her finger to trace the pattern of either an 'H' or an 'X' with a horizontal line through the middle; deviations in eye movement are noted • In the unconscious patient, the oculocephalic reflex (doll's eyes) can be assessed once the cervical spine has been checked and the neck can be safely manipulated; the patient's head is turned side to side with the eyes held open; normally, the eyes should move in the opposite direction to the head; eyes that remain in a fixed position indicate dysfunction of the midbrain/pontine region, which houses the nuclei of cranial nerves III, IV, and VI

VII. Facial (sensory and motor)	Cell body located in the pons. Supplies sensory fibres to the anterior two-thirds of the tongue and soft palate; supplies motor fibres to the muscles of the face	Taste and sensation for the anterior two-thirds of the tongue and soft palate; serves as the primary motor nerve for facial expression	• Facial expression is tested by having the patient puff out the cheeks, smile/show the teeth, tightly close the eyes, and lift the eyebrows; asymmetry is noted • Taste is rarely tested
VIII. Acoustic (sensory)	Cell body located in the pons Cochlear sensory fibres originate in the ganglia of the cochlea, transmitting auditory sensation to the organ of Corti in the ear, pons, and temporal lobe Vestibular sensory fibres originate in the semicircular canals of the ear and vestibular ganglion, terminating in the pons	Hearing Equilibrium	• Whispered-word testing may be considered • In the unconscious patient, the oculovestibular reflex (ice water caloric testing) may determine brainstem integrity. The III, IV, VI, and VIII nerves are stimulated through injection of iced water into the ear canal whilst the head is kept in a midline/neutral position with the eyes held open. Confirm that the tympanic membrane is intact prior to performing the procedure. The normal response is a conjugate nystagmus with deviation in the direction of the irrigated ear with a slow rhythmic quality. Absent eye movement or dysconjugate movement indicates brainstem injury. This procedure may produce nausea and vomiting in the conscious patient
IX. Glossopharyngeal (sensory and motor)	Cell body located in the medulla oblongata Sensory divisions transmit stimuli from the external ear, tympanic membrane, upper pharynx, and posterior one-third of the tongue to the medulla Motor divisions supply voluntary control of the stylopharyngeus muscle and innervate the parotid gland	Stylopharyngeus muscle elevation for swallowing and speech Parotid gland secretion General sensory (pain, touch, temperature) function as specified	• The IX and X nerves are commonly tested together • Assess for symmetrical elevation of the palate, posterior pharynx, and uvula • Palpate the larynx during swallowing, assessing for symmetrical laryngeal elevation • Have the patient repeat a word with a 'K' sound (e.g. 'kitty cat') and listen for complete/discrete pronunciation of the 'K' • Assess gag reflex

(continued)

TABLE 2.7 Cranial nerve anatomy, physiology, and assessment (*continued*)

Cranial nerve	Anatomy	Physiology	Assessment
X. Vagus (sensory and motor)	The major parasympathetic nerve of the body, 'vagus' is Latin for 'wandering'; it originates in the medulla oblongata and travels as far as the splenic flexure of the colon. Motor components supply the pharynx, larynx, and thoracic and abdominal viscera; sensory components transmit larynx, oesophagus, trachea, carotid bodies, and thoracic and abdominal viscera, as well as stretch and chemoreceptors from the aorta	Provides the majority of parasympathetic innervation to the regions specified. Effects include digestion, defaecation, slowing of heart rate, and reduction of contraction strength	
XI. Spinal accessory (motor)	Cell body located in the medulla oblongata with two roots: cranial and spinal Cranial root innervates muscles of the larynx and pharynx; spinal root innervates trapezius and sternocleidomastoid muscles	Plays a role in swallowing and phonation. Innervates the muscles that turn the head and elevate the shoulders (shoulder shrug)	• Have the patient shrug his or her shoulders against resistance whilst pushing them downward • Have the patient turn his or her head against resistance whilst pushing on one side of the face; repeat with resistance applied to the opposite side
XII. Hypoglossal (motor)	Cell body located in the medulla oblongata. Sends off motor fibres to the tongue	Tongue movement	• Have the patient push his or her tongue into a cheek whilst applying resistance against the cheek; repeat with resistance applied to the other cheek • Have the patient stick his or her tongue out and move it side to side • Have the patient repeat a word with an 'L' sound (e.g. 'lollypop', 'la-la-la') and listen for complete/discrete pronunciation of the 'L'

TABLE 2.8   Brainstem function examination techniques

Clinical examination
Cranial nerves III–XII (see Table 2.7)
Dysphagia testing
Level of consciousness: • Alert = awake • Lethargic = sleepy, dull, indifferent • Obtunded = deeply sleeping • Stuporous = arousable to noxious stimuli (localises or withdraws) • Comatose = unresponsive with absent or reflex response (decorticate, decerebrate, or spinal cord reflex arc) to noxious stimuli
Voluntary motor function: • 0/5 = No movement • 1/5 = Flicker of movement • 2/5 = Cannot overcome gravity • 3/5 = Cannot overcome resistance • 4/5 = Weak power • 5/5 = Normal power
Pin-prick
Touch
Vibration
Respiratory pattern, heart rate, and blood pressure

Note: Cerebellar dysfunction commonly occurs alongside brainstem dysfunction.

sensory stimuli throughout the cerebral cortex; additionally, it activates the hypothalamus, resulting in diffuse cortical and autonomic stimulation. Injury to the thalamic or hypothalamic RAS pathways may result in impaired consciousness [15]. Table 2.8 presents the clinical examination pertinent to the brainstem.

2.5   Standardised Instruments for Acute Neurological Assessment

All assessments and supporting instruments require appropriate training to produce reliable assessment findings. A number of instruments have been constructed to support clinicians in conducting an acute neurological assessment, including:

- the Glasgow Coma Scale (GCS) [20];
- the Intracerebral Haemorrhage Score (ICHS) [21];
- the Hunt and Hess (H-H) Score [12]; and
- the National Institutes of Health Stroke Scale (NIHSS) [22].

2.5.1 Glasgow Coma Scale (GCS)

The GCS is the most widely utilised neurological assessment instrument. It tests three categories of functioning to gauge level of consciousness (LOC): eye opening, best verbal response, and best motor response (Table 2.9). Each category should be reported separately; the highest possible total score is 15, and the lowest is 3, with scores of 7 or less indicating significant LOC dysfunction. Commonly used across a wide variety of diagnoses, it is not a substitute for complete neurological assessment. Additionally, those using the GCS should bear in mind that it was developed to gauge severity in patients with traumatic brain injury [20], which explains its limited 'fit' with stroke presentation. Importantly, the GCS is insensitive to detection of focal neurological deficit and is based on recording the patient's best response; because of this, the tool will fail to capture deficits limited to one side of the body or fluctuating signs [23]. Scores of verbal response

TABLE 2.9 Glasgow Coma Scale (GCS). E + M + V = 3–15

	Activity	Score	Characteristics
Eye opening	None	1	Even to supra-orbital pressure
	To pain	2	Pain from sternum/limb/supra-orbital pressure
	To speech	3	Non-specific response, not necessarily to command
	Spontaneous	4	Eyes open, not necessarily aware
Motor response	None	1	To any pain; limbs remain flaccid
	Extension	2	Shoulder adducted and shoulder and forearm internally rotated
	Flexor response	3	Withdrawal response or assumption of hemiplegic posture
	Withdrawal	4	Arm withdraws to pain, shoulder abducts
	Localises pain	5	Arm attempts to remove supra-orbital/chest pressure
	Obeys commands	6	Follows simple commands
Verbal response	None	1	No verbalisation of any type
	Incomprehensible	2	Moans/groans, no speech
	Inappropriate	3	Intelligible, no sustained sentences
	Confused	4	Converses but confused, disoriented
	Oriented	5	Converses and oriented

TABLE 2.10   **Intracerebral Haemorrhage Score (ICHS)**

Component	Score
Glasgow Coma Scale score	
GCS = 3–4	2
GCS = 5–12	1
GCS = 13–15	0
ICH volume (cm³)	
ICH ≥30 ml	1
ICH <30 ml	0
Intraventricular component?	
Yes – intraventricular component present	1
No – no intraventricular haemorrhage	0
Infratentorial origin of ICH?	
Yes –infratentorial in origin	1
No – not infratentorial in origin	0
Age in years	
≥80 yr	1
<80 yr	0
Total score	*0–6*

are confounded by endotracheal intubation. The GCS was validated for use in traumatic brain injury, yet it is used as a measure of LOC in haemorrhagic stroke [11].

2.5.2 Intracerebral Haemorrhage Score (ICHS)

The ICHS was developed to support acute trials in therapies for IPH [11, 21]. It consists of five components: GCS score, volume of the haemorrhage, presence of intraventricular haemorrhage, infratentorial bleed location, and patient age (Table 2.10). Scores of 3 have been associated with 70% mortality, whilst scores of 4 or more have been associated with 90–100% mortality.

2.5.3 Hunt and Hess (H-H) Score

The H-H Score is used to grade the clinical severity of non-traumatic SAH [12]. The score consists of five grades ranging from minimal (grade 1) to severe (grade 5) (Table 2.11).

TABLE 2.11 **Hunt and Hess (H-H) Score**

Grade	Clinical features
1	Asymptomatic, mild headache, slight nuchal rigidity
2	Moderate to severe headache, nuchal rigidity
	No neurological deficit other than cranial nerve palsy
3	Drowsiness/confusion; mild focal neurological deficit
4	Stupor; moderate–severe hemiparesis
5	Coma; decerebrate posturing

2.5.4 National Institutes of Health Stroke Scale (NIHSS)

The NIHSS was developed to support acute ischaemic stroke treatment trials and has reliability when used by appropriately trained clinicians [22]. It is considered the only valid tool to assess stroke deficit severity [2, 23]. The NIHSS consists of a total of 14 categories that test LOC, extraocular movement, visual fields, facial expression, arm and leg motor function, cerebellar function, sensory function, language fluency, speech articulation, and neglect or extinction (Table 2.12) [24]. Total possible score ranges from 0 (no neurological deficit) to 42 (severe neurological deficit). Each item within the scale must be scored unless it is deemed 'untestable'. Whilst the NIHSS appears complex on first glance, experience with the instrument may result in rapid completion, taking 5–7 minutes. The NIHSS is mandated as an assessment supporting practice by US stroke guidelines, the US Centers for Medicare and Medicaid, and accrediting agencies for US Stroke Centers, because it provides a common language for gauging stroke severity and improvement following treatment with intravenous thrombolysis or intra-arterial rescue therapies.

Other instruments to assess stroke-related impairment are also used; for example, the Scandinavian Stroke Scale provides an index of overall stroke impairment severity, the Barthel Index provides a broad measure of disability, and the Action Research Arm Test provides a focused view of effects in one limb. In addition, a range of broader tools have been employed, such as the Medical Outcomes Study Short Form 36 (SF-36) and the Stroke-Specific Quality of Life tool, which examine the effects of stroke within a whole-life context.

2.6 Conclusion

This chapter provides a brief overview of normal anatomy and physiology, disease processes associated with development of a stroke, and tools commonly used to gauge the severity and detail of the physiological impact of the stroke on the individual. It offers the basic and fundamental knowledge essential for all clinicians involved with stroke patients, enabling them to understand the disease process as a first step towards care and treatment of the person.

TABLE 2.12   National Institutes of Health Stroke Scale (NIHSS)

1a. *Level of consciousness*. The investigator must choose a response, even if a full evaluation is prevented by such obstacles as an endotracheal tube, language barrier, or orotracheal trauma/bandages. A 3 is scored only if the patient makes no movement (other than reflexive posturing) in response to noxious stimulation	1a: —— 0 = Alert; keenly responsive 1 = Not alert, but arousable by minor stimulation to obey, answer, or respond 2 = Not alert, requires repeated stimulation to attend, or is obtunded and requires strong or painful stimulation to make movements (not stereotyped) 3 = Responds only with reflex motor or autonomic effects or is totally unresponsive, flaccid, and areflexic
1b. *LOC questions*. The patient is asked the month and his or her age. The answer must be correct – there is no partial credit for being close. Aphasic and stuporous patients who do not comprehend the questions will score 2. Patients unable to speak because of endotracheal intubation, orotracheal trauma, severe dysarthria from any cause, a language barrier, or any other problem not secondary to aphasia are given a 1. It is important that only the initial answer be graded and that the examiner not 'help' the patient with verbal or non-verbal cues	1b: —— 0 = Answers both questions correctly 1 = Answers one question correctly 2 = Answers neither question correctly
1c. *LOC commands*. The patient is asked to open and close the eyes and then to grip and release the non-paretic hand. Substitute another one-step command if the hands cannot be used. Credit is given if an unequivocal attempt is made but not completed due to weakness. If the patient does not respond to command, the task should be demonstrated to them (pantomime) and the result scored (i.e. follows none, one, or two commands). Patients with trauma, amputation, or other physical impediments should be given suitable one-step commands. Only the first attempt is scored	1c: —— 0 = Performs both tasks correctly 1 = Performs one task correctly 2 = Performs neither task correctly

(continued)

TABLE 2.12 National Institutes of Health Stroke Scale (NIHSS) (*continued*)

2. *Best gaze.* Only horizontal eye movements will be tested. Voluntary or reflexive (oculocephalic) eye movements will be scored but caloric testing is not done. If the patient has a conjugate deviation of the eyes that can be overcome by voluntary or reflexive activity, the score will be 1. If a patient has an isolated peripheral nerve paresis (CN III, IV, or VI), score a 1. Gaze is testable in all aphasic patients. Patients with ocular trauma, bandages, pre-existing blindness, or other disorder of visual acuity or fields should be tested with reflexive movements and a choice should be made by the investigator. Establishing eye contact and then moving about the patient from side to side will occasionally clarify the presence of a partial gaze palsy	0 = Normal 1 = Partial gaze palsy. This score is given when gaze is abnormal in one or both eyes, but where forced deviation or total gaze paresis is not present 2 = Forced deviation, or total gaze paresis not overcome by the oculocephalic manoeuvre	2: ____
3. *Visual.* Visual fields (upper and lower quadrants) are tested by confrontation, using finger counting or visual threat as appropriate. Patient must be encouraged, but if they look at the side of the moving fingers appropriately, this can be scored as normal. If there is unilateral blindness or enucleation, visual fields in the remaining eye are scored. Score 1 only if a clear-cut asymmetry, including quadrantanopia, is found. If patient is blind from any cause, score 3. Double simultaneous stimulation (DSS) is performed at this point. If there is extinction, score a 1 and use the results to answer point 11	0 = No visual loss 1 = Partial hemianopia 2 = Complete hemianopia 3 = Bilateral hemianopia (blind, including cortical blindness)	3: ____
4. *Facial palsy.* Ask or use pantomime to encourage the patient to show the teeth or raise the eyebrows and close the eyes. Score symmetry of grimace in response to noxious stimuli in the poorly responsive or non-comprehending patient. If facial trauma/bandages, orotracheal tube, tape, or another physical barrier obscures the face, this should be removed to the extent possible	0 = Normal symmetrical movement 1 = Minor paralysis (flattened nasolabial fold, asymmetry on smiling) 2 = Partial paralysis (total or near-total paralysis of lower face) 3 = Complete paralysis of one or both sides (absence of facial movement in the upper and lower face)	4: ____

5 and 6. *Motor arm and leg*. Place the limb in the appropriate position: extend the arms (palms down) 90° (if sitting) or 45° (if supine) and the leg 30° (always tested supine). Score drift if the arm falls before 10 seconds or the leg before 5 seconds. Encourage the aphasic patient using vocal urgency and pantomime, but not noxious stimulation. Test each limb in turn, beginning with the non-paretic arm. Only in the case of amputation or joint fusion at the shoulder or hip may the score be 9, and the examiner must clearly write the explanation for not scoring	0 = No drift, limb holds 90° (or 45°) for full 10 seconds 1 = Drift, limb holds 90° (or 45°) but drifts down before full 10 seconds; does not hit bed or other support 2 = Some effort against gravity, limb cannot get to or maintain (if cued) 90° (or 45°), drifts down to bed, but has some effort against gravity 3 = No effort against gravity, limb falls 4 = No movement 9 = Amputation, joint fusion. Explain: _____	5a. L Arm: ____ 5b. R Arm: ____ 6a. L Leg: ____ 6b. R Leg: ____
7. *Limb ataxia*. This item is aimed at finding evidence of a unilateral cerebellar lesion. Test with eyes open. In case of visual defect, ensure testing is done in intact visual field. Perform the finger–nose–finger and heel–shin tests on both sides, and score ataxia only if present out of proportion to weakness. Ataxia is absent in the patient who cannot understand or is paralysed. Only in the case of amputation or joint fusion may the item be scored 9, and the examiner must clearly write the explanation for not scoring. In case of blindness, test by touching nose from extended arm position	0 = Absent 1 = Present in one limb 2 = Present in two limbs. If present, is ataxia in: Right arm? 1 = Yes, 2 = No 9 = Amputation or joint fusion. Explain: _____ Left arm? 1 = Yes, 2 = No 9 = Amputation or joint fusion. Explain: _____ Right leg? 1 = Yes, 2 = No 9 = amputation or joint fusion. Explain: _____ Left leg? 1 = Yes, 2 = No 9 = Amputation or joint fusion. Explain: _____	7: ____

(continued)

TABLE 2.12 National Institutes of Health Stroke Scale (NIHSS) (continued)

		8: ___
8. *Sensory.* Sensation or grimace to pin-prick when tested, or withdrawal from noxious stimulus in the obtunded or aphasic patient. Only sensory loss attributed to stroke is scored as abnormal, and the examiner should test as many body areas (arms [not hands], legs, trunk, face) as needed to accurately check for hemisensory loss. A score of 2, 'severe or total', should only be given when a severe or total loss of sensation can be clearly demonstrated. Stuporous and aphasic patients will therefore probably score 1 or 0. The patient with brainstem stroke who has bilateral loss of sensation is scored 2. If the patient does not respond and is quadriplegic, score 2. Patients in a coma (item 1a = 3) are automatically given a 2 on this item	0 = Normal; no sensory loss 1 = Mild to moderate sensory loss; patient feels pinprick is less sharp or is dull on the affected side, or there is a loss of superficial pain with pinprick but patient is aware he or she is being touched 2 = Severe to total sensory loss; patient is not aware of being touched in the face, arm, and leg	

		9: ___
9. *Best language.* A great deal of information about comprehension will be obtained during the preceding sections of the examination. The patient is asked to describe what is happening in the attached picture, to name the items on the attached naming sheet, and to read from the attached list of sentences. Comprehension is judged from responses here as well as to all of the commands in the preceding general neurological exam. If visual loss interferes with the tests, ask the patient to identify objects placed in the hand, repeat, and produce speech. The intubated patient should be asked to write. The patient in coma (question 1a = 3) will arbitrarily score 3 on this item. The examiner must choose a score in the patient with stupor or limited cooperation but a score of 3 should be used only if the patient is mute and follows no one-step commands (The patient's language will be tested by having the patient identify standard groups of objects and by reading a series of sentences. Comprehension of language should be judged as the physician performs the entire neurologic examination. The physician should give the patient adequate time to identify the objects on the sheet of paper. Only the first response is measured. If the patient misidentifies the object and later corrects him or herself, the response is still considered abnormal. The physician should then give the patient a sheet of paper with the series of sentences. The examiner should ask the patient to read at least three sentences. The first attempt to read the sentence is measured. If the patient misreads the sentence and later corrects him or herself, the response is still considered abnormal. If the patient's visual loss precludes visual identification of objects or reading, the examiner should ask the patient to identify objects placed in his or her hand and the examiner should judge the patient's spontaneous speech and ability to repeat sentences. If the examiner judges these responses as normal, the score should be 0. If the patient is intubated or is unable to speak, the examiner should check the patient's writing)	0 = No aphasia, normal 1 = Mild to moderate aphasia; some obvious loss of fluency or facility of comprehension, without significant limitation on ideas expressed or form of expression. Reduction of speech or comprehension, but without making conversation about provided material impossible. For example, in conversation about provided materials, examiner can identify picture or naming card from patient's response 2 = Severe aphasia; all communication is through fragmentary expression; great need for inference, questioning, and guessing by the listener. Range of information that can be exchanged is limited; listener carries burden of communication. Examiner cannot identify materials provided from patient response 3 = Mute, global aphasia; no usable speech or auditory comprehension	

10. *Dysarthria*. If patient is thought to be normal, an adequate sample of speech must be obtained by asking patient to read or repeat words from the attached list. If the patient has severe aphasia, the clarity of articulation of spontaneous speech can be rated. Only if the patient is intubated or has other physical barrier to producing speech may the item be scored '9', and the examiner must clearly write an explanation for not scoring. The patient should not be told why he or she is being tested. (The primary method of examination is to ask the patient to read and pronounce a standard list of words from a sheet of paper. If the patient is unable to read the words because of visual loss, the physician may say them aloud and ask the patient to repeat them. If the patient has severe aphasia, the clarity of articulation of spontaneous speech should be rated. If the patient is mute or comatose (item 9, Best Language = 3) or has an endotracheal tube, this item can be rated as 9 – untestable)	10: ____ 0 = Normal 1 = Mild to moderate; patient slurs at least some words and, at worst, can be understood with some difficulty 2 = Severe; patient's speech is so slurred as to be unintelligible in the absence of or out of proportion to any dysphasia, or is mute/anarthric 9 = Intubated or other physical barrier. Explain: ____
11. *Extinction and inattention (formerly Neglect)*. Sufficient information to identify neglect may be obtained during the prior testing. If the patient has a severe visual loss preventing visual double simultaneous stimulation, and the cutaneous stimuli are normal, the score is normal. If the patient has aphasia but does appear to attend to both sides, the score is normal. The presence of visual spatial neglect or anosognosia may also be taken as evidence of abnormality. Since the abnormality is scored only if present, the item is never untestable	11: ____ 0 = No abnormality 1 = Visual, tactile, auditory, spatial, or personal inattention or extinction to bilateral simultaneous stimulation in one of the sensory modalities 2 = Profound hemi-inattention or hemi-inattention to more than one modality. Does not recognise own hand or orients to only one side of space ____

References

1. UK Stroke Forum Education & Training. About the SSEF. Available from: http://www.stroke-education.org.uk/about [30 November 2018].
2. Jauch, E.C., Saver, J.L., Adams, H.P.J. et al. (2013). Guidelines for the early management of patients with acute ischemic stroke: a guideline for healthcare professionals from the American Heart Association/American Stroke Association. Stroke 44 (3): 870–947.
3. Adams, H.P., Bendixen, B.H., Kappelle, L.J. et al. (1993). Classification of subtype of acute ischemic stroke. Definitions for use in a multicenter clinical trial. Stroke 24 (1): 35–41.
4. Foulkes, M.A., Wolf, P.A., Price, T.R. et al. (1988). The Stroke Data Bank: design, methods, and baseline characteristics. Stroke 19 (5): 547–554.
5. Cabanes, L., Mas, J.L., Cohen, A. et al. (1993). Atrial septal aneurysm and patent foramen ovale as risk factors for cryptogenic stroke in patients less than 55 years of age. A study using transesophageal echocardiography. Stroke 24 (12): 1865–1873.
6. Lechat, P., Lascault, G., Mas, J.L. et al. (1989). Prevalence of patent foramen ovale in young patients with ischemic cerebral complications. Archives des Maladies due Couer et des Vaisseaux 82 (6): 847–852.
7. Webster, M.W.I., Smith, H.J., Sharpe, D.N. et al. (1988). Patent foramen ovale in young stroke patients. The Lancet 332 (8601): 11–12.
8. Ciconte, G., Giacopelli, D., and Pappone, C. (2017). The role of implantable cardiac monitors in atrial fibrillation management. Journal of Atrial Fibrillation 10 (2): 1–7.
9. Bernstein, R.A., Di Lazzaro, V., Rymer, M.M. et al. (2015). Infarct topography and detection of atrial fibrillation in cryptogenic stroke: results from CRYSTAL AF. Cerebrovascular Diseases 40 (1–2): 91–96.
10. Brachmann, J., Morillo, C.A., Sanna, T. et al. (2016). Uncovering atrial fibrillation beyond short-term monitoring in cryptogenic stroke patients. Three-year results from the cryptogenic stroke and underlying atrial fibrillation trial. Stroke 9 (1): 1–9.
11. Hemphill, J.C., Greenberg, S.M., Anderson, C.S. et al. (2015). Guidelines for the management of spontaneous intracerebral hemorrhage. A guideline for healthcare professionals from the American Heart Association/American Stroke Association. Stroke 46 (7): 2032–2060.
12. Bederson, J.B., Connolly, E.S., Batjer, H.H. et al. (2009). Guidelines for the management of aneurysmal subarachnoid hemorrhage. A statement for healthcare professionals from a special writing group of the Stroke Council, American Heart Association. Stroke 40 (3): 994–1025.
13. Goldstein, L.B., Bushnell, C.D., Adams, R.J. et al. (2011). Guidelines for the primary prevention of stroke. A guideline for healthcare professionals from the American Heart Association/American Stroke Association. Stroke 42 (2): 517–584.
14. Standring, S. (2016). Gray's Anatomy: The Anatomical Basis for Clinical Practice, 41e. Philadelphia: Elsevier.
15. Hall, J.E. (2016). Guyton and Hall Textbook of Medical Physiology, 13e. Philadelphia: Elsevier.
16. Alexandrov, A.V. (2003). Cerebrovascular Ultrasound in Stroke Prevention and Treatment. Armonk: Blackwell-Futura.
17. Alexandrov, A.W. (2012). Core Curriculum for Neurovascular Nursing. Phoenix: Association of Neurovascular Clinicians.
18. Gloor, P. (1997). The Temporal Lobe and Limbic System. New York: Oxford University Press.
19. Patestas, M.A. and Gartner, L.P. (2007). A Textbook of Neuroanatomy, 2e. New York: Wiley Blackwell.

20. Teasdale, G. and Jennett, B. (1974). Assessment of coma and impaired consciousness: a practical scale. The Lancet 304 (7872): 81–84.
21. Hemphill, J.C., Bonovich, D.C., Besmertis, L. et al. (2001). The ICH score: a simple, reliable grading scale for intracerebral hemorrhage. Stroke 32 (4): 891–897.
22. Goldstein, L.B. and Samsa, G.P. (1997). Reliability of the National Institutes of Health Stroke Scale-Extension to non-neurologists in the context of a clinical trial. Stroke 28 (2): 307–310.
23. Nye, B.R., Hyde, C.E., Tsivgoulis, G. et al. (2012). Slim strokes for assessing patients with acute stroke: ease of use or loss of valuable assessment data? American Journal of Critical Care 21 (6): 442–448.
24. National Institute of Neurological Disorders and Stroke. Stroke information page. Available from: https://www.ninds.nih.gov/Disorders/All-Disorders/Stroke-Information-Page [30 November 2018].

CHAPTER 3

Reducing the Risk of Stroke

Josephine Gibson and Stephanie Jones
School of Nursing, University of Central Lancashire, Preston, UK

KEY POINTS

- Stroke is an increasingly important public health issue because of the ageing of the population and the rising prevalence of major risk factors such as obesity and type 2 diabetes.
- Public awareness of stroke risk factors, and of the signs and symptoms of stroke, is poor, especially in those at higher risk.
- Primary prevention, via identifying and addressing risk factors before stroke or transient ischaemic attack (TIA) occurs, is a major part of many primary care initiatives, but is challenging to implement successfully.
- The management of anticoagulation to reduce stroke risk in atrial fibrillation (AF) is evolving rapidly with the advent of direct oral anticoagulants, but many people with AF are still undiagnosed or untreated.
- After stroke or TIA, an individualised plan for secondary prevention should be implemented immediately and continued long-term to reduce the risk of future stroke and other vascular events.
- Carotid endarterectomy is an important measure to reduce the risk of stroke after TIA, but is an adjunct to – not a replacement for – concurrent and long-term risk factor management via appropriate medication and behaviour modification.

Stroke Nursing, Second Edition. Edited by Jane Williams, Lin Perry, and Caroline Watkins.
© 2020 John Wiley & Sons Ltd. Published 2020 by John Wiley & Sons Ltd.

This chapter maps to criteria within the following sections of the Stroke-Specific Education Framework (SSEF):

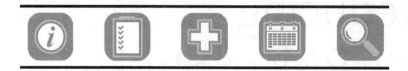

I'd never heard of TIA and assumed I'd had a stroke until I saw 'TIA' written on the discharge letter I was given. No one mentioned it to me, never mind explaining what it was, or that it increased my stroke risk. I was told that someone who could give me lifestyle advice would get in contact but it never happened. I was given no information about diet or other ways to reduce my risk and I've since taken it upon myself to switch to low-fat milk and olive oil spread instead of butter. When healthcare staff promise to follow up, they should get in contact.

(Janet, aged 77) [2]

3.1 Introduction

Stroke is a major public health issue: despite a fall in incidence, it is still the third most common cause of death and the leading cause of adult-onset disability in high-income countries (HICs). Therefore, even a small reduction in stroke incidence may result in major public health gains. Reducing stroke risk – for individuals or whole populations – is challenging for many reasons. Stroke risk is multifactorial, so strategies to reduce stroke incidence require management of medical and behavioural factors which are not always treatable. Furthermore, those at highest risk of stroke may also face the greatest challenges in reducing their risk. Stroke risk reduction is therefore an important component of practice for nurses and other health professionals working with patients across the stroke pathway, including pre-stroke care. These reflect SSEF elements of managing risk, information, transient ischaemic attack (TIA) assessment and treatment, long-term care, and review.

We will discuss measures to reduce stroke risk and impact on several levels: population measures aimed at reducing stroke risk and raising stroke awareness; primary prevention for those at risk of stroke; and secondary prevention to reduce risk of recurrent stroke. We consider interventions to address common medical and behavioural risk factors for stroke, challenges to reducing stroke risk for populations and individuals, interventions for specific medical conditions for both primary and secondary prevention, and management of ongoing stroke risk where no specific cause has been identified.

3.2 Primary Prevention

3.2.1 An Epidemiological Perspective

Stroke incidence has been greater in HICs compared to low- and middle-income countries (LMICs), but with some within-country variations. The incidence of stroke in LMICs now exceeds that in HICs. LMICs also have greater case fatality and a younger age of stroke onset, factors that contribute to a high stroke burden. Incidence rates are affected by the population age profiles and several behavioural factors.

The world's population is ageing: the proportion aged over 60 is projected to increase from 12% in 2013 to 21% in 2050 [3]. In the United Kingdom, the proportion aged over 60 is projected to increase from 19.4% in 2012 to 29.3% by 2032 [4]. As stroke risk rises with age, there are clear implications for stroke incidence.

Important modifiable risk factors for stroke are smoking, obesity and the consequent development of type 2 diabetes mellitus (DM), as well as hypertension and atrial fibrillation (AF). Whilst tobacco smoking uptake and prevalence rates are falling in HICs, in LMICs they are rising. Tobacco smoking trebles the risk of stroke compared to non-smokers [5]. Obesity is increasing in many countries, with an associated epidemic of type 2 DM. This is a major public health concern due to the increased risk of vascular diseases, including stroke.

Within countries, socioeconomic inequalities confer an increased stroke risk. It is estimated that people in social class 5 (unskilled workers) have around 2.5 times the stroke risk of those in social class 1 (professional and managerial workers), even after adjusting for confounding variables such as tobacco smoking, lack of exercise, and dietary factors [6].

3.2.2 Population Approaches to Reducing Stroke Risk and Raising Awareness

Although stroke risk factors are well understood by health professionals, public awareness varies. The ability to name one or more risk factors when unprompted ranges between 18 and 94% [7]. Recognition of major risk factors is poor: when responding to open-ended questions, only 24% of the public were able to identify high blood pressure (BP) as a stroke risk factor [8]. Those with lower levels of education tend to have poorer knowledge of stroke [9, 10]. Age and ethnicity also affect knowledge, with older people having poorer knowledge of stroke risk factors [11–13] and symptoms [14]. People at high risk of stroke, including stroke survivors, have similar levels of knowledge about stroke risk as the general population [15]. This warrants further attention, particularly as these groups are, by definition, at higher risk of stroke than the general population.

Lack of knowledge of stroke risk factors has potential to compromise the effectiveness of risk-reduction approaches. Consider the example of the National Health Service (NHS) 'Health Checks' programme in England and Wales. This population approach to addressing stroke risk aims to identify people at higher risk of developing vascular conditions, including stroke, and to offer them support to address risk factors through behavioural modification and appropriate medical treatment. The scheme invites people aged 40–74 years without existing vascular conditions to have a test battery including fasting glucose and lipids blood tests, BP, and weight, and discussion of tobacco and alcohol use, diet, and physical activity. However, there is little evidence the scheme is more effective than opportunistic case-finding [16]. Uptake of health checks is also poor, with less than half of those invited attending [17].

Public knowledge is also important in relation to help-seeking behaviour for stroke and TIA symptoms, especially given the time-critical nature of stroke treatment. Evidence from systematic reviews has demonstrated that calling for an ambulance leads to more timely triage and management of acute stroke [18, 19]. Achieving rapid patient presentation to a healthcare provider relies mainly on the patient's family member or a bystander recognising stroke and TIA symptoms and immediately contacting emergency medical services [20, 21]. Emergency stroke calls are rarely (~2%) made by the patient themselves [22–25]. Family members, bystanders, and patients must appreciate the urgency of seeking help and the seriousness of stroke symptoms. The Stroke Association (UK) highlighted this in its Face, Arm, Speech, Time to call (FAST) campaign, as has the US Brain Attack Coalition and the Stroke Foundation in Australia. The United Kingdom's National Clinical Guidelines for Stroke [26] highlight the need for more research on improving awareness and appropriate response behaviour [19].

Delays in accessing treatment may also arise within the healthcare system itself. There may be delays in primary care, for example if the health professional assessing the patient does not correctly diagnose a stroke or TIA, or fails to refer the patient appropriately. There may be problems at the point of referral from primary to secondary care or within secondary care, if the patient is referred swiftly but investigation and treatment is delayed. The longer the delay, the greater the risk of irremediable damage or further stroke. These factors pose practical difficulties in identifying patients with TIA, and investigating and treating them swiftly. Since the risk of subsequent stroke is highest in the first days and weeks after onset of TIA or stroke symptoms, the potential benefit of secondary prevention reduces the longer the patient survives event-free; for example, if carotid endarterectomy (CEA) is delayed, the risks of the procedure may outweigh the benefits.

Even for those who access appropriate services after stroke or TIA, their understanding of the importance of symptoms, acute treatment, and the effectiveness of secondary prevention can fall short of what is required to ensure optimal uptake of specialist stroke care. Primary and secondary care need to work together, with specific written and verbal individualised instructions provided to every patient [27].

3.3   Primary Prevention – Medical Considerations

3.3.1   Diabetes Mellitus

The presence of DM (type 1 or type 2) is an independent risk factor for stroke; in type 1 but not type 2 DM, there is strong evidence that stroke risk is increased by poor glycaemic control [28, 29]. Poor glycaemic control is an important risk factor for other DM complications. Most people with type 2 diabetes are overweight, and obesity worsens the associated metabolic and physiological abnormalities. The increased stroke risk for people with diabetes may be related to their higher incidence of hypertension and hyperlipidaemia compared with people without diabetes [30]. Aggressive treatment of raised BP and cholesterol is essential [31–33] and can reduce stroke risk [34]. The National Institute for Health and Care Excellence (NICE) [35] advocates that for primary prevention, target clinic BP for people with diabetes should be under 140/90 mmHg for those aged under 80 and 150/90 mmHg for those over 80. However, many people with type 2 DM – perhaps as many as one in two – are undiagnosed, making risk factor management problematic. In those identified as 'at risk' of developing DM, diet and exercise (principally caloric restriction if overweight, low fat (especially saturated fat), high carbohydrate, and increased fibre intake; exercise averaging at least 150 minutes per week of activities such as brisk walking, cycling, or jogging) have been shown to reduce DM incidence by 37% [36].

3.3.2 Hypertension

Hypertension (BP above 150/80 mmHg) is the single most important modifiable risk factor for stroke, doubling the long-term risk for every 10–12 mmHg rise in systolic BP or 7–8 mmHg rise in diastolic BP [37]. Treating hypertension is the most important factor for preventing stroke. As with some other risk factors, hypertension is usually asymptomatic and is often only identified by opportunistic screening.

Lifestyle measures recommended for hypertension management include smoking cessation, reduced alcohol consumption, avoiding excessive caffeine intake, reducing dietary sodium intake, and relaxation therapies. Most people with hypertension also require drug therapy to reduce their BP to below the target (140/80 or 150/80 mmHg for those aged under/over 80 years).

The choice of medication to treat hypertension depends on age and ethnicity. For people aged over 55 and Black people of African or Caribbean ethnic origin of any age, first-line treatment should be a calcium-channel blocker (CCB) or a thiazide-like diuretic (if CCBs are contraindicated). For those under 55 years of any other family origin, the recommended first-line therapy is an angiotensin-converting enzyme (ACE) inhibitor or a low-cost angiotensin-II receptor blocker (ARB) [35]. A combination of drugs may be needed if first-line therapy is ineffective, but it is important to check whether the patient is actually taking their medication as prescribed before adding additional drugs.

3.3.3 Dyslipidaemia

Statins are the mainstay of lipid-lowering therapy, and should be offered to anyone who has been identified using the QRISK2 algorithm [38] as being at 10% or greater 10-year risk of developing vascular disease [39]. It is, however, important to do this in conjunction with lifestyle modification and optimisation of other modifiable risk factors [39]. Statins act as inhibitors of the enzyme HMG-CoA reductase, which controls the rate-limiting step of cholesterol synthesis in the liver. They also exert an additional protective effect by stabilising atheromatous plaque in arteries, thus reducing risk of plaque rupture, subsequent embolisation, and thrombosis. Statins are occasionally associated with the development of myotoxicity, manifested as muscle pain or weakness, but this risk can be overstated, and patients may attribute unrelated aches and pains to their statin medication.

Appropriate lifestyle measures to reduce vascular risk may include dietary measures: limiting fat intake, substitution of saturated fat (e.g. animal fats) with mono- or unsaturated products (e.g. olive or rapeseed oils), and increased activity levels. These measures are helpful even in people without dyslipidaemia. Despite their commercial popularity, there is no evidence for the use of dietary supplements (e.g. plant stanols and sterols) in reducing vascular events, and they should not be recommended [39]. Such products might be erroneously used as a substitute for appropriate dietary changes which could have a real impact on vascular health.

Increased recognition of vascular risk has led to a rise in the prescribing of common combinations of drug therapy, such as statins, antihypertensives, and aspirin. This increases treatment burden for patients. Simplification of medication regimes can improve uptake and adherence [40]. A 'polypill' containing combination drug therapy has been trialled and shown to achieve reductions in vascular risk [41], although reductions in mortality and morbidity were not demonstrated.

3.3.4 Atrial Fibrillation, Anticoagulant, and Antiplatelet Therapy

People with AF have a high stroke risk because incomplete ejection of blood from the atria's due to inadequate contraction allows the formation of cardiac thrombus with subsequent distal embolisation into the cerebral circulation. Strokes arising from cardiac thrombus in untreated or poorly managed AF are often serious: AF-related ischaemic strokes are nearly twice as likely to be fatal, and confer an increased chance of severe disability and stroke recurrence compared with non-AF ischaemic strokes [42, 43].

The incidence of AF increases with age and, since the condition itself is often asymptomatic, its detection and treatment present a challenge for stroke prevention. Undiagnosed AF is estimated to be present in nearly 25% of patients with stroke or TIA [44]. Mass screening around age 75 detects previously undiagnosed AF in 3.0% of those screened, and prompts initiation of treatment in people with diagnosed but untreated AF [45]. Opportunistic screening in people aged 65 and over may be as effective as systematic screening for detection of undiagnosed AF in primary care, and is much cheaper per case detected [46]. Opportunistic screening may be carried out readily at any clinical contact via simple pulse palpation or using a medical device designed for the purpose. Automated BP machines may miss opportunities to detect AF because they do not require pulse palpation or auscultation, although some automated machines highlight pulse irregularity.

The mainstay of treatment for asymptomatic AF is oral anticoagulation (OAC). OAC with a vitamin K antagonist (warfarin) significantly reduces stroke risk (odds ratio versus placebo: 0.3). It also increases haemorrhage risk, however, but this does not outweigh the benefits of reduced stroke risk [47]. Aspirin is not recommended for stroke prevention in AF as it is much less effective than OAC but still has a significant bleeding risk.

Direct oral anticoagulants (DOACs – also called novel oral anticoagulants, NOACs) licensed for use in AF include apixaban, dabigatran, and rivaroxaban. They appear as effective as warfarin for stroke prevention and confer similar risk of major bleeding when used in AF [48]. The main difference is that International Normalised Ratio (INR) monitoring and dose adjustment are not required with DOACs as they are with warfarin. In cohort studies, although the benefits of dabigatran and warfarin were similar, warfarin appeared to confer a lower risk of gastrointestinal bleeding but a higher risk of intracranial bleeding [49]. However, the bleeding risks associated with warfarin were reduced with optimal monitoring and INR control [50]. Current national guidelines recommend continuation of warfarin in people with stable INR, and that the choice of warfarin or DOAC for those starting OACs should be made on an individual basis by the clinician and patient [51].

Decisions about OAC in AF entail a trade-off between stroke risk and bleeding risk [52]. Stroke risk can be calculated using the CHADS2 score, or its refinement CHADS2VASC [53]. Bleeding risk can be estimated using HAS-BLED. The use of these scores enables the clinician and patient to have an informed discussion about the risks and benefits of anticoagulation. Decisions about anticoagulation may also take into account other factors – such as the patient's social circumstances and past medication-taking behaviours – which are not included in these scoring systems [54]. Prescribers may tend to be 'risk-averse' with regard to the possibility of bleeding with OACs, often overestimating this risk and failing to weigh this against the often much higher risk of a major stroke without OAC therapy [55].

There is often reluctance from both clinicians and patients to commence or continue anticoagulation treatment [56]. Patients' reasons include the burden of regular INR monitoring, dose adjustment, and restrictions on alcohol intake with warfarin, whilst clinicians may worry about patient safety, adherence, and bleeding risk. The use of an audit tool such as Guidance on Risk Assessment and Stroke Prevention in Atrial Fibrillation (GRASP-AF) may be an effective method of identifying and facilitating clinical review with the 40% of patients with known AF who are not on anticoagulants [57].

Antiplatelet agents such as aspirin and clopidogrel are only recommended for primary stroke prevention in people with ischaemic heart disease or peripheral vascular disease [30]. Clopidogrel and aspirin have never been compared head-to-head, but clopidogrel may achieve slightly greater long-term risk reduction [58]. A combination of aspirin and clopidogrel does not confer any significant benefit in reducing vascular events; it does, however, increase the risk of haemorrhage compared with clopidogrel alone [59].

3.4 Secondary Medical Prevention After TIA or Stroke

3.4.1 Early Post-Event Preventive Care

Secondary risk reduction is an important part of reducing the burden of stroke mortality and morbidity, and is flagged in clinical practice guidelines. As survival rates for stroke have improved, the proportion of people requiring secondary prevention measures has increased. However, stroke risk factors are often inadequately controlled post-stroke or TIA [60, 61], even in specialist neurovascular clinics [62].

All acute stroke or TIA patients should have an individualised plan for stroke risk reduction implemented within 7 days of the event [26, 63]. Factors which need to be considered in ischaemic stroke or TIA include behavioural changes (smoking, exercise, diet and weight control, reducing salt and alcohol intake), BP management, antithrombotic treatment, OACs for people with AF, lipid-lowering therapy, assessment and treatment of carotid stenosis, and stopping hormone replacement therapy. After haemorrhagic stroke, stroke risk reduction requires BP management and behavioural changes; statin therapy and antithrombotic treatment are ineffective and may increase risk of recurrence. It is therefore imperative that the cause of stroke is investigated to initiate an appropriate treatment plan.

After an ischaemic stroke or TIA, all patients should commence antiplatelet therapy unless they are prescribed anticoagulants. The mainstay of treatment for many years, aspirin plus dipyridamole, has now been superseded in both efficacy and cost by generic clopidogrel [58]. If clopidogrel is contraindicated or not tolerated, the combination of aspirin and dipyridamole (or one of them alone, if the other is not tolerated) is recommended [26].

A stroke or TIA is sometimes accompanied by a diagnosis of type 2 DM, although the individual may have had the condition for some time. Whether it is newly diagnosed or longstanding, it is common for blood glucose to be elevated in acute stroke, and this is associated with higher mortality. Thus, monitoring and adjustment of hypoglycaemic therapy is needed, especially in acute stroke, where intravenous glucose and insulin may be necessary.

Dyslipidaemia may be identified during the stroke presentation, even though longstanding. For those with ischaemic stroke or TIA, statin therapy reduces risk of stroke recurrence even where the lipid profile is within normal laboratory limits. After haemorrhagic stroke, however, statin therapy does not reduce stroke risk in those with a normal lipid profile, and may even increase it. Decisions about statin therapy therefore depend on brain imaging to determine stroke aetiology.

It is common to find that BP is elevated in acute stroke, but there is little evidence to guide its management. Patients already taking oral antihypertensives should continue them (unless they have dysphagia). Guidelines recommend initiation of antihypertensive therapy in ischaemic stroke only when there is a hypertensive emergency or other serious condition which may be worsened by hypertension, such as aortic dissection or pre-eclampsia. In intracerebral haemorrhage, BP should be treated if the systolic is above 200 mmHg. In ischaemic stroke, BP should be reduced to 185/110 mmHg or lower in people eligible for thrombolysis.

Some patients present with stroke with known AF but with poorly controlled or no anticoagulation. Others are diagnosed with AF for the first time only when they present with stroke. The identification of AF in acute stroke is challenging. Whilst some patients may be in permanent AF, others have paroxysmal (intermittent) AF which is not always identified on a single pulse check or an electrocardiogram [44]. Longer-term monitoring in cryptogenic stroke results in detection of more cases of AF [64], but there is currently no consensus about how AF is best identified in patients who do not have it on presentation but for whom no cause of ischaemic stroke has been identified.

Where AF has been diagnosed immediately after acute stroke, anticoagulation should be started only when brain imaging has excluded haemorrhage. For TIA, it can then be commenced immediately, using an agent with rapid onset – either low-molecular-weight heparin or a DOAC. After an ischaemic stroke, anticoagulation should be delayed for 2 weeks, to reduce the risk of haemorrhagic transformation of the infarct. An antiplatelet agent may be used in the interim.

3.4.2 Long-Term Preventive Care

Although the risk of recurrent stroke is highest early after an initial event, elevated risk persists for many years [65]. To reduce long-term mortality, risk factors must continue to be addressed. The UK stroke guidelines recommend review at 6 weeks and 6 months post-stroke. This may be undertaken by specialist stroke staff or in primary care. People who have sustained a stroke or TIA should be on their general practitioner's (GP's) 'Stroke Register' to facilitate ongoing review of risk factor management. As a minimum, stroke and TIA survivors need annual checks of BP, blood tests for lipids and glucose, review of behavioural factors (e.g. diet, weight management, alcohol and smoking), and review of medication. More frequent review and support may be needed and should be individually tailored.

3.4.3 Adherence and Persistence

The World Health Organization (WHO) estimates that, in long-term conditions, only about 50% of prescribed medication is taken as intended [66]. Stroke and TIA are no exception. Factors which may make medication persistence (continuance of a prescription for the intended duration of treatment) and adherence (actually taking the medication as intended) especially problematic after stroke include the 'preventive' nature of the treatment (with no obvious relief of symptoms) and its long-term or indefinite nature. Commonly reported predictive factors for poor medication adherence after stroke include treatment concerns, lack of support with medications, polypharmacy, higher levels of disability, and more severe stroke [67]. Perhaps surprisingly, older age, comorbidities, and the complexity of the medication regime do not appear to be strongly associated with poorer medication adherence. However, people with AF tend to be more likely to discontinue their medication. This might be because of the complexity of dosing and monitoring with vitamin K antagonists such as warfarin. It is unclear whether medication adherence and persistence are better or worse with DOACs, which do not require the same monitoring and dose modification, than with vitamin K antagonists [68, 69].

For medication adherence, it is not enough to just give information about drug dosages and duration of treatment; patients need to understand what their medication is for – being clear that it is to reduce risk of a future stroke rather than to relieve present symptoms. The long-term nature of medication needs to be explained, so that patients understand that they need to continue to take a statin (for example) even if their cholesterol (for example) returns to normal. Any specific barriers to taking medication, such as cognitive or physical impairments, need to be identified. In some cases, a simplified medication regimen may be needed. Health providers need to adopt a collaborative approach, utilising the skills of medical, pharmacy, nursing and social care staff, and informal carers, to identify and support those having difficulty managing their medicines.

There is a high prevalence of depression and other psychological disorders post-stroke; better identification and management of these conditions may improve medication adherence. It is vital that healthcare providers adopt a nonjudgmental approach when discussing possible medication adherence problems. Barriers may be related to the healthcare team/health system, therapy, condition, patient, and social and economic situation [66], and the patient's difficulties must be understood in this context.

3.4.4 Secondary Prevention of Stroke in Less Common Aetiologies and Patient Groups

3.4.4.1 Intracerebral Haemorrhage Identification of stroke aetiology is essential to reducing the risk of recurrent intracerebral haemorrhage. Several underlying conditions may lead to intracerebral haemorrhage, including hypertension leading to the rupture of micro-aneurysms, cerebral amyloid angiopathy in older people (particularly in association with dementia), arteriovenous malformations, vasculitis, bleeding into tumours, haematological disorders, Moyamoya disease, and cerebral vein thrombosis. Other factors which may precipitate intracerebral haemorrhage include drug use (e.g. amphetamines), excess alcohol intake, and use of prescribed medication such as oral anticoagulants and thrombolytic agents [70]. Reduction of recurrence needs to be directed at the primary cause. If no other cause is identified, treatment of BP and advice about alcohol intake are necessary.

3.4.4.2 Stroke in Those Aged Under 45 Years Although stroke is rare in those aged under 45 years, its incidence is rising [71]. The most common causes of stroke or TIA at young age are cardioembolic disease and cervical artery dissection: each accounts for about 25% of strokes in this age group. A further 25% are due to numerous other rare causes of stroke [72], but the final 25% are idiopathic. Young stroke is rarely due to atheromatous disease [73]. All younger stroke or TIA patients need thorough expert assessment to exclude differential diagnoses, for identification of rare causes (such as genetic neurological conditions, e.g. cerebral autosomal-dominant arteriopathy with subcortical infarcts and leuko-encephalopathy [74]) and implementation of appropriate risk-reduction measures [75].

3.4.4.3 Young Women and Pregnancy Women with a history of stroke should not take oral contraceptives as they increase the risk of recurrent stroke. If a stroke survivor becomes pregnant, however, there is a low risk of recurrence during the pregnancy and puerperium. The risk is higher in those with stroke where a cause has been identified and in the puerperium rather than during pregnancy itself [76]. Prior stroke should not normally be a bar to subsequent pregnancies.

3.4.4.4 Cerebral Venous Thrombosis This rare cause of stroke can occur at any age, including in pre- or full-term neonates [77]. It may be due to haematological or prothrombotic conditions, infection or inflammatory disease, tumours, the puerperium, oral contraceptive use, or head injury. Anticoagulation, usually short-term, may be used to prevent progression [78] and seems to be beneficial even in those with haemorrhagic infarction.

3.5 Interventions for Secondary Prevention After TIA or Recovered Stroke

3.5.1 TIA Assessment and Risk Management

TIA has conventionally been defined as 'a sudden, focal neurologic deficit that lasts for less than 24 hours, is of presumed vascular origin, and which is confined to an area of the brain or eye perfused by a specific artery' [79]. However, most TIAs resolve well within this time – around 50% in under 30 minutes – and improvements in cerebral imaging techniques have shown that most people who have symptoms lasting longer than one hour do in fact have a cerebral infarct [80]. TIA has therefore been redefined as 'a transient episode of neurological dysfunction caused by focal brain, spinal cord, or retinal ischemia, without acute infarction' [81]. It is vital to distinguish TIA from stroke and from other differential diagnoses because treatments for acute stroke, notably thrombolysis or mechanical clot retrieval, should be administered early for greatest benefit [82]. Revising the definition of TIA means that the diagnosis is clarified earlier, enabling prompt treatment decisions. The proposed new definition is thus both a closer reflection of the underlying pathology, and a pragmatic step towards improving access to acute stroke treatment. In practice, many people with TIA do not seek medical advice for several hours or days post-onset of symptoms, particularly if their symptoms are mild or have resolved within minutes. Patients tend not to seek medical advice via emergency routes, and those who experience symptoms 'out of hours' delay seeking medical advice for significantly longer than those who notice TIA symptoms during GP surgery opening hours [83].

After a TIA, the speed of implementation of secondary preventative measures is a crucial factor in the prevention of further strokes. A TIA, like stroke, must be considered a medical emergency. Those at greatest risk of an early further stroke are those with large artery atherosclerosis, usually carotid stenosis, whereas those with small vessel disease, usually subcortical or lacunar, have the lowest risk of early recurrence [84]. The EXPRESS Study [85] demonstrated that improving the speed of initiation of secondary prevention measures after TIA significantly reduces the incidence of subsequent stroke. In particular, the immediate administration of aspirin in both stroke and TIA substantially reduces the risk of early recurrent stroke (see Case Studies 3.1 and 3.2) [86].

Case Study

Case 3.1 Vernon

Vernon is a 78-year-old retired man who lives with his wife. He is a non-smoker, is not known to have diabetes or hypertension, and is in good health. One day, whilst he was driving home from shopping, his wife noticed that his driving was 'erratic' and 'jerky'. Vernon had not noticed a problem, but 10 minutes after returning home, he found he could not move his right leg. This lasted for 20 minutes. He did not feel a need to seek advice, but his wife phoned the GP, who saw him and referred him to hospital. His BP on presentation was 170/90 mmHg.

Questions

a. What is Vernon's ABCD2 score (Table 3.1)?

b. What further investigations does Vernon need?

Vernon's blood tests were within normal ranges, with a total cholesterol of 4.6 mmol l⁻¹. His ECG was normal. He had a duplex scan of the carotid arteries and was found to have a 1–14% right internal carotid artery stenosis and a 15–49% left internal carotid artery stenosis.

c. What further treatment and medication will Vernon need?

d. What other advice and long-term follow-up will be needed?

TABLE 3.1 The ABCD2 score [87, 88]

		Score
Age	≥60 yr	1
BP	Systolic ≥140 and/or diastolic ≥90	1
Clinical	Unilateral motor weakness	2
	Speech disturbance without weakness	1
	Other, e.g. amaurosis fugax	0
Duration of TIA	≥60 min	2
	10–59 min	1
	<10 min	0
Diabetes	Yes	1
	No	0
Total (maximum)		7

Answers

a. The ABCD2 score is 5 (age = 1; BP = 1; clinical symptoms = 2; duration = 1; diabetes = 0). This indicates a need for immediate assessment and implementation of secondary prevention measures within 48 hours.

b. Vernon will need full neurological assessment, blood tests including glucose and cholesterol, further assessment of BP, ECG, and carotid duplex scan.

c. Vernon will need to commence long-term antihypertensive medication, a statin, and clopidogrel 75 mg daily (or aspirin 75 mg daily plus dipyridamole 200 mg twice daily). Carotid endarterectomy is not advised as the degree of internal carotid stenosis is moderate (15–49%).

d. Vernon must be educated about the symptoms of stroke and TIA, and advised to seek immediate medical help if these symptoms recur. He must not drive for 4 weeks. Follow-up should be arranged according to local service arrangements to ensure he is taking his medication correctly and that his risk factors (e.g. hypertension) are controlled. He will be entered into the GP's Stroke Register to facilitate long-term follow-up.

Case Study

| Case 3.2 | Colin |

Colin is a 50-year-old man who runs a local restaurant and works long hours. He smokes 15 cigarettes per day and is not overweight. He feels in good health, takes no regular medication, and rarely consults a doctor.

Colin had a transient episode of left-sided weakness, lasting only moments, which he ignored and later described as a 'little wobble'. Two days later, whilst at work, he had a further and more severe episode of left-sided weakness, and fell to the floor. He had slurred speech. A colleague phoned for an ambulance, and he went to the emergency department (ED) for further assessment. On arrival at hospital, his symptoms had resolved.

Colin had urgent carotid imaging, which showed a stenosis of the right internal carotid artery of 80–89% and one of the left internal carotid artery of 15–49%. His cholesterol was raised at $5.7 \, \text{mmol} \, \text{l}^{-1}$, and his BP was 160/70.

Questions

a. What is Colin's diagnosis and ABCD2 score (Table 3.1)?

b. What can be done to expedite further investigations?

c. What is Colin's risk of stroke over the next 3 years with best medical treatment or with urgent carotid endarterectomy in addition to best medical treatment?

d. In addition to prescribed medication and surgical treatment, what further action can Colin take to reduce his risk of stroke?

Answers

a. Colin's ABCD2 score is 5 (age = 0; BP = 1; clinical symptom = 2; duration = 2 (recurrent event); diabetes = 0.) The diagnosis on arrival at hospital is recurrent TIA, as this is the second event within 2 days.

b. Colin needs to be admitted to hospital, preferably to the stroke unit, to facilitate urgent investigations and treatment.

c. Colin's 3-year risk of stroke on best medical treatment is estimated at 16.8%. With carotid endarterectomy, this is reduced to 2.8%, but with an additional 7.5% surgical stroke/death rate (figures from European Carotid Surgery Trial, ECST). Local audit data for stroke/death after carotid endarterectomy may vary from this.

d. Colin must stop smoking, and may need advice and support to achieve this. Although he is not overweight, his long working hours and the nature of his job may mean that he needs to undertake some dietary changes. He may need to reduce stress by modifying his busy lifestyle and to take exercise.

3.5.2 Carotid Intervention

The first surgical CEA was performed by DeBakey in 1953 [89]. CEA was widely used from the 1960s to the mid-1980s, intended to reduce the risk of stroke in patients with asymptomatic or recently symptomatic carotid stenosis. It is estimated that about 1 million people worldwide had the operation between 1974 and 1985 [90, 91]. However, CEA itself confers a small but important risk of perioperative stroke, which could outweigh the effectiveness of the operation in reducing future stroke risk.

The first randomised trial of CEA [92] had high perioperative mortality and morbidity rates. Subsequently, two major trials were conducted with recently symptomatic patients: the European Carotid Surgery Trial (ECST) [93, 94] and the North American Symptomatic Carotid Endarterectomy Trial (NASCET) [95]. Both trials found that for patients with ipsilateral internal carotid stenosis of 70–99%, surgery was more effective than best medical treatment alone in reducing the long-term stroke/surgical death rate, even taking into account the risk of perioperative stroke or death (7.5% in ECST; 5.8% in NASCET). For patients in ECST with stenosis of less than 30%, surgery was found to be less effective than best medical treatment, whilst for patients in both studies with 30–69% stenosis, the outcomes of either treatment were evenly balanced.

Further analysis of the final results of both trials has suggested some additional refinements. Factors which confer a higher likelihood of benefit from CEA include: male sex, age more than 75 years, higher degree of stenosis (90–99%), hemispheric symptoms (sensorimotor TIA) rather than ocular symptoms, contralateral occlusion, carotid plaque irregularity, and other comorbidities [96]. Whilst some of these factors (e.g. older age) also confer a higher surgical risk of stroke or death, this is outweighed by the higher baseline risk of stroke with medical treatment alone in these patients.

CEA for symptomatic carotid stenosis has subsequently been evaluated in a Cochrane review [97], which suggests that CEA may be of benefit for

50–69% symptomatic stenosis and is highly beneficial for 70–99% stenosis without near-occlusion. In carotid near-occlusion, benefit is marginal in the short term and uncertain in the long term. Delays in treatment after the onset of TIA, whether due to delayed presentation, referral, or surgery, may reduce or eliminate the potential benefits that can be gained from surgery, because the risk of the procedure will outweigh the diminished underlying risk of recurrent stroke.

An important concern for implementing study results in present-day practice is that best medical treatment has changed since ECST and NASCET reported their results. A further trial [98] is assessing whether optimised medical treatment (OMT) in patients with carotid stenosis at low and intermediate risk for stroke is as effective in the long-term prevention of cerebral infarction and myocardial infarction (MI) as revascularisation and OMT combined. The trial uses a risk model based on clinical characteristics to stratify patients as at high risk (=15%), intermediate risk (7.5–15%), or low risk (<7.5%) of future stroke.

The outcomes of CEA under loco-regional anaesthesia have been compared with those for general anaesthesia. There is no difference in clinical outcomes [99], but local anaesthesia normally means a reduced length of hospital stay and greater cost–benefit, and is also more acceptable to many patients.

Amongst the criticisms of the ECST and NASCET trials was the lack of assessment of quality of life, anxiety, and depression. These were important factors to consider for these patients, who were faced with undergoing potentially harmful surgery for a currently asymptomatic condition, with no guarantee of long-term benefit [100]. CEA is performed to reduce the risk of future stroke, but patients might not weigh up the risks of surgical and non-surgical treatment in the same way as clinicians. A 5% risk of perioperative stroke may be perceived as a serious threat, even though their overall long-term risk of stroke will be reduced. Patients may perceive that the benefits of CEA include not just a reduction in risk of stroke, but the eradication of anxiety about that risk [101].

All patients who have had a non-disabling carotid territory event should be offered assessment and treatment of carotid stenosis by duplex scanning, followed by CEA if surgery is indicated. A review of imaging techniques to detect carotid stenoses indicated magnetic resonance angiography (MRA) with contrast enhancement as the most accurate, non-invasive imaging method, although there was little to choose between duplex ultrasound, computerised tomography angiography (CTA), and MRA [102]. Inter and intraobserver variability for the measurement of carotid stenosis is probably more important than differences in imaging technique [103]. The UK National Stroke Strategy (NSS) Imaging Guide emphasises the importance of swift access to high-quality audited services [104], whichever modality is used. The UK NSS [105] stated that CEA should be performed within 48 hours in patients with ABCD2 scores of 4 or more and within 7 days in other patients in order to have the maximum effect on reducing the number of patients who go on to have a completed stroke after a carotid territory event. The NICE guidelines [106] take a more conservative approach and recommend CEA within 2 weeks of the event.

People who have not had previous symptoms of stroke or TIA but who have a carotid stenosis are also at increased risk of subsequent stroke. Current optimal medical management is likely to be equally as effective as CEA in reducing stroke incidence, and is three to eight times more cost-effective [107]. The potential benefit of CEA for asymptomatic carotid disease is limited by the difficulty of identifying patients who have a severe carotid stenosis but who have not had any carotid territory symptoms. Asymptomatic carotid disease is usually detected opportunistically; screening for the condition is not recommended [108].

Carotid stenting is a less invasive procedure than CEA, but it is unclear whether it is a safe and durable alternative. Meta-analysis of carotid stenting has found a higher risk of periprocedural stroke when compared to CEA [109]. Stenting may be appropriate for some patients who have a high risk of surgical complications, but more trials are required to address the complications of the procedure and its long-term durability.

Continuing audit of individuals', centres', and collective results in CEA is necessary. In a systematic review of 51 studies of the outcome of CEA, the risk of stroke and death was found to range from 2.3 to 7.7%, although the mean risk was 5.6%, consistent with ECST and NASCET [110]. In the light of this variability, those performing CEA should advise patients of their own track record, based on rigorous clinical audit, rather than quoting data from the clinical trials.

3.6 Conclusion

There are many measures to reduce the risk of stroke, whether via primary or secondary prevention (see Cases 3.1 and 3.2 for examples). However, the processes of enabling people first to identify themselves as being at risk of cerebrovascular disease and second to access the help they need in order to reduce their stroke risk are far from straightforward. Interventions need to be tailored to the individual, initiated as soon as possible after the increased risk is identified, and continued long-term with regular review.

There is strong evidence that timely investigation and implementation of the interventions described in this chapter substantially reduce individuals' risk of first or subsequent stroke. It is, however, important to remember that patients who have had a TIA, or who have apparently fully recovered from a stroke, have other healthcare needs apart from secondary prevention. TIA or stroke itself generates anxiety and affects individuals' perceptions of their health and health status. It is a distressing syndrome in its own right, not just because of its implication that the patient is at risk of a first or further stroke.

References

1. UK Stroke Forum Education & Training. Stroke-Specific Education Framework, United Kingdom: UK Stroke Forum 2010. Available from: http://www.stroke-education.org.uk/about. [30 November 2018]
2. Stroke Association (2014. Available from: http://www.stroke.org.uk/resources/not-just-funny-turn). Not Just a Funny Turn. London: The Stroke Association [30 November 2018].

3. World Population Ageing 2013. ST/ESA/SER.A/348. (2013) United Nations, Department of Economic and Social Affairs, Population Division.
4. Office for National Statistics (2014). National Population Projections 2014-Based Statistical Bulletin. London: Office for National Statistics.
5. Hankey, G. (1999). Smoking and risk of stroke. Journal of Cardiovascular Risk 6 (4): 207–211.
6. McFadden, E., Luben, R., Wareham, N. et al. (2009). Social class, risk factors, and stroke incidence in men and women. Stroke 40 (4): 1070–1077.
7. Reeves, M., Hogan, J., and Rafferty, A. (2002). Knowledge of stroke risk factors and warning signs among Michigan adults. Neurology 59 (10): 1547–1552.
8. Das, K., Mondal, G.P., Dutta, A.K. et al. (2007). Awareness of warning symptoms and risk factors of stroke in the general population and in survivors stroke. Journal of Clinical Neuroscience 14 (1): 12–16.
9. Yoon, S., Heller, R., Levi, C. et al. (2001). Knowledge of stroke risk factors, warning symptoms, and treatment among an Australian urban population. Stroke 32 (8): 1926–1930.
10. Müller-Nordhorn, J., Nolte, C., Rossnagel, K. et al. (2006). Knowledge about risk factors for stroke. Stroke 37 (4): 946–950.
11. Samsa, G., Cohen, S., Goldstein, L. et al. (1997). Knowledge of risk among patients at increased risk for stroke. Stroke 28 (5): 916–921.
12. Pancioli, A., Broderick, J., Kothari, R. et al. (1998). Public perception of stroke warning signs and knowledge of potential risk factors. Journal of the American Medical Association 279 (16): 1288–1292.
13. Segura, T., Vega, G., López, S. et al. (2003). Public perception of stroke in Spain. Cerebrovascular Diseases 16 (1): 21–26.
14. Kothari, R., Sauerbeck, L., Jauch, E. et al. (1997). Patients' awareness of stroke signs, symptoms, and risk factors. Stroke 28 (10): 1871–1875.
15. Jones, S., Jenkinson, A., Leathley, M., and Watkins, C. (2010). Stroke knowledge and awareness: an integrative review of the evidence. Age and Ageing 39 (1): 11–22.
16. Caley, M., Chohan, P., Hooper, J., and Wright, N. (2014). The impact of NHS health checks on the prevalence of disease in general practices: a controlled study. British Journal of General Practice 64 (625): e516–e521.
17. Public Health England. NHS Health Check Overview 2015. Available from: http://fingertips.phe.org.uk/profile/nhs-health-check-detailed/data [30 November 2018]
18. Sprigg, N., Machili, C., Otter, M. et al. (2009). A systematic review of delays in seeking medical attention after transient ischaemic attack. Journal of Neurology, Neurosurgery & Psychiatry 80 (8): 871–875.
19. Lecouturier, J., Murtagh, M., Thomson, R. et al. (2010). Response to symptoms of stroke in the UK: a systematic review. BMC Health Services Research 10 (1): 157.
20. Ferro, J., Melo, T., Oliveira, V. et al. (1994). An analysis of the admission delay of acute strokes. Cerebrovascular Diseases 4 (2): 72–75.
21. Harraf, F., Sharma, A., Brown, M. et al. (2002). A multicentre observational study of presentation and early assessment of acute stroke. British Medical Journal 325 (7354): 17.
22. Porteous, G., Corry, M., and Smith, W. (1999). Emergency medical services dispatcher identification of stroke and transient ischemic attack. Prehospital Emergency Care 3 (3): 211–216.
23. Wein, T., Staub, L., Felberg, R. et al. (2000). Activation of emergency medical services for acute stroke in a nonurban population. Stroke 31 (8): 1925–1928.
24. Mosley, I., Nicol, M., Donnan, G. et al. (2007). Stroke symptoms and the decision to call for an ambulance. Stroke 38 (2): 361–366.
25. Jones, S., Carter, B., Ford, G. et al. (2013). The identification of acute stroke: an analysis of emergency calls. International Journal of Stroke 8 (6): 408–412.
26. Intercollegiate Stroke Working Party. (2012). National Clinical Guideline for Stroke. London: Royal College of Physicians.

27. Maasland, L., Koudstaal, P., Habbema, J., and Dippel, D. (2007). Knowledge and understanding of disease process, risk factors and treatment modalities in patients with a recent TIA or minor ischemic stroke. Cerebrovascular Diseases 23 (5–6): 435–440.

28. Epidemiology of Diabetes Interventions and Complications (EDIC) Study Research Group (2016). Intensive diabetes treatment and cardiovascular outcomes in type 1 diabetes: the DCCT/EDIC study 30-year follow-up. Diabetes Care 39 (5): 686–693.

29. UK Prospective Diabetes Study Group (1998). Intensive blood-glucose control with sulphonylureas or insulin compared with conventional treatment and risk of complications in patients with type 2 diabetes (UKPDS 33). The Lancet 352 (9131): 837–853.

30. Straus, S.E., Majumdar, S.R., and McAlister, F.A. (2002). New evidence for stroke prevention: scientific review. Journal of the American Medical Association 288 (11): 1388–1395.

31. Costa, J., Borges, M., David, C., and Carneiro, A.V. (2006). Efficacy of lipid lowering drug treatment for diabetic and non-diabetic patients: metaanalysis of randomised controlled trials. British Medical Journal 332 (7550): 1115–1124.

32. Investigators HOPES (2000). Effects of ramipril on cardiovascular and microvascular outcomes in people with diabetes mellitus: results of the HOPE study and MICRO-HOPE substudy. The Lancet 355 (9200): 253–259.

33. Reckless, J. (2006). Diabetes and lipid lowering: where are we?: We're now sure that statins cut cardiovascular risks in type 2 diabetes. British Medical Journal 332 (7550): 1103–1104.

34. UK Prospective Diabetes Study Group (1998). Tight blood pressure control and risk of macrovascular and microvascular complications in type 2 diabetes: UKPDS 38. British Medical Journal 317: 703–713.

35. National Institute for Health and Care Excellence (NICE) (2011). Hypertension in Adults: Diagnosis and Management. London: National Institute for Health and Care Excellence.

36. Orozco, L., Buchleitner, A., Gimenez-Perez, G. et al. (2008). Exercise or exercise and diet for preventing type 2 diabetes mellitus. Cochrane Database of Systematic Reviews 3 (Art. No.: CD003054). https://doi.org/10.1002/14651858.CD003054.pub3.

37. Lawes, C., Bennett, D., Feigin, V., and Rodgers, A. (2004). Blood pressure and stroke. Stroke 35 (3): 776–785.

38. Hippisley-Cox, J., Coupland, C., Vinogradova, Y. et al. (2008). Predicting cardiovascular risk in England and Wales: prospective derivation and validation of QRISK2. British Medical Journal 336 (1475): 1–15.

39. National Institute for Health and Care Excellence (NICE) (2014). Cardiovascular Disease: Risk Assessment and Reduction, Including Lipid Modification. London: National Institute for Health and Care Excellence.

40. van Dulmen, S., Sluijs, E., van Dijk, L. et al. (2007). Patient adherence to medical treatment: a review of reviews. BMC Health Services Research 7 (1): 55.

41. PILL Collaborative Group (2011). An international randomised placebo-controlled trial of a four-component combination pill ('polypill') in people with raised cardiovascular risk. PLoS One 6 (5): 1–11.

42. Lin, H., Wolf, P., Kelly-Hayes, M. et al. (1996). Stroke severity in atrial fibrillation. Stroke 27 (10): 1760–1764.

43. Kimura, K., Minematsu, K., and Yamaguchi, T. (2005). Atrial fibrillation as a predictive factor for severe stroke and early death in 15 831 patients with acute ischaemic stroke. Journal of Neurology, Neurosurgery & Psychiatry 76 (5): 679–683.

44. Sposato, L., Cipriano, L., Saposnik, G. et al. (2015). Diagnosis of atrial fibrillation after stroke and transient ischaemic attack: a systematic review and meta-analysis. The Lancet Neurology 14 (4): 377–387.

45. Svennberg, E., Engdahl, J., Al-Khalili, F. et al. (2015). Mass screening for untreated atrial fibrillation: the STROKESTOP study. Circulation 131 (25): 2176–2184.

46. Moran, P., Teljeur, C., Ryan, M., and Smith, S. (2016). Systematic screening for the detection of atrial fibrillation. Cochrane Database of Systematic Reviews 6 (Art. No.: CD009586). https://doi.org/10.1002/14651858.CD009586.pub3.

47. Aguilar, M.I. and Hart, R.G. (2006). Antiplatelet therapy for preventing stroke in patients with non-valvular atrial fibrillation and no previous history of stroke or transient ischemic attacks. Stroke 37 (1): 274–275.

48. Sardar, P., Chatterjee, S., Lavie, C. et al. (2015). Risk of major bleeding in different indications for new oral anticoagulants: insights from a meta-analysis of approved dosages from 50 randomized trials. International Journal of Cardiology 179 (2015): 279–287.

49. Romanelli, R., Nolting, L., Dolginsky, M. et al. (2016). Dabigatran versus warfarin for atrial fibrillation in real-world clinical practice. Circulation: Cardiovascular Quality and Outcomes 9 (2): 126–134.

50. Chan, P., Li, W., Hai, J. et al. (2015). Gastrointestinal hemorrhage in atrial fibrillation patients: impact of quality of anticoagulation control. European Heart Journal-Cardiovascular Pharmacotherapy 1 (4): 265–272.

51. National Institute for Health and Care Excellence (NICE) (2014). Atrial Fibrillation: Management. London: National Institute for Health and Care Excellence.

52. Lip, G.Y., Andreotti, F., Fauchier, L. et al. (2011). Bleeding risk assessment and management in atrial fibrillation patients. Thrombosis and Haemostasis 106 (6): 997–1011.

53. Yarmohammadi, H., Varr, B., Puwanant, S. et al. (2012). Role of CHADS 2 score in evaluation of thromboembolic risk and mortality in patients with atrial fibrillation undergoing direct current cardioversion (from the ACUTE Trial Substudy). American Journal of Cardiology 110 (2): 222–226.

54. Decker, C., Garavalia, L., Garavalia, B. et al. (2012). Exploring barriers to optimal anticoagulation for atrial fibrillation: interviews with clinicians. Journal of Multidisciplinary Healthcare 5: 129–135.

55. Sen, S. and Dahlberg, K. (2014). Physician's fear of anticoagulant therapy in nonvalvular atrial fibrillation. American Journal of the Medical Sciences 348 (6): 513–521.

56. Xuereb, C.B., Shaw, R.L., and Lane, D.A. (2012). Patients' and health professionals' views and experiences of atrial fibrillation and oral-anticoagulant therapy: a qualitative meta-synthesis. Patient Education and Counseling 88: 330–337.

57. Shantsila, E., Wolff, A., Lip, G., and Lane, D. (2015). Optimising stroke prevention in patients with atrial fibrillation: application of the GRASP-AF audit tool in a UK general practice cohort. British Journal of General Practice 65 (630): e16–e23.

58. National Institute for Health and Care Excellence (NICE) (2010). Clopidogrel and Modified-Release Dipyridamole for the Prevention of Occlusive Vascular Events (Review of Technology Appraisal Guidance 90). London: National Institute for Health and Care Excellence.

59. Diener, H., Bogousslavsky, J., Brass, L. et al. (2004). Aspirin and clopidogrel compared with clopidogrel alone after recent ischaemic stroke or transient ischaemic attack in high-risk patients (MATCH): randomised, double-blind, placebo-controlled trial. The Lancet 364 (9431): 331–337.

60. Joseph, L., Babikian, V., Allen, N., and Winter, M. (1999). Risk factor modification in stroke prevention. Stroke 30 (1): 16–20.

61. Sappok, T., Faulstich, A., Stuckert, E. et al. (2001). Compliance with secondary prevention of ischemic stroke: a prospective evaluation. Stroke 32: 1884–1889.

62. Mouradian, M., Majumdar, S., Senthilselvan, A. et al. (2002). How well are hypertension, hyperlipidemia, diabetes, and smoking managed after a stroke or transient ischemic attack? Stroke 33 (6): 1656–1659.

63. National Institute for Health and Care Excellence (NICE) (2008). Stroke: The Diagnosis and Acute Management of Stroke and Transient Ischaemic Attacks. London: National Institute for Health and Care Excellence.

64. Dussault, C., Toeg, H., Nathan, M. et al. (2015). Electrocardiographic monitoring for detecting atrial fibrillation after ischemic stroke or transient ischemic attack: a systematic review and meta-analysis. Circulation: Arrhythmia and Electrophysiology 8 (2): 263–269.

65. Mohan, K.M., Wolfe, C.D., Rudd, A.G. et al. (2011). Risk and cumulative risk of stroke recurrence: a systematic review and meta-analysis. Stroke 42 (5): 1489–1494.

66. Sabaté, E. (2003). Adherence to Long-Term Therapies: Evidence for Action. Geneva: World Health Organization.

67. Al AlShaikh, S., Quinn, T., Dunn, W. et al. (2016). Predictive factors of non-adherence to secondary preventative medication after stroke or transient ischaemic attack: a systematic review and meta-analyses. European Stroke Journal 1 (2): 65–75.

68. Nelson, W., Song, X., Coleman, C. et al. (2014). Medication persistence and discontinuation of rivaroxaban versus warfarin among patients with non-valvular atrial fibrillation. Current Medical Research and Opinion 30 (12): 2461–2469.

69. Zhou, M., Chang, H.-Y., Segal, J.B. et al. (2015). Adherence to a novel oral anticoagulant among patients with atrial fibrillation. Journal of Managed Care and Specialty Pharmacy 21 (11): 1054–1062.

70. Steiner, T., Kaste, M., Forsting, M. et al. (2006). Recommendations for the management of intracranial haemorrhage-part I: spontaneous intracerebral haemorrhage. The European Stroke Initiative Writing Committee and the Writing Committee for the EUSI Executive Committee. Cerebrovascular Diseases (Basel, Switzerland) 22 (4): 294.

71. Béjot, Y., Delpont, B., and Giroud, M. (2016). Rising stroke incidence in young adults: more epidemiological evidence, more questions to be answered. Journal of the American Heart Association 5 (5): 1–3.

72. Nedeltchev, K., der Maur, T., Georgiadis, D. et al. (2005). Ischaemic stroke in young adults: predictors of outcome and recurrence. Journal of Neurology, Neurosurgery & Psychiatry 76 (2): 191–195.

73. Bogousslavsky, J. (2001). Uncommon Causes of Stroke. Cambridge: Cambridge University Press.

74. Taylor, M. and Doody, G. (2008). CADASIL: a guide to a comparatively unrecognised condition in psychiatry. Advances in Psychiatric Treatment 14 (5): 350–357.

75. Martin, P., Young, C., Enevoldson, T., and Humphrey, P. (1997). Overdiagnosis of TIA and minor stroke: experience at a regional neurovascular clinic. Quarterly Journal of Medicine 90 (12): 759–763.

76. Lamy, C., Hamon, J., Coste, J., and Mas, J. (2000). Ischemic stroke in young women: risk of recurrence during subsequent pregnancies. Neurology 55 (2): 269–274.

77. Bousser, M.G. and Ferro, J.M. (2007). Cerebral venous thrombosis: an update. The Lancet Neurology 6 (2): 162–170.

78. Stam, J. (2005). Thrombosis of the cerebral veins and sinuses. New England Journal of Medicine 352 (17): 1791–1798.

79. National Institutes of Health (1975). A classification and outline of cerebrovascular diseases II. Stroke 6 (5): 564–616.

80. Levy, D. (1988). How transient are transient ischemic attacks? Neurology 38 (5): 674–677.

81. Easton, J., Saver, J., Albers, G. et al. (2009). Definition and evaluation of transient ischemic attack. Stroke 40 (6): 2276–2293.

82. Hacke, W., Kaste, M., Bluhmki, E. et al. (2008). Thrombolysis with alteplase 3 to 4.5 hours after acute ischemic stroke. New England Journal of Medicine 359 (13): 1317–1329.

83. Lasserson, D., Chandratheva, A., Giles, M. et al. (2008). Influence of general practice opening hours on delay in seeking medical attention after transient ischaemic attack (TIA) and minor stroke: prospective population based study. British Medical Journal 337: a1569.

84. Lovett, J., Coull, A., and Rothwell, P. (2004). Early risk of recurrence by subtype of ischemic stroke in population-based incidence studies. Neurology 62 (4): 569–573.

85. Rothwell, P., Giles, M., Chandratheva, A. et al. (2007). Effect of urgent treatment of transient ischaemic attack and minor stroke on early recurrent stroke (EXPRESS study): a prospective population-based sequential comparison. The Lancet 370 (9596): 1432–1442.

86. Rothwell, P., Algra, A., Chen, Z. et al. (2016). Effects of aspirin on risk and severity of early recurrent stroke after transient ischaemic attack and ischaemic stroke: time-course analysis of randomised trials. The Lancet 388 (10042): 365–375.

87. Rothwell, P., Giles, M., Flossmann, E., and Nielsen, E. (2006). A simple score (ABCD) to identify individuals at high early risk of stroke after transient ischemic attack. Journal of Emergency Medicine 30 (2): 251–252.

88. Johnston, K.C. and Mayer, S.A. (2003). Blood pressure reduction in ischemic stroke: a two-edged sword? Neurology 61 (8): 1030–1031.

89. DeBakey, M.E. (1975). Successful carotid endarterectomy for cerebrovascular insufficiency: nineteen-year follow-up. Journal of the American Medical Association 233 (10): 1083–1085.

90. Barnett, H. (1991). Evaluating methods for prevention in stroke. Annals of the Royal College of Physicians and Surgeons of Canada 24 (1): 33–42.

91. Barnett, H. (1990). Symptomatic carotid endarterectomy trials. Stroke 21 (11 Suppl.): III2–III5.

92. Fields, W., Maslenikov, V., Meyer, J. et al. (1970). Joint study of extracranial arterial occlusion: V. Progress report of prognosis following surgery or nonsurgical treatment for transient cerebral ischemic attacks and cervical carotid artery lesions. Journal of the American Medical Association 211 (12): 1993–2003.

93. Warlow, C. (1991). MRC European Carotid Surgery Trial: interim results for symptomatic patients with severe (70-99%) or with mild (0-29%) carotid stenosis. The Lancet 337 (8752): 1235–1243.

94. Godwin, J. (1998). Randomised trial of endarterectomy for recently symptomatic carotid stenosis: final results of the MRC European Carotid Surgery Trial (ECST). The Lancet 351 (9113): 1379–1387.

95. Collaborators NASCET (1991). Beneficial effect of carotid endarterectomy in symptomatic patients with high-grade carotid stenosis. The New England Journal of Medicine 325: 445–453.

96. Naylor, A.R., Rothwell, P.M., and Bell, P.R. (2003). Overview of the principal results and secondary analyses from the European and North American randomised trials of endarterectomy for symptomatic carotid stenosis. European Journal of Vascular and Endovascular Surgery 26 (2): 14.

97. Rerkasem, K. and Rothwell, P. (2011). Carotid endarterectomy for symptomatic carotid stenosis. Cochrane Database of Systematic Reviews 4 (Art. No.: CD001081). https://doi.org/10.1002/14651858.CD001081.pub2.

98. Second European Carotid Surgery Trial (ECST-2). Protocol 2015. Protocol Version 3.1. Available from: http://s489637516.websitehome.co.uk/ECST2/downloads/ECST-2%20Protocol%20v%203_1.pdf [30 November 2018]

99. GALA Trial Collaborative Group (2009). General anaesthesia versus local anaesthesia for carotid surgery (GALA): a multicentre, randomised controlled trial. The Lancet 372 (9656): 2132–2142.

100. Rose, G. (1981). Strategy of prevention: lessons from cardiovascular disease. British Medical Journal (Clinical Research Edition) 282 (6279): 1847.

101. Gibson, J. and Watkins, C. (2013). The use of formal and informal knowledge sources in patients' treatment decisions in secondary stroke prevention: qualitative study. Health Expectations 16 (3): e13–e23.

102. Wardlaw, J., Chappell, F., Best, J. et al. (2006). Non-invasive imaging compared with intra-arterial angiography in the diagnosis of symptomatic carotid stenosis: a meta-analysis. The Lancet 367 (9521): 1503–1512.

103. Young, G., Sandercock, P., Slattery, J. et al. (1996). Observer variation in the interpretation of intra-arterial angiograms and the risk of inappropriate decisions about carotid endarterectomy. Journal of Neurology, Neurosurgery & Psychiatry 60 (2): 152–157.
104. Department of Health (2008). Implementing the National Stroke Strategy – An Imaging Guide. London: Department of Health.
105. Department of Health (2007). National Stroke Strategy. London: Department of Health.
106. National Collaborating Centre for Chronic Conditions (NICCC) (2008). National Clinical Guideline for Diagnosis and Initial Management of Acute Stroke and Transient Ischaemic Attack (TIA). London: Royal College of Physicians.
107. Abbott, A. (2009). Medical (nonsurgical) intervention alone is now best for prevention of stroke associated with asymptomatic severe carotid stenosis: results of a systematic review and analysis. Stroke 40 (10): e573–e583.
108. LeFevre, M.L. (2014). Screening for asymptomatic carotid artery stenosis: US Preventive Services Task Force recommendation statement. Annals of Internal Medicine 161 (5): 356–362.
109. De Rango, P., Brown, M.M., Chaturvedi, S. et al. (2015). Summary of evidence on early carotid intervention for recently symptomatic stenosis based on meta-analysis of current risks. Stroke 46 (12): 3423–3436.
110. Rothwell, P., Slattery, J., and Warlow, C. (1996). A systematic review of the risks of stroke and death due to endarterectomy for symptomatic carotid stenosis. Stroke 27 (2): 260–265.

CHAPTER 4

Acute Stroke Nursing Management

Anne W. Alexandrov

Health Outcomes Institute, Fountain Hills, AZ, USA

University of Tennessee Health Science Center at Memphis, Memphis, TN, USA

University of Tennessee – Memphis Mobile Stroke Unit, Memphis, TN, USA

KEY POINTS

- Historically, stroke care comprised only supportive care and rehabilitation, but those days are past.
- Timely initiation of appropriate interventions can make the difference between life and death, independence and dependence – 'time is brain'.
- Hyper-acute and acute stroke care entails identification of stroke aetiology and proactive management to achieve haemodynamic stability, reperfusion, arrest, or evacuation of haemorrhage.
- Ongoing priorities include prevention of complications and initiation of rehabilitation.
- Education of patients and families and preparation for hospital discharge and life after stroke are priorities.

This chapter maps to criteria within the following sections of the Stroke-Specific Education Framework (SSEF):

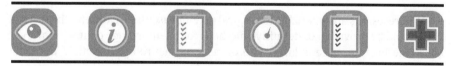

> *Your mission when caring for stroke patients is to 'find reasons to treat',
> instead of hiding behind non-evidence-based reasons 'not to treat'. Life with
> severe disability provides incentive to reverse stroke symptoms ... just do it!*
> (F.C., Stroke Coordinator, San Jose, California, USA)

4.1 Introduction

As detailed in Chapter 2, stroke may result from a number of different pathogenic mechanisms, and swift diagnosis and treatment is essential for the best patient outcomes. This chapter provides an overview of priority-driven acute stroke care, and discusses the evidence which supports best-practice diagnostic and treatment processes. It identifies where changes are required in stroke care systems to support rapid management. Mechanisms supporting ongoing quality improvement will be highlighted, including guideline recommendations for governmental and accreditation requirements aimed at improving acute stroke outcomes.

4.2 Priorities in Acute Stroke Management

Management of acute stroke patients is organised around priorities that include rapid diagnosis, stabilisation, and ensuring patient safety. In ischaemic stroke, this necessitates providing reperfusion therapies aimed at recanalisation of occluded arterial vessels, thereby restoring brain perfusion and minimising disability. Improved function and rates of independence are associated with both intravenous (IV) thrombolysis [2, 3] and endovascular thrombectomy [4–7]; patients eligible for reperfusion therapies who present at hospitals unable to provide these procedures must be rapidly transferred to a suitable facility [8]. Once reperfusion therapy has been considered and completed, the next priority is determination of pathogenic mechanism (discussed in Chapter 2). This is achieved through a comprehensive work-up to determine the probable cause of ischaemic stroke or transient ischaemic attack (TIA); findings inform appropriate secondary prevention.

In haemorrhagic stroke, there are two almost simultaneous priorities:

- Determination of haemorrhage mechanism (e.g. hypertensive intraparenchymal; anticoagulation-related, aneurysmal subarachnoid haemorrhage (aSAH), vascular malformation, or traumatic mimicking acute stroke).
- Prevention of haemorrhagic expansion to limit neurological disability.

Where lesions are amenable to surgical or endovascular treatment, the focus of care should be provision of definitive methods for haemorrhage control. However, where the haemorrhage is large with devastating neurological deficit, the focus may shift to palliative care.

For both ischaemic and haemorrhagic stroke, secondary prevention and therapies to prevent complications associated with neurological disability, as well as evaluation for type and level of rehabilitation services, are also early priorities. The duration of acute stage hospitalisation varies both internationally and regionally and is associated with severity of neurological deficit, development of complications, and the structure and capabilities of health services, including payment mechanisms.

4.3 Hyper-acute Stroke Management

4.3.1 Pre-hospital and Emergency Evaluation

Whilst systems and personnel requirements vary throughout the world, most countries offer some system of emergency response, stabilisation, and transport of patients to hospitals for definitive diagnosis and treatment. Accurate recognition of stroke is prerequisite for early initiation of treatment; valid and reliable pre-hospital stroke scales have been shown to improve accuracy (Table 4.1) [9–11].

TABLE 4.1 **Valid and reliable stroke scales**

Stroke scale	Scale elements				
Los Angeles Pre-hospital Stroke Scale (LAPSS)	Last time patient known to be symptom free: Date_____Time_____				
	Screening criteria:				
	Age ≥45 yr:		Yes	Unknown	No
	No history of seizures or epilepsy:		Yes	Unknown	No
	Symptoms present ≤24 h:		Yes	Unknown	No
	Not previously bedridden or wheelchair-bound:		Yes	Unknown	No
	If all above elements are 'unknown' or 'yes':				
	Blood glucose 60–400 mg dl^{-1}:		Yes	No	
	Examination:				
	Facial smile grimace:	Normal	Right droop	Left droop	
	Grip:	Normal	Right weak	Left weak	
		No right grip	No left grip		
	Arm strength:	Normal	Right drift	Left drift	
		Right falls	Left falls		
	Based on examination, patient has unilateral weakness:		Yes	No	
	If items are yes or unknown, meets criteria for stroke				
Cincinnati	Facial droop:				
Pre-hospital Stroke Scale (CPSS Scale)	Normal – both sides of face move equally				

(continued)

TABLE 4.1 Valid and reliable stroke scales (*continued*)

Stroke scale	Scale elements
	Abnormal – one side of face does not move as well as the other
	Arm drift:
	Normal – both arms move the same or both arms do not move at all
	Abnormal – one arm either does not move or drifts down compared to the other
	Speech:
	Normal – says correct words with no slurring
	Abnormal – slurs words, says the wrong words, or is unable to speak
	Time:
	Onset time of stroke symptoms:_____
	Transport FAST to Stroke Centre Hospital
Recognition of Stroke in the Emergency Room (ROSIER)	GCS E = M = V= BP= ᵃBG=
	ᵃ**If BG < 3.5 mmol l⁻¹, treat urgently and reassess once blood glucose normal**
	Has there been loss of consciousness or syncope? Y(−1) N(0)
	Has there been seizure activity? Y(−1) N(0)
	Is there a NEW ACUTE onset (or on awakening from sleep)?
	I. Asymmetric facial weakness Y(+1) N(0)
	II. Asymmetric arm weakness Y(+1) N(0)
	III. Asymmetric leg weakness Y(+1) N(0)
	IV. Speech disturbance Y(+1) N(0)
	V. Visual field defect Y(+1) N(0)
	Total Score (−2 to +5)=
	Provisional diagnosis
	Stroke [ ] Non-stroke [ ] (specify)
	Stroke is unlikely but not completely excluded if total scores are ≤0
	BG, blood glucose; BP, blood pressure (mmHg); GCS, Glasgow Coma Scale; E, eye; M, motor; V, verbal component

Note: These scales have been validated within either the US pre-hospital environment (LAPSS and CPSS) or UK emergency departments (ROSIER). Other valid and reliable stroke screening scales may be available in different countries worldwide.

Use of pre-hospital standardised protocols (Table 4.2) further benefits pre-hospital care by outlining priorities, limiting the time spent on scene, and expediting rapid transport of suspected stroke patients to hospitals capable of delivering acute stroke treatment [9, 12–15]. Collectively, these scales and protocols increase the number of stroke patients eligible for reperfusion therapies.

	American Stroke Association guidelines for pre-hospital
TABLE 4.2	**management of suspected acute ischaemic stroke [9]**

Category	Components
Components of the medical history recommended for collection in the pre-hospital setting	• Symptom onset time • Recent medical problems: stroke; myocardial infarction (MI); trauma; surgery; bleeding • Comorbid diseases: hypertension; diabetes mellitus • Medications: anticoagulants; insulin; antihypertensives
Recommended pre-hospital management	• Manage airway, breathing, and circulation • Monitor cardiac rhythm • Obtain IV access • Supplemental oxygen • Assess blood glucose • Nil orally • Notify receiving emergency department of en route status • Rapidly transfer to the nearest 'stroke capable' emergency department; spend minimal time on scene
Practices NOT recommended in the pre-hospital environment	• Do *NOT* use dextrose-containing IV fluids unless there is evidence of hypoglycaemia • Do *NOT* lower blood pressure • Do *NOT* administer excessive IV fluid

Within the emergency department (ED), interdisciplinary staff must be alert to the recognition of acute stroke patients because, for various reasons including knowledge deficits amongst the population, a significant number of acute stroke patients arrive by private transport, not ambulance [12, 16–18]. Use of simple scales such as the Face, Arm, Speech Test (FAST) [19] or the Recognition of Stroke in the Emergency Room (ROSIER) [20] (Table 4.1) in the triage area of the ED may result in rapid identification of patients with possible stroke or TIA [11].

Emergency triage of an acute stroke or TIA patient using the Emergency Severity Index (ESI) typically locates the patient in category 2 (Box 4.1), although concurrent airway, breathing, and/or haemodynamic instability will trigger triage to category 1 [21, 22]. All suspected stroke and TIA patients with or without current neurological deficit should be rapidly identified in the triage area [23].

Evidence from studies of patients with TIA and minor strokes indicates that very early intervention (within 24 hours) can avert stroke recurrence [24], with the risk of a definitive stroke event after TIA being 'front-loaded': highest in the first few hours to days after an initial TIA event. Whilst some countries favour discharge of TIA patients from the ED with definitive work-up for cause of stroke performed within 24–48 hours in the outpatient setting [24], others insist that TIA as a warning sign for stroke mandates short-term hospital admission so that work-up can commence immediately [9]. All patients suspected of stroke should be admitted for diagnosis, with reperfusion therapy if indicated.

Box 4.1 | The Emergency Severity Index (ESI) in Relation to Triage of Acute Stroke

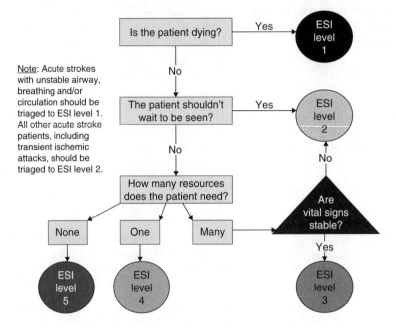

Note: Acute strokes with unstable airway, breathing and/or circulation should be triaged to ESI level 1. All other acute stroke patients, including transient ischemic attacks, should be triaged to ESI level 2.

- Call a 'Code Stroke' alert in the hospital so that the stroke team is mobilised to the ED, if this has not been automatically triggered by ambulance call to the ED.
- If needed, administer oxygen in doses necessary to treat hypoxia.
- Establish two 0.9% (normal) saline IV lines.
- Order and draw initial blood samples (e.g. for complete blood count, blood chemistry and glucose, coagulation profile, and cardiac enzymes).
- If indicated, order and collect a drug screen panel and pregnancy test.
- Order an immediate non-contrast computed tomography (CT) scan of the head, along with computed tomography angiogram (CTA) to examine the extra- and intracranial vasculature.
- Complete the National Institutes of Health Stroke Scale (NIHSS; see Table 2.12, Chapter 2) whilst en route to CT scan.
- Complete a 12-lead electrocardiogram.
- If indicated by airway or oxygenation assessment findings, order an upright chest X-ray.

Establishing time of stroke symptom onset, or time the patient was last seen symptom-free, is a high priority for both pre-hospital and triage personnel. To expedite emergency management of suspected stroke patients, many EDs have implemented standing orders that empower nurses to institute care prior to assessment by an emergency physician [23].

The Brain Attack Coalition (BAC) Guidelines [25, 26] first identified the need for physician evaluation of an acute stroke patient within 10 minutes of arrival to the ED, completion of a non-contrast CT within 25 minutes of hospital arrival, and CT diagnostic interpretation within 45 minutes of hospital arrival, culminating in delivery of intravenous tissue-type plasminogen activator (IV-tPA) within 60 minutes of hospital arrival. However, Meretoja et al. [27, 28] challenged the notion that a full 60 minutes was necessary to complete these assessments and tests, influencing how most designated stroke centres provide care today. These investigators showed that it was unnecessary to wait for a physician to assess the patient when prompt pre-hospital notification was provided because the stroke team can be at the ED door to conduct this evaluation, and it is safe to take patients with intact airway/breathing directly to CT instead of taking them first to ED and then moving them to a scanner.

Meretoja et al. [27, 28] further challenged the norm of delivering alteplase tPA only within the setting of the stroke unit or ED, showing that the stroke team can safely deliver the tPA bolus and start the infusion whilst the patient is on the CT scanning bed, after completion of the non-contrast CT and once blood pressure (BP) is controlled, immediately prior to initiation of CTA. Table 4.3 provides an

TABLE 4.3   'Stroke On the Run' methods to improve door-to-treatment times

Process	Methods
Notification	• Ambulance pre-notifies ED; stroke team paged to the ambulance entrance door *prior to* ambulance arrival
	• Statistics kept by stroke team personnel of ambulance diagnostic accuracy, including mimic diagnoses, used to educate ambulance personnel
	• CT notified of an incoming stroke so that the CT table can be made immediately available
Stroke 'On the Go' tools	• Dedicated 'ED stroke nurses' are available 24/7/365 to provide mobile care
	• ED stroke nurses meet the patient at the ED door with the stroke team; if airway, breathing, and circulation are intact/stable, the patient is taken directly to the CT scan from the ambulance or triage entrance
	• Stroke team or ED stroke nurse completes the NIHSS en route to the CT scan
	• A pre-assembled backpack containing the following items accompanies the team to the CT:
	o IV line start kits
	o Blood lab tubes for required samples
	o Point-of-care glucose and International Normalised Ratio (INR) testing equipment (INR tested only with a history of anticoagulation medication)
	o Antihypertensive medication (continuous IV infusions preferred)
	o Alteplase tPA medication with admix components
	o IV pump tubing (two sets)
	o 10 ml syringe to draw up IV-tPA bolus
	o 30 ml syringe to draw off excess alteplase tPA dose for discarding
	• Two IV pumps (or one dual-chamber pump) kept in CT scan at all times to manage antihypertensive drip and tPA infusion

(continued)

TABLE 4.3	'Stroke On the Run' methods to improve door-to-treatment times *(continued)*
Process	**Methods**

Imaging, treatment, and transfer protocols	• Non-contrast CT performed rapidly, typically started within 5–10 min of ED arrival
	
	• Alteplase tPA bolus and infusion commenced on CT scanning bed after completion of non-contrast CT, once blood pressure is controlled
	
	• CTA performed immediately after start of tPA infusion
	
	• Transfer:
	  ○ Ischemic stroke:
	    ○ If the CTA is negative for vascular occlusion (i.e. small-vessel or lacunar stroke), the patient is transported to the stroke unit for continued management
	    ○ If CTA documents large vessel occlusion (LVO), the patient is triaged directly to the catheter lab for mechanical thrombectomy
	  ○ Haemorrhagic stroke:
	    ○ If CTA documents structural lesion (aneurysm; vascular malformation), neurosurgery is consulted and the patient is triaged either directly to the catheter lab for digital subtraction angiography (DSA) and interventional occlusion or to the neuro-intensive care unit (NICU) for evaluation for surgery
	    ○ If CTA documents expansive bleeding (presence of a 'spot sign'), measures are initiated to control BP, and the patient is transferred to the NICU

overview of 'Stroke On the Run' rapid diagnosis and treatment methods based on the work of Meretoja et al. [27, 28]. As 'time is brain', hospitals throughout the world focus on performance measures to reduce their hospital arrival (door) to tPA treatment (needle) times, with most designated stroke centres instituting an Emergency Stroke Care Quality Scorecard based on either the BAC Guidelines [26, 29] or Meretoja's Model [27, 28] (see Box 4.1) to drive and support ongoing improvement of ED systems and processes.

Using methods proposed by Meretoja, the neurological examination is completed rapidly, most commonly whilst en route to the CT scan, using a valid tool (e.g. NIHSS) [30–37]. Of paramount importance is whether neurologic impairment follows neurovascular territory in the brain (clinical localisation), because ischaemic stroke is a clinical diagnosis. Non-contrast CT is then performed, which is highly sensitive to the presence of blood, allowing practitioners to identify haemorrhage and so exclude reperfusion therapies from the treatment plan [9]. In the case of ischaemic stroke (symptoms occurring within 6–8 hours prior to hospital arrival), the non-contrast CT is expected to be normal or to contain only early infarct signs such as sulcal effacement, blurring of grey and white matter interface, or a hyperdense artery sign [38].

Use of CTA to image vessel occlusion is unnecessary to make a tPA treatment decision, but is essential to differentiate large vessel occlusions (LVOs) from small-vessel/lacunar stroke [8]. Attempts have been made to use the NIHSS, or scores based on cortical sign components of the NIHSS, to identify LVO through clinical assessment alone; these methods notoriously misclassify on average 20% of LVO cases, disadvantaging patients who should have received mechanical thrombectomy (MT) and wrongly classifying cases as LVO only to find no occlusion once catheter angiography is commenced [39–43]. Additionally, CTA is essential in the determination of stroke mechanism, so should be completed during hospitalisation; moving this test to the admission/diagnosis phase of management benefits both emergency treatment and secondary prevention decision-making.

Additional neuroimaging technologies may complement the diagnostic work-up. Transcranial Doppler (TCD) may provide evidence of LVO [44]. Magnetic resonance imaging (MRI) is usually impractical within the hyper-acute phase, except in advanced stroke centres where rapid MRI protocols have been established with maximum 20-minute scanning times [8, 9]. For patients arriving within the 4.5-hour window for thrombolysis or the 6-hour window for thrombectomy, computed tomography perfusion (CTP) is not recommended in favour of expert non-contrast CT interpretation using the Alberta Stroke Program Early Computed Tomography Score (ASPECTS) [8]. In the case of haemorrhagic stroke, CTA provides information about structural causes of haemorrhage such as aneurysms and vascular malformations, as well as whether an intraparenchymal haemorrhage is actively expanding (evidenced by presence of a 'spot sign' [45, 46]). Use of catheter angiography (digital subtraction angiography, DSA), provides gold-standard vascular imaging, with the ability to extend the procedure to definitive treatment such as MT or aneurysm coiling [8, 9, 47].

4.3.2 Delivery of Reperfusion Therapies and Early Treatment in Hyper-acute Ischaemic Stroke

In hyper-acute LVO patients, particularly those eligible for reperfusion therapies, appropriate head positioning may play an important role in ensuring stability until treatment can be commenced and completed. Several small but adequately powered studies have shown that patients diagnosed with hyper-acute LVO ischaemic stroke should be positioned with the head of bed placed at 0° level, as this has been shown to increase blood flow into the ischaemic territory by 20% [48–50]. This finding is theoretically consistent with passive large artery dilation caused by vasomotor relaxation within energy-depleted penumbral zones, allowing blood flow to be directed by gravity towards zones of ischaemia, thereby optimising collateralisation. Development of increased intracranial pressure (ICP) is not a concern in hyper-acute stroke, in that oedema is generally only evident at 36–48 hours, and the risk for malignant oedema is small due to cerebral atrophy with age leaving room inside the skull. Additionally, use of 0° head positioning has been shown to be safe when patients are positioned on their side, with low rates of pneumonia reported [51, 52].

Note that 0° positioning has only been found beneficial in hyper-acute LVO ischaemic stroke – in patients with severe strokes, 0° head positioning should be used only as a temporary neuroprotective rescue procedure whilst definitive treatment with thrombolysis or thrombectomy is commenced. The HeadPoST cluster randomised clinical trial examined whether head positioning could impact outcome at 3 months in different types of stroke [52]. HeadPoST was powered using blood flow and real-time proximal clinical improvement data derived exclusively from hyper-acute LVO patients and tPA thrombolysis studies; investigators then assumed similar findings could be obtained through head positioning alone, measuring a 3-month outcome not previously validated in pilot work [53]. HeadPoST included both intracerebral haemorrhage (ICH) and ischaemic stroke, but did not require vascular imaging to ensure accuracy in determination of LVO and small-vessel/lacunar subtypes. The study's sample group was primarily patients with small-vessel minor ischaemic strokes (median NIH Stroke Scale score of 4) who were late into onset of stroke symptoms, and HeadPoST found no difference in 3-month outcomes in this group [52]. The ongoing ZODIAC trial aims to determine the contribution of 0° positioning to preventing proximal worsening in patients with CTA-confirmed hyper-acute LVO [54].

4.3.3 Thrombolysis

Ischaemic stroke patients arriving within 4.5 hours of symptom onset who meet current criteria for tPA treatment should be rapidly thrombolysed with IV-tPA [8, 9]. In US hospitals, administration of IV-tPA does not require written consent because patients with acute stroke are at significant risk for severe neurological disability, warranting emergency medical treatment with available approved therapies. In the United Kingdom and Australia, IV-tPA is a recognised and licensed treatment, so only explanation and verbal agreement is required – or a medical 'best interests' decision, if the patient cannot participate in decision-making. Good practice entails providing appropriate information to patients and relatives. The waiver of written consent for IV-tPA treatment in ischaemic stroke mirrors that applied to major traumatic injury requiring emergency surgery or acute myocardial infarction (MI) warranting emergency reperfusion. Additionally, neurological disability may preclude a stroke patient's ability to sign written consent; waiting to obtain consent from the legally designated family member may prevent timely administration of IV-tPA, thereby worsening subsequent neurological disability.

Numerous studies have demonstrated the safety and benefit of IV-tPA in acute ischaemic stroke [2, 3, 55–59]. A potentially serious adverse event of IV-tPA is symptomatic intracerebral haemorrhage (sICH), defined as an increase of four or more points on the NIHSS associated with a post-treatment finding of a large parenchymal haematoma type 2 (PH-2) on non-contrast CT [9]. However, in the hands of well-trained, experienced stroke teams, sICH is a relatively rare event. Stroke teams with high IV-tPA treatment rates typically have sICH rates lower than the 6.4% observed in the NIH National Institutes of Neurological Disorders and Stroke (NINDS) tPA trial that led to national drug approval in the United States in 1996; in the most recent large trials of tPA, rates of sICH have not exceeded 3% [2, 59], suggesting that experience with IV-tPA administration reduces treatment complications.

It is also important to consider the risk of sICH in relation to the risk of significant neurological disability. For example, from the data from the NINDS tPA trial [3], about 6 of 100 patients treated with IV-tPA were at risk for development of an sICH; applying the data from the phase IV European Safe Implementation of Thrombolysis in Stroke Monitoring Study (SITSMOST) [59], this becomes 2 of 100 patients. Additionally, in the NINDS tPA trial [3], 39%

of patients receiving IV-tPA – compared to only 26% of placebo patients – achieved a modified Rankin Score (mRS) of 0–1 by 3 months, and they had a 30% greater chance of sustaining either minimal or no neurological disability at 3 months. Interestingly, SITS-MOST data also demonstrated that 39% of subjects receiving tPA had attained an mRS of 0–1 by 3 months [59], providing significant validation of both the safety and the benefit of IV-tPA in the treatment of acute ischaemic stroke patients.

Clearly, the odds of significant neurological improvement with reduction of devastating neurological disability outweigh the risks associated with IV-tPA treatment. Where resistance to the use of IV-tPA for ischaemic stroke remains, it may be related to the challenges of updating emergency systems that have slow approaches to stroke care, practitioners who may be unwilling to take on the practice of emergency stroke management, and/or health systems with significant financial constraints to the costs of swift diagnostic imaging, emergency medical and nursing management, and IV-tPA. However, it is important to recognise that hyper-acute stroke practice today equates to 'stat' (immediate) emergency management, and is likely to continue down this path as researchers explore methods to enhance or restore brain perfusion to ward off neurological disability.

Adherence to an evidence-based protocol for administration of IV-tPA is closely tied to patient outcome. Whilst optimal, weighing ischaemic stroke patients in the ED is rarely undertaken, and was not undertaken in any of the IV-tPA trials. Instead, patients or family are asked to provide approximate weight; where they cannot, weight is estimated by the stroke team. Dosage of IV-tPA is then calculated at 0.9 mg of tPA per 1 kg of patient weight. The total dose should never exceed 90 mg, so when the calculated dose exceeds this level, it is dropped back to the 90 mg limit. Once the total dose has been calculated, 10% is given as an IV bolus over 1 minute, and the remaining 90% is infused over the next 60 minutes.

The recent ENCHANTED trial aimed to determine if use of the 0.9 mg kg^{-1} tPA dose was safe in Asian patients, compared to 0.6 mg kg^{-1} dosing. It reported that the standard 0.9 mg kg^{-1} dose tPA produced a 'safe' 2.1% rate of sICH. In the 0.6 mg kg^{-1} group, sICH rates were only 1%; however, rates of significant permanent disability were 28.9% with low-dose tPA versus 26.3% with standard-dose tPA [60]. Given that the aim of tPA treatment is to reduce stroke disability, current recommendations in the United States, Australia, and Europe do not support treatment with a lower dose of alteplase. Safety measures to ensure that the exact amount of tPA ordered is given are set out in Box 4.2.

Prior to administration of the bolus, throughout the tPA infusion, and for 24 hours post-infusion, it is paramount that BP is accurately measured and controlled to maintain the parameters in Table 4.4 [9]. These parameters were developed to support the NINDS rt-PA study [3] by consensus amongst trial investigators. Evidence is lacking to support recommendations for upper and lower limits of BP during and post-thrombolysis, but uncontrolled high BP is the most common reason associated with sICH in IV-tPA-treated patients. Therefore, all deviations from the current upper BP limit must be immediately treated with IV antihypertensive agents. Pharmaceutical agents that allow for rapid, precise, non-aggressive BP reduction are best, because dropping the BP too low may decrease blood flow through residual arteries, which may worsen perfusion within the ischaemic penumbra [9, 61, 62].

Box 4.2 | Safety Measures to Ensure Exact tPA Dosing

- Double check and verify amongst stroke team members the estimated patient weight used in the calculation of total tPA dose.
- Double check the total dose calculation.
- Withdraw and discard from the tPA vial the amount of drug that exceeds the total dose. (Clinical example: Each vial of tPA contains a total of 100 mg/100 ml fluid once reconstituted. If the total dose to be given is 68 mg, the stroke team nurse should withdraw and discard 32 ml of the reconstituted tPA, leaving only the 68 ml in the vial for infusion.)
- Withdraw with a 10 ml syringe a 10% bolus dose. (Clinical example: If the total dose to be given is 68 mg, the 10% bolus dose amounts to 6.8 mg or 6.8 ml.)
- Administer the bolus dose over 1 minute via the IV line that will be dedicated to the tPA infusion.
- Attach the IV tubing to the tPA bottle or other administration device (e.g. syringe driver) and clear the line of air; ensure that no tPA is wasted whilst clearing air from the line.
- Attach the tPA infusion to an infusion pump (or prepare the syringe driver) and set for 60 minutes to deliver the drug remaining in the vial.
- Ensure that once the infusion is complete, all tPA remaining in the tubing reaches the patient before the infusion is discontinued. (Note: Most IV tubing contains about 23 ml of fluid; if this is wasted, it amounts to cutting the dose of tPA by 23 mg.)
- Once discontinued, flush the IV line with 3–5 ml normal saline.

TABLE 4.4 **Control of blood pressure in IV-tPA-treated patients**

Phase of management	Blood pressure control guidelines
Preparing for tPA administration	*If BP is >185 mmHg systolic or >110 mmHg diastolic, administer:*
	• Labetalol 10–20 mg IV over 1–2 min, may repeat once; or
	• Nicardipine infusion, 5 mg h^{-1}; titrate up by 0.25 mg h^{-1} at 5–15 min intervals, maximum dose 15 mg h^{-1}
	If BP remains >185 mmHg systolic or >110 mmHg diastolic, do NOT give tPA bolus
During and after tPA treatment	• Monitor BP every 15 min during treatment
	• Immediately post-treatment, vital signs frequency for the next 24 h should be: every 15 min for 2 h; every 30 min for 6 h; every hour for 16 h
	• Maintain systolic BP <180 mmHg and diastolic BP <105 mmHg
	If BP > 180 mmHg and diastolic BP > 105 mmHg, administer:
	• Labetalol 10 mg IV over 1–2 min, may repeat every 10–20 min to a total of 300 mg (consider labetalol infusion if repeated injections are necessary); or
	• Nicardipine infusion, 5 mg h^{-1}; titrate up by 0.25 mg h^{-1} at 5–15 min intervals, maximum dose 15 mg h^{-1}

Source: Adapted from the American Stroke Association 2013 Guidelines [9].

4.3.4 Monitoring

Use of non-invasive oscillometric automatic blood pressure (NIBP) cuffs was originally thought to be dangerous in IV-tPA-treated patients, because intense mechanical compression of the arm might cause bruising. However, no study has been undertaken to investigate this, and these devices are regularly used in many facilities without harmful effects. Future investigation may assist in quantifying safety concerns with these devices during and post-treatment with IV-tPA.

Elevated glucose levels should also be identified in the hyper-acute phase due to their association with poor neurological outcome; when present, elevated glucose should be treated and infusion of glucose-potassium-insulin may be required. An intensive approach to the maintenance of tight glycaemic control (between 4.0 and 7.5 mmol l^{-1}) is not recommended [63, 64]. Consensus management recommendations vary: in the United Kingdom, the aim is to maintain blood glucose levels in the range of 5–15 mmol l^{-1} in the first 24–72 hours post-stroke; in Australia, an upper limit at 10 mmol l^{-1} is suggested [65, 66].

Fever in acute stroke patients is also associated with poor outcome, and these patients should be rapidly returned to normothermic levels using routine measures such as paracetamol or cooling blankets [9, 67–73]. The Quality in Acute Stroke Care cluster randomised trial by Middleton et al. found that when nurses utilise protocols for measurement and management of fever and hyperglycaemia, along with strict bedside screening of dysphagia and cautious management of oral intake, a significant improvement in 3-month outcomes [74] and a 20% decrease in adjusted long-term mortality rates may be realised [75]. However, the intense focus on rapid diagnostic imaging and delivery of reperfusion treatment in hyper-acute stroke patients may overshadow practitioners' vigilant attention to both glucose and temperature monitoring and management; a recent study reported no temperature measurement in 39% of patients arriving to five US Comprehensive Stroke Centres, with poor glucose and temperature control common early after acute stroke admission [76].

Other nursing priorities during and after delivery of IV-tPA include close monitoring for neurological change using an objective quantifiable tool (e.g. NIHSS) to alert clinicians to improvement or deterioration warranting repeat of a 'stat' non-contrast CT to rule out sICH. Sudden onset of neurological deterioration in the first 24 hours from treatment with IV-tPA is associated with either sICH (rare) or, more commonly, arterial reocclusion, which may occur in up to 22% of patients [77]. By closely assessing patients for neurological change, reocclusion can be immediately identified and acted on by means of MT. Finally, nurses and other clinicians involved in the care of patients treated with IV-tPA must remember that once the drug has been administered, invasive procedures should be withheld for the next 24 hours unless there is a life-threatening need AND only when the invasive procedure is performed in a compressible or surgically controlled manner. Case Study 4.1 provides an example of expected diagnosis and treatment of an ischaemic stroke patient.

4.3.5 Mechanical Clot Removal

For ischaemic stroke patients with LVO evident on neuroimaging, endovascular MT with a retrievable stent has been shown to improve 3-month outcomes

Case Study

Case 4.1   Maureen

Maureen is a 94-year-old female who is witnessed by her family members suddenly falling to the right and losing the ability to speak whilst cooking breakfast at 08.10. Her 89-year-old brother activates the local ambulance service, who arrive at 08.25. They immediately perform the CPSS, finding a flattened right nasolabial fold, a flaccid right arm, and loss of comprehension and verbal language skills. They also note that Maureen has lost almost all right leg motor function; only a flicker of movement is detected. She has no previous stroke history but smokes and has hypertension for which she is non-compliant with medications; on occasion, she takes aspirin for headache, but no other medications. Immediately suspecting stroke, the ambulance team notifies the local Stroke Centre Hospital.

On arrival to the hospital at 08.55, the stroke team is present in the ED; with Maureen breathing on her own, and with a BP of 196/110 mmHg, they take her immediately to the CT suite, completing the NIHSS score en route and totalling 23 points (2 = questions, 2 = commands, 1 = left gaze preference, 2 = right homonymous hemianopia, 2 = weak lower right face, 4 = flaccid right arm, 3 = weak right leg, 2 = dense right hemi-sensory loss, 3 = muteness, 2 = right hemi-neglect). An additional large-bore antecubital IV is placed in the left arm, and point-of-care testing confirms a normal blood glucose.

Non-contrast CT is completed within 1 minute and read on the CT console by the stroke team. A decision is made to treat Maureen with IV-tPA, and the clinical pharmacist begins mixing the drug in CT for administration whilst the physician discusses treatment with her family. The stroke team nurses initiate antihypertensive treatment and control Maureen's BP to 168/88 mmHg. The tPA bolus is given on the CT scanning bed at 09.10 and the infusion is subsequently started. Maureen then immediately undergoes CTA, which reveals a proximal M1 occlusion of the left middle cerebral artery.

whether pre-treated with alteplase tPA or not, in cases outside the tPA window [4–7, 78, 79]. Retrievable stents (stentrievers) are devices that expand upon deployment, pushing the clot into its wire mesh and rapidly restoring blood flow to the affected large artery. After several minutes of recovery time have passed, the interventionalist retrieves the stent, withdrawing it from the artery, and the clot trapped within the mesh of the stent is pulled out with it. Whilst other devices and methods remain available for use in the catheterisation lab, stentrievers are acknowledged in the US stroke guidelines as the superior device for use in a MT procedure [8].

Arterial access is typically achieved through canalising the femoral artery. Serial angiograms are taken to diagnose the problem, determine the treatment, and, once treatment is complete, evaluate the outcome. Few patients undergoing endovascular MT require intubation, and the procedure is faster than in previous years where general anaesthesia was standard. Once it is concluded, patients often go directly to MRI so final infarct size can be determined. Nursing care of patients undergoing MT is outlined in Box 4.3. Case Study 4.2 describes the management of Maureen as she proceeds to MT.

In patients with large infarction affecting the cerebral hemispheres, particularly in young patients who lack the space within the cranial vault associated with atrophic age-related changes, hemicraniectomy (removal of a large section of skull over an affected region of infarction) may be considered as a life-saving technique where

---

Box 4.3 | Nursing Care of Patients Undergoing MT Includes

- Airway management for conscious sedation cases.
- Weaning and extubation, if intubated.
- Monitoring and control of BP before, during, and after the procedure, using the parameters stipulated for IV-tPA; when recanalisation has occurred, maintenance of normotension must be ensured.
- Management of intraprocedural sedation.
- Assessment of the groin arterial puncture site for haematoma development, with assessment of pulses distal to the puncture.
- Ongoing neurological monitoring with a quantifiable tool (e.g. NIHSS) to determine change from baseline scores, using the parameters recommended for IV-tPA.

Case Study

Case 4.2   Maureen (Cont.)

Maureen is kept laid flat after CTA and rapidly transferred back to the ED stretcher whilst the stroke team physician contacts the interventional team. At 09.25, she is en route to the interventional suite. The stroke team physician rapidly explains to her family that this is the best plan of care, and uses data from clinical trials to explain the likelihood of a favourable outcome if MT is performed immediately after IV-tPA treatment.

Maureen is transferred on to the angiography suite bed and kept in a 0° head position. The team preps and drapes her for the procedure. The stroke team nurse remains with Maureen through the procedure to hold her hands and keep her still; no intubation with additional sedation is given since she is very disabled and time is of the essence. Vascular access is obtained at 09.33 and the first angiographic run is displayed as a roadmap for the interventionalist at 09.40. The interventionalist advances the retrievable stent and is successful in establishing complete recanalisation by 09.53.

Serial clinical examinations of Maureen over the next hour show remarkable improvement in her NIHSS score, with a score of zero achieved by 11.15. The cause of Maureen's stroke is determined to be atrial fibrillation (AF), which was noted on the monitor during her time in the hospital. She is eventually started on anticoagulation prior to discharge home, although there is concern amongst the family and staff over her compliance with this treatment regimen. She will be followed up in the outpatient clinic at 3 months post-discharge.

---

intracranial mass effects risk herniation [9, 80]. Craniectomy may also be employed to treat cerebellar infarctions that risk compromise of brainstem structures due to oedema and obstructive hydrocephalus. Cautious patient selection and early timing for craniectomy procedures are important. Post-procedural serial assessments using the NIHSS are important and should be accompanied by non-contrast CT to determine response to therapy. Bone removed during hemicraniectomy procedures for large middle cerebral artery strokes may be either stored in a bone bank or sewn into a pouch made in the patient's abdomen, whereas bone removed for cerebellar stroke is discarded; reserved bone is replaced at around 3 months from the time of the brain infarction, and until then the patient needs to wear a helmet.

4.4 Hyper-acute Treatment of Haemorrhagic Stroke

Non-contrast CT is used to differentiate haemorrhagic from ischaemic stroke. Often, a CTA is also completed to determine the mechanism for the haemorrhage and to document active bleeding within a haematoma (CTA 'spot sign') [81]. In patients with structural causes of haemorrhage (e.g. aSAH or vascular malformations), definitive treatment of arterial anomalies using endovascular occlusion (e.g. detachable coils) or surgical procedures is an early consideration to reduce the risk for rebleeding. Serial monitoring is important in patients with haemorrhagic stroke, as haemorrhage expansion is common and is associated with life-threatening clinical deterioration. The validity of the NIHSS as a quantitative tool to capture neurological disability in haemorrhagic stroke has not yet been studied, but this tool may be suitable since it does provide more complete neurological assessment data than the Glasgow Coma Scale (GCS). Use of the GCS is also considered acceptable in haemorrhagic stroke, but by itself this instrument does not capture key elements of the neurological examination other than the 'best response' of factors most closely aligned with consciousness. The Intracerebral Haemorrhage Score (ICHS) should also be calculated in patients with intraparenchymal haemorrhage (Table 4.5), because it provides a useful estimate of outcome [82]. In cases of large haemorrhagic stroke with coma, the stroke team must cautiously decide what measures are in the patient's best interest, and consider consulting with family members about palliative care.

Once non-contrast CT evidence of haemorrhage has been obtained, the patient is usually positioned with the head of the bed at 30° elevation, because of the potential for development of increased ICP secondary to intracranial haemorrhage. The HeadPoST study showed that intraparenchymal haemorrhage patients maintained at 0° did not differ in 90-day outcomes from those positioned at 30° [52], but lack of serial monitoring in the hyper-acute phase of haemorrhage limits our understanding of subtle changes. Medical treatment of haemorrhagic stroke is closely associated with haemorrhage subtype: intraparenchymal (hypertensive, coagulopathic or amyloid origins), aSAH or arteriovenous malformation (AVM) (Table 4.5).

4.4.1 Intraparenchymal Haemorrhage (IPH)

Intraparenchymal haemorrhage (IPH) is the most common form of haemorrhagic stroke, producing bleeding into brain tissues. In hypertensive IPH, the most vulnerable areas of the brain include the basal ganglia, thalami, and occasionally the pons and cerebellum [81]. It is not known whether hypertension occurs in response to haemorrhage expansion with increased ICP, or whether prolonged elevation of BP is responsible for haemorrhagic expansion. The two processes are clearly related, with the risk for haemorrhage expansion and clinical deterioration ranging from 14 to 38% within the first 24 hours of the initial bleed [81, 83, 84].

Coagulopathic IPH due to anticoagulation or antiplatelet agents may occur in a variety of locations depending on whether concurrent head trauma is a

TABLE 4.5   **Intracerebral Haemorrhage (ICH) Score**

Finding	Score
Glasgow Coma Scale score	
3–4	2
5–12	1
13–15	0
ICH volume	
≥ 30 cc	1
< 30 cc	0
Intraventricular haemorrhage	
Yes	1
No	0
Infratentorial origin	
Yes	1
No	0
Age:	
≥ 80 yr	1
< 80 yr	0
Total score	0–6

factor, and whether there is also amyloid angiopathy or hypertension [81, 85]. Management aims to reverse the coagulopathy, and treatment strategies vary due to the agent/mechanism involved. The Neurocritical Care Society (NCS) and the Society of Critical Care Medicine (SCCM) have developed international guidelines that detail these treatment strategies, serving as the major resource for these complex cases [86]. Pure amyloid-related IPH most commonly occurs in the convexities of the grey matter, and this type of IPH is more common with older age and genetic predisposition.

IPH continues to challenge stroke practitioners, with surgical treatment no more effective than conservative non-surgical approaches [87] and no drug therapy showing a difference in 3-month outcomes [81]. Considerations in the medical management of IPH include:

- close monitoring and control of BP;
- rapid or early detection and reversal of coagulopathies;
- identification of non-communicating hydrocephalus resulting from ventricular clot obstruction; and
- ongoing neurological assessment, and in some cases palliative care [81].

Intensive BP reduction has been thought to be beneficial in preventing expansion of haematomas and improving 3-month outcomes. Whilst the INTER-ACT-2 study showed a trend (p = 0.06) towards improved 3-month outcomes in the intensive BP-lowering group [88], 66% of patients in this group never achieved intensive lowering of BP, and study management has been questioned. The ATACH-2 study [89] used rigorous, standardised BP management methods, but was stopped prematurely for futility, as no difference in 3-month outcome was found between intensive BP-lowering and control groups. Nonetheless, most practitioners favour some degree of BP lowering (to less than 160 or 140 mmHg systolic), although it remains unclear what parameters best support patient management.

Serial non-contrast CT is important in IPH to document stability or expansion of haemorrhage, especially when significant clinical change is identified. In the case of subcortical or pontine IPH, extension into or obstruction of the ventricular system may occur and make insertion of ventriculostomy necessary for drainage of cerebrospinal fluid [81]. Once the haemorrhage size has stabilised, instilling small amounts of tPA into intraventricular catheters has been shown to be safe and effective for catheter clearance to facilitate ventricular blood clot dissolution and drainage [90, 91]; it may reduce the need for permanent shunting [91], but it has not been shown to make a difference in 3-month functional outcomes. Once inserted, ventricular drains should be levelled and zero-balanced to the foramen of Monro; ICP should be monitored closely, with the system open to drainage and a consistent head height maintained at 30° elevation. Standard measures for treatment of increased ICP should be employed as indicated. Neurological status should be closely observed, since haemorrhage enlargement is associated with poor clinical outcome and death.

4.4.2 Aneurysmal Subarachnoid Haemorrhage (aSAH)

In aSAH, once the aneurysm has been occluded by endovascular (most commonly) or surgical means, priorities shift to prevention of delayed secondary ischaemic stroke associated with refractory vasospasm. Medical strategies to prevent delayed secondary ischaemic stroke include induced hypertension and intra-arterial angioplasty or instillation of vasodilatory agents into the spastic arterial segment, although clear differences in clinical outcome have not been observed between these techniques [92]. Use of 'triple H' therapy (hypertension, hypervolaemia, and haemodilution) is no longer considered acceptable management. Nimodipine is now widely acknowledged to have no direct effect on reduction of vasospasm, but probably increases the tolerance of ischaemia within brain tissues subjected to vasospasm. Dihydropyridine-class calcium channel blockers such as nicardipine have recently emerged as promising strategies for the prevention and treatment of vasospasm, and also provide likely neuroprotective effects through elevation of tissue thresholds to ischaemic insult. However, data from large trials are lacking. They are delivered by direct surgical implantation after open surgical flushing of the basal cisterns [93] or by intra-arterial infusion during direct intracranial arterial canalisation.

aSAH is also associated with stunning of the myocardium [94, 95], which challenges the use of induced hypertension, placing patients at risk for development of heart failure due to significant left ventricular afterload and elevated preload. Judicious use of volume- and pressure-driven therapies is paramount. Development of non-communicating hydrocephalus is common in aSAH, requiring management by ventriculostomy and often long-term shunt placement. As early surgical or endovascular treatment is now standard care for aSAH, development of increased ICP in patients with aSAH is most commonly associated with either hydrocephalus that has not been properly identified and treated by ventriculostomy or delayed secondary ischaemic stroke with malignant oedema.

4.5   Acute Stroke Management

4.5.1   General Management Priorities

Once the hyper-acute phase of stroke management is complete, priorities shift to:

- identifying aetiological stroke mechanisms;
- developing individualised secondary stroke prevention measures;
- prevention of complications;
- evaluation of rehabilitation needs; and
- patient and family preparation for discharge from acute care services.

4.5.2   Routine Monitoring

BP control continues during the acute phase of hospitalisation for stroke, but goals may vary when haemodynamic factors suggest the need for higher pressures (e.g. persisting extracranial or intracranial vessel occlusions). By 24 hours, oral antihypertensive agents or those that may be given through enteral feeding tubes are commenced and patients are progressively weaned from IV antihypertensive agents. Multiple agents are often required to achieve adequate BP control and should be added slowly and adjusted to achieve the therapeutic effect over the course of hospitalisation [9, 81, 96]. Selection of antihypertensive drugs should be based on factors such as underlying renal function, history of MI, Diabetes Mellitus, left ventricular dysfunction, baseline cardiac rhythm, and genetic factors. For example, clinical trial data suggest that people of Black ethnic origin may respond better to calcium channel blockers in combination with thiazide diuretics compared to angiotensin-converting enzyme (ACE) inhibitors or angiotensin-II receptor blockers (ARBs), due to their lower rates of renin-based hypertension [96].

Blood glucose levels should continue to be closely monitored and controlled. Temperature should also be monitored, as hyperthermia has been associated with poor neurological outcome and may also indicate an underlying infectious process requiring management [9, 74].

4.5.3 Swallowing

Swallow integrity must be assessed in all stroke patients, with the patient kept 'nil orally' (NPO/NBM) until the ability to safely manage oral intake has been adequately assessed [9, 74]. Chapter 5 provides a detailed overview of the measures used to screen and diagnose swallow dysfunction in stroke patients, alongside recommendations for nutritional support and rehabilitation. The risk of aspiration is high in patients with dysphagia and/or strokes that are associated with a decreased level of consciousness. Vigilant nursing assessment of airway patency, breathing pattern, breath sounds, and gas exchange is important in the prevention and early detection of aspiration. In cases where the patient was found on the ground and unconscious, aspiration may have occurred prior to hospitalisation, and this should be noted in their record.

4.5.4 Sleep Apnoea

The prevalence of sleep apnoea in stroke patients ranges from 30 to 70% [97, 98]. It remains unclear how often sleep apnoea in stroke patients is of central, obstructive, or mixed aetiology, and whilst all patients suspected of this disorder should receive formal sleep studies, the early identification and management of sleep-disordered breathing should be promptly undertaken by stroke practitioners. The 'reversed Robin Hood syndrome' entails the intravascular 'steal' of blood from neurovascular territories associated with stroke, which need optimal perfusion, to normal vascular territories during apnoeic episodes [99]. Use of non-invasive modes of ventilation with continuous positive airway pressure (CPAP) have been shown to improve and maintain steady arterial flow through neurovascular territories in patients with sleep apnoea, whilst improving and maintaining clinical outcome [98]. Nurses working with stroke patients will need to become expert in non-invasive ventilation, with its growing use to combat sleep-disordered breathing problems.

4.5.5 Venous Thromboembolism

As in many other conditions, prolonged immobility contributes to the risk of venous thromboembolism (VTE), pneumonia with reduced systemic perfusion, skin breakdown, physical deconditioning, lethargy, and mental confusion [9, 29, 100]. It is important to emphasise that once the hyper-acute stage has ended (and there are no medical contraindications), patients should be moved to a mobilisation protocol that includes moving out of bed to a chair, range of motion, and progressive ambulation. Patients should be thoroughly assessed for their rehabilitation needs by members of the interdisciplinary stroke team [9, 29]. However, it should be emphasised that early mobilisation within the first 24 hours is not beneficial (associated with a number needed to harm of 25 [101]; see Chapter 7 for more details). Given that stroke is a disease of vascular insufficiency (similar to MI, which is treated with a slow, steady approach to mobilisation), it is not surprising that early exercise should be considered with caution.

Development of VTE is a significant concern where stroke is associated with prolonged immobility [9, 29, 81, 102, 103]. Prophylactic measures to prevent VTE are standard throughout most of the world, with a variety of strategies recommended in evidence-based guidelines. By far the best prophylaxis against VTE is anticoagulation [9, 104, 105]. Rates of serious bleeding in patients receiving anticoagulation prophylaxis are relatively low [104, 106], and long-term management with oral agents after hospital is well tolerated, particularly with newer-generation anticoagulants that require a single standard dose without blood monitoring. For prevention of symptomatic pulmonary embolism – a rarer complication than lower-limb VTE – the potential benefit of anticoagulation in recent stroke does not outweigh the risk of symptomatic haemorrhagic transformation [107], and as a result some guidelines recommend that anticoagulation is not used. In patients with acute IPH, use of anticoagulation may cause high risk of haemorrhagic expansion [108], and alternative strategies are recommended until bleeding has ceased and stabilised. The safety of anticoagulation for VTE prophylaxis in IPH has not been established by clinical trials, although many experts assert that once the haemorrhage has stabilised – at approximately 36–72 hours from stroke onset – anticoagulation is probably safe and should be considered given its superiority to other prophylactic measures, with sequential compression used prior to this time [81]. Sequential compression devices (SCDs) have been shown to be efficacious at preventing VTE compared to thigh-length compression stockings [109]. Compression stockings may cause serious limb ischaemia and skin breakdown, are ineffective at preventing VTE in acute stroke patients, and are no longer recommended in the American, Australian, or European guidelines. In the United Kingdom, the National Clinical Guideline for Stroke states: 'Patients with immobility after acute stroke should not be routinely given low molecular weight heparin or graduated compression stockings (either full-length or below-knee) for the prevention of deep vein thrombosis' [65]. VTE prophylaxis using subcutaneous heparin is not recommended in UK guidelines, although it is still recommended in US and Australian ones [65, 110, 111].

4.5.6   Urinary Catheters

The routine insertion of urinary catheters in acute stroke patients should be discouraged. Chapter 9 provides detailed information related to continence. Within the context of this chapter, urinary catheters should only be considered when very close monitoring of intake and output takes precedence or when urinary retention is a concern; they should not be routinely used as incontinence management. When patients are admitted with urinary tract infection (UTI), this should be clearly documented to exclude a diagnosis of hospital-acquired UTI.

4.5.7   Secondary Prevention

In ischaemic stroke, treatment with antithrombotic (anticoagulation or antiplatelet) agents is important for secondary prevention of future stroke. For documented cardioembolic stroke (AF, left ventricular thrombus, concurrent congestive heart failure, or right-to-left intracardiac shunt with documentation of embolic source), anticoagulation is started with oral agents such as warfarin – or direct oral anti-coagulants (DOACs) if AF is the documented cause – to reduce the risk of future stroke. IV heparin is rarely if ever used during acute hospitalisation, in favour of oral agents. When warfarin is used, the target for most patients is an International Normalised Ratio (INR) of 2–3, although patients with prosthetic heart valves are managed with a target INR of 2.5–3.5. For non-cardioembolic ischaemic stroke, antiplatelet agents such as aspirin and clopidogrel are started.

Patients who smoke should be counselled to reduce the risk of another stroke event and cardiac disease [9]. It is essential that family and significant others be involved in this process, because smoking cessation requires all those close to the patient to quit smoking as well, in order to ensure long-term sustainability. Use of nicotine patches or varenicline (Chantix/Champix) may complement a smoking cessation plan. Chapter 3 provides more information about smoking cessation.

Throughout their hospital admission, patients and their family members should also receive ongoing education on:

- ischaemic and haemorrhagic stroke disease processes;
- warning signs;
- rapid access to a hospital delivering hyper-acute stroke care, including use of emergency medical transport systems;
- personal risk factors for stroke and their modification;
- stroke treatment;
- stroke recovery;
- prevention of complications; and
- hospital discharge planning and societal reintegration [9].

4.6 Conclusion

Hyper-acute stroke management requires a rapid response by stroke team members to reduce disability and death; the focus of acute management subsequently shifts to prevention of worsening due to stroke progression or complications and initiation of secondary stroke prevention strategies. Hyper-acute and acute stroke nurses must embrace the challenge of supporting rapid diagnosis and treatment, whilst exploring methods to further improve our multidisciplinary approach to stroke management.

References

1. UK Stroke Forum Education & Training. Stroke-Specific Education Framework, United Kingdom: UK Stroke Forum 2010. Available from: http://www.stroke-education.org.uk/about. [30 November 2018]
2. Hacke, W., Kaste, M., Bluhmki, E. et al. (2008). Thrombolysis with alteplase 3 to 4.5 hours after acute ischemic stroke. New England Journal of Medicine 359 (13): 1317–1329.

3. The National Institute of Neurological Disorders Stroke rt-PA Stroke Study Group (1995). Tissue plasminogen activator for acute ischemic stroke. New England Journal of Medicine 333 (24): 1581–1588.

4. Berkhemer, O.A., Fransen, P.S.S., Beumer, D. et al. (2015). A randomized trial of intraarterial treatment for acute ischemic stroke. New England Journal of Medicine 372 (1): 11–20.

5. Goyal, M., Demchuk, A.M., Menon, B.K. et al. (2015). Randomized assessment of rapid endovascular treatment of ischemic stroke. New England Journal of Medicine 372 (11): 1019–1030.

6. Campbell, B.C.V., Mitchell, P.J., Kleinig, T.J. et al. (2015). Endovascular therapy for ischemic stroke with perfusion-imaging selection. New England Journal of Medicine 372 (11): 1009–1018.

7. Jovin, T.G., Chamorro, A., Cobo, E. et al. (2015). Thrombectomy within 8 hours after symptom onset in ischemic stroke. New England Journal of Medicine 372 (24): 2296–2306.

8. Powers, W.J., Derdeyn, C.P., Biller, J. et al. (2015). 2015 American Heart Association/American Stroke Association focused update of the 2013 guidelines for the early management of patients with acute ischemic stroke regarding endovascular treatment. A guideline for healthcare professionals from the American Heart Association/American Stroke Association. Stroke 46 (10): 3020–3035.

9. Jauch, E.C., Saver, J.L., Adams, H.P.J. et al. (2013). Guidelines for the early management of patients with acute ischemic stroke: a guideline for healthcare professionals from the American Heart Association/American Stroke Association. Stroke 44 (3): 870–947.

10. Kidwell, C.S., Starkman, S., Eckstein, M. et al. (2000). Identifying stroke in the field: prospective validation of the Los Angeles Prehospital Stroke Screen (LAPSS). Stroke 31 (1): 71–76.

11. Kothari, R.U., Pancioli, A., Liu, T. et al. (1999). Cincinnati prehospital stroke scale: reproducibility and validity. Annals of Emergency Medicine 33 (4): 373–378.

12. Morris, D.L., Rosamond, W., Madden, K. et al. (2000). Prehospital and emergency department delays after acute stroke. The Genentech stroke presentation survey. Stroke 31 (11): 2585–2590.

13. Rossnagel, K., Jungehülsing, G.J., Nolte, C.H. et al. (2004). Out-of-hospital delays in patients with acute stroke. Annals of Emergency Medicine 44 (5): 476–483.

14. Silliman, S.L., Quinn, B., Huggett, V., and Merino, J.G. (2003). Use of a field-to-stroke center helicopter transport program to extend thrombolytic therapy to rural residents. Stroke 34 (3): 729–733.

15. Ramanujam, P., Castillo, E., Patel, E. et al. (2009). Prehospital transport time intervals for acute stroke patients. Journal of Emergency Medicine 37 (1): 40–45.

16. Schroeder, E.B., Rosamond, W.D., Morris, D.L. et al. (2000). Determinants of use of emergency medical services in a population with stroke symptoms. The second Delay in Accessing Stroke Healthcare (DASH II) Study. Stroke 31 (11): 2591–2596.

17. Schwamm, L.H., Pancioli, A., Acker, J.E. et al. (2005). Recommendations for the establishment of stroke systems of care. Recommendations from the American Stroke Association's task force on the development of stroke systems. Stroke 36 (3): 690–703.

18. Wojner-Alexandrov, A.W., Alexandrov, A.V., Rodriguez, D. et al. (2005). Houston paramedic and emergency stroke treatment and outcomes study (HoPSTO). Stroke 36 (7): 1512–1518.

19. Harbison, J., Hossain, O., Jenkinson, D. et al. (2003). Diagnostic accuracy of stroke referrals from primary care, emergency room physicians, and ambulance staff using the face arm speech test. Stroke 34 (1): 71–76.

20. Nor, A.M., McAllister, C., Louw, S.J. et al. (2004). Agreement between ambulance paramedic- and physician-recorded neurological signs with Face Arm Speech Test (FAST) in acute stroke patients. Stroke 35 (6): 1355–1359.

21. Tanabe, P., Gimbel, R., Yarnold, P.R. et al. (2004). Reliability and validity of scores on the Emergency Severity Index version 3. Academic Emergency Medicine 11 (1): 59–65.
22. Tanabe, P., Travers, D., Gilboy, N. et al. (2005). Refining Emergency Severity Index triage criteria. Academic Emergency Medicine 12 (6): 497–501.
23. Middleton, S., Grimley, R., and Alexandrov, A.W. (2015). Triage, treatment, and transfer. Evidence-based clinical practice recommendations and models of nursing care for the first 72 hours of admission to hospital for acute stroke. Stroke 46 (2): e18–e25.
24. National Collaborating Centre for Chronic Conditions (NICCC) (2008). National Clinical Guideline for Diagnosis and Initial Management of Acute Stroke and Transient Ischaemic Attack (TIA). London: Royal College of Physicians.
25. Alberts, M.J., Hademenos, G., Latchaw, R.E. et al. (2000). Recommendations for the establishment of primary stroke centers. Journal of the American Medical Association 283 (23): 3102–3109.
26. Alberts, M.J., Latchaw, R.E., Selman, W.R. et al. (2005). Recommendations for comprehensive stroke centers. A Consensus Statement From the Brain Attack Coalition 36 (7): 1597–1616.
27. Meretoja, A., Strbian, D., Mustanoja, S. et al. (2012). Reducing in-hospital delay to 20 minutes in stroke thrombolysis. Neurology 79 (4): 306–313.
28. Meretoja, A., Weir, L., Ugalde, M. et al. (2013). Helsinki model cut stroke thrombolysis delays to 25 minutes in Melbourne in only 4 months. Neurology 81 (12): 1071–1076.
29. Alberts, M.J., Hademenos, G., Latchaw, R.E. et al. (2000). Recommendations for the establishment of primary stroke centers. JAMA 283 (23): 3102–3109.
30. Dewey, H.M., Donnan, G.A., Freeman, E.J. et al. (1999). Interrater reliability of the NIHSS: rating by neurologists and nurses in a community-based stroke incidence study. Cerebrovascular Diseases 9 (6): 323–327.
31. Domínguez, R., Vila, J.F., Augustovski, F. et al. (2006). Spanish cross-cultural adaptation and validation of the NIHSS: Mayo clinic proceedings. Stroke 81 (4): 476–480.
32. Josephson, S.A., Hills, N.K., and Johnston, S.C. (2006). NIH Stroke Scale reliability in ratings from a large sample of clinicians. Cerebrovascular Diseases 22 (5–6): 389–395.
33. Kasner, S.E. (2006). Clinical interpretation and use of stroke scales. The Lancet Neurology 5 (7): 603–612.
34. Lyden, P., Brott, T., Tilley, B. et al. (1994). Improved reliability of the NIH Stroke Scale using video training. NINDS TPA Stroke Study Group. Stroke 25 (11): 2220–2226.
35. Lyden, P., Lu, M., Jackson, C. et al. (1999). Underlying structure of the National Institutes of Health Stroke Scale. Results of a Factor Analysis 30 (11): 2347–2354.
36. Lyden, P., Raman, R., Liu, L. et al. (2005). NIHSS training and certification using a new digital video disk is reliable. Stroke 36 (11): 2446–2449.
37. Goldstein, L.B. and Samsa, G.P. (1997). Reliability of the National Institutes of Health Stroke Scale – extension to non-neurologists in the context of a clinical trial. Stroke 28 (2): 307–310.
38. Patel, S.C., Levine, S.R., Tilley, B.C. et al. (2001). Lack of clinical significance of early ischemic changes on computed tomography in acute stroke. Journal of the American Medical Association 286 (22): 2830–2838.
39. Katz, B.S., McMullan, J.T., Sucharew, H. et al. (2015). Design and validation of a prehospital scale to predict stroke severity. Cincinnati Prehospital Stroke Severity Scale 46 (6): 1508–1512.
40. Hastrup, S., Damgaard, D., Johnsen, S.P., and Andersen, G. (2016). Prehospital acute stroke severity scale to predict large artery occlusion: design and comparison with other scales. Stroke 47 (7): 1772–1776.
41. Heldner, M.R., Hsieh, K., Broeg-Morvay, A. et al. (2016). Clinical prediction of large vessel occlusion in anterior circulation stroke: mission impossible? Journal of Neurology 263 (8): 1633–1640.

42. Turc, G., Maïer, B., Naggara, O. et al. (2016). Clinical scales do not reliably identify acute ischemic stroke patients with large-artery occlusion. Stroke 47 (6): 1466–1472.

43. Pérez de la Ossa, N., Carrera, D., Carrera, D. et al. (2014). Design and validation of a prehospital stroke scale to predict large arterial occlusion. Stroke 45 (1): 87–91.

44. Alexandrov, A.W. (2011). Transcranial Doppler Monitoring. In: AACN's Procedure Manual for Critical Care, 6e (ed. D.L.-M. Wiegand), 849. Philadelphia: WB Saunders.

45. Dowlatshahi, D., Brouwers, H.B., Demchuk, A.M. et al. (2016). Predicting intracerebral hemorrhage growth with the spot sign: the effect of onset-to-scan time. Stroke 47 (3): 695–700.

46. Rodriguez-Luna, D., Coscojuela, P., Rubiera, M. et al. (2016). Ultraearly hematoma growth in active intracerebral hemorrhage. Neurology 87 (4): 357–364.

47. Connolly, E.S., Rabinstein, A.A., Carhuapoma, J.R. et al. (2012). Guidelines for the management of aneurysmal subarachnoid hemorrhage: a guideline for healthcare professionals from the American Heart Association/ American Stroke Association. Stroke 43 (6): 1711–1737.

48. Wojner-Alexander, A.W., Garami, Z., Chernyshev, O.Y., and Alexandrov, A.V. (2005). Heads down. Flat positioning improves blood flow velocity in acute ischemic stroke. Neurology 64 (8): 1354–1357.

49. Olavarría, V.V., Arima, H., Anderson, C.S. et al. (2014). Head position and cerebral blood flow velocity in acute ischemic stroke: a systematic review and meta-analysis. Cerebrovascular Diseases 37 (6): 401–408.

50. Hunter, A.J., Snodgrass, S.J., Quain, D. et al. (2011). HOBOE (Head-of-Bed Optimization of Elevation) study: association of higher angle with reduced cerebral blood flow velocity in acute ischemic stroke. Physical Therapy 91 (10): 1503–1512.

51. Palazzo, P., Brooks, A., James, D. et al. (2016). Risk of pneumonia associated with zero-degree head positioning in acute ischemic stroke patients treated with intravenous tissue plasminogen activator. Brain and Behavior 6 (2): e00425.

52. Anderson, C.S. (ed.) (2017). Final Results of the HeadPoST Trial. American Heart Association/American Stroke Association, Stroke on Demand. Dallas: American Heart Association/American Stroke Association.

53. Muñoz-Venturelli, P., Arima, H., Lavados, P. et al. (2015). Head Position in Stroke Trial (HeadPoST) – sitting-up vs lying-flat positioning of patients with acute stroke: study protocol for a cluster randomised controlled trial. Trials 16 (1): 256.

54. Zodiac. Zero degree head positioning. In Hyperacute Ischemic Stroke Trial 2017. Available from: http://www.zodiac-stroke.com [30 November 2018].

55. Albers, G.W., Bates, V.E., Clark, W.M. et al. (2000). Intravenous tissue-type plasminogen activator for treatment of acute stroke: the standard treatment with alteplase to reverse stroke (stars) study. Journal of the American Medical Association 283 (9): 1145–1150.

56. Hacke, W., Kaste, M., Fieschi, C. et al. (1998). Randomised double-blind placebo-controlled trial of thrombolytic therapy with intravenous alteplase in acute ischaemic stroke (ECASS II). The Lancet 352 (9136): 1245–1251.

57. Hill, M.D. and Buchan, A.M. (2005). Thrombolysis for acute ischemic stroke: results of the Canadian Alteplase for Stroke Effectiveness Study. Canadian Medical Association Journal 172 (10): 1307–1312.

58. Steiner, T., Bluhmki, E., Kaste, M. et al. (1998). The ECASS 3-hour cohort. Cerebrovascular Diseases 8 (4): 198–203.

59. Wahlgren, N., Ahmed, N., Dávalos, A. et al. (2007). Thrombolysis with alteplase for acute ischaemic stroke in the Safe Implementation of Thrombolysis in Stroke-Monitoring Study (SITS-MOST): an observational study. The Lancet 369 (9558): 275–282.

60. Anderson, C.S., Robinson, T., Lindley, R.I. et al. (2016). Low-dose versus standard-dose intravenous alteplase in acute ischemic stroke. New England Journal of Medicine 374 (24): 2313–2323.

61. Castillo, J., Leira, R., García, M.M. et al. (2004). Blood pressure decrease during the acute phase of ischemic stroke is associated with brain injury and poor stroke outcome. Stroke 35 (2): 520–526.
62. Johnston, K.C. and Mayer, S.A. (2003). Blood pressure reduction in ischemic stroke: a two-edged sword? Neurology 61 (8): 1030–1031.
63. Bellolio, M.F., Gilmore, R.M., and Ganti, L. (2014). Insulin for glycaemic control in acute ischaemic stroke. Cochrane Database of Systematic Reviews 1 (Art. No.: CD005346). https://doi.org/10.1002/14651858.CD005346.pub4.
64. Ntaios, G., Papavasileiou, V., Bargiota, A. et al. (2014). Intravenous insulin treatment in acute stroke: a systematic review and meta-analysis of randomized controlled trials. International Journal of Stroke 9 (4): 489–493.
65. Intercollegiate Stroke Working Party (2016). National Clinical Guideline for Stroke, 5e. London: Royal College of Physicians.
66. Stroke Foundation (2017). Clinical Guidelines for Stroke Management. Melbourne: Stroke Foundation.
67. Azzimondi, G., Bassein, L., Nonino, F. et al. (1995). Fever in acute stroke worsens prognosis. A Prospective Study 26 (11): 2040–2043.
68. Castillo, J., Dávalos, A., Marrugat, J., and Noya, M. (1998). Timing for fever-related brain damage in acute ischemic stroke. Stroke 29 (12): 2455–2460.
69. Ginsberg, M.D. and Busto, R. (1998). Combating hyperthermia in acute stroke: a significant clinical concern. Stroke 29 (2): 529–534.
70. Hajat, C., Hajat, S., and Sharma, P. (2000). Effects of poststroke pyrexia on stroke outcome: a meta-analysis of studies in patients. Stroke 31 (2): 410–414.
71. Reith, J., Jrgensen, H.S., Pedersen, P.M. et al. (1996). Body temperature in acute stroke: relation to stroke severity, infarct size, mortality, and outcome. The Lancet 347 (8999): 422–425.
72. Wang, Y., Lim, L.L.-Y., Levi, C. et al. (2000). Influence of admission body temperature on stroke mortality. Stroke 31 (2): 404–409.
73. Zaremba, J. (2004). Hyperthermia in ischemic stroke. Medical Science Monitor 10 (6): RA148–RA153.
74. Middleton, S., McElduff, P., Ward, J. et al. (2011). Implementation of evidence-based treatment protocols to manage fever, hyperglycaemia, and swallowing dysfunction in acute stroke (QASC): a cluster randomised controlled trial. The Lancet 378 (9804): 1699–1706.
75. Middleton, S., Coughlan, K., Mnatzaganian, G. et al. (2017). Mortality reduction for fever, hyperglycemia, and swallowing nurse-initiated stroke intervention: QASC Trial (Quality in Acute Stroke Care) follow-up. Stroke 48 (5): 1331–1336.
76. Biby, S., Palazzo, P., Grove, M. et al. (In press). Early control of glucose and temperature in acute stroke: an opportunity for improvement. Interventional Neurology.
77. Alexandrov, A.V., Molina, C.A., Grotta, J.C. et al. (2004). Ultrasound-enhanced systemic thrombolysis for acute ischemic stroke. New England Journal of Medicine 351 (21): 2170–2178.
78. Saver, J.L., Goyal, M., Bonafe, A. et al. (2015). Stent-retriever thrombectomy after intravenous t-PA vs. t-PA alone in stroke. New England Journal of Medicine 372 (24): 2285–2295.
79. Nogueria RG, Jovan TG. DAWN trial results demonstrate a 73% reduction in disability in stroke patients treated up to 24 hours. European Stroke Organization Conference. Kalamazoo: PR Web eBooks; 2017.
80. Vahedi, K., Hofmeijer, J., Juettler, E. et al. (2007). Early decompressive surgery in malignant infarction of the middle cerebral artery: a pooled analysis of three randomised controlled trials. The Lancet Neurology 6 (3): 215–222.
81. Broderick, J., Connolly, S., Feldmann, E. et al. (2007). Guidelines for the management of spontaneous intracerebral hemorrhage in adults: 2007 update: a guideline from the American Heart Association/American Stroke Association Stroke Council, High Blood Pressure Research Council, and the Quality of Care and Outcomes in Research Interdisciplinary Working Group. Stroke 38 (6): 2001–2023.

82. Hemphill, J.C., Bonovich, D.C., Besmertis, L. et al. (2001). The ICH score: a simple, reliable grading scale for intracerebral hemorrhage. Stroke 32 (4): 891–897.

83. Brott, T., Broderick, J., Kothari, R. et al. (1997). Early hemorrhage growth in patients with intracerebral hemorrhage. Stroke 28 (1): 1–5.

84. Kazui, S., Naritomi, H., Yamamoto, H. et al. (1996). Enlargement of spontaneous intracerebral hemorrhage: incidence and time course. Stroke 27 (10): 1783–1787.

85. Flibotte, J.J., Hagan, N., O'Donnell, J. et al. (2004). Warfarin, hematoma expansion, and outcome of intracerebral hemorrhage. Neurology 63 (6): 1059–1064.

86. Frontera, J.A., Lewin Iii, J.J., Rabinstein, A.A. et al. (2016). Guideline for reversal of antithrombotics in intracranial hemorrhage. Neurocritical Care 24 (1): 6–46.

87. Mendelow, A.D., Gregson, B.A., Rowan, E.N. et al. (2013). Early surgery versus initial conservative treatment in patients with spontaneous supratentorial lobar intracerebral haematomas (STICH II): a randomised trial. The Lancet 382 (9890): 397–408.

88. Anderson, C.S., Heeley, E., Huang, Y. et al. (2013). Rapid blood-pressure lowering in patients with acute intracerebral hemorrhage. New England Journal of Medicine 368 (25): 2355–2365.

89. Qureshi, A.I., Palesch, Y.Y., Barsan, W.G. et al. (2016). Intensive blood-pressure lowering in patients with acute cerebral hemorrhage. The New England Journal of Medicine 375 (11): 1033–1043.

90. Hanley, D.F., Lane, K., McBee, N. et al. (2017). Thrombolytic removal of intra-ventricular haemorrhage in treatment of severe stroke: results of the randomised, multicentre, multiregion, placebo-controlled CLEAR III trial. The Lancet 389 (10069): 603–611.

91. Staykov, D., Kuramatsu, J.B., Bardutzky, J. et al. (2017). Efficacy and safety of combined intraventricular fibrinolysis with lumbar drainage for prevention of permanent shunt dependency after intracerebral hemorrhage with severe ventricular involvement: a randomized trial and individual patient data meta-analysis. Annals of Neurology 81 (1): 93–103.

92. Zwienenberg-Lee, M., Hartman, J., Rudisill, N. et al. (2008). Effect of prophylactic transluminal balloon angioplasty on cerebral vasospasm and outcome in patients with fisher grade III subarachnoid hemorrhage. Results of a phase II multicenter, randomized, clinical trial. Stroke 39 (6): 1759–1765.

93. Barth, M., Capelle, H.-H., Weidauer, S. et al. (2007). Effect of nicardipine prolonged-release implants on cerebral vasospasm and clinical outcome after severe aneurysmal subarachnoid hemorrhage: a prospective, randomized, double-blind phase IIa study. Stroke 38 (2): 330–336.

94. Lee, V.H., Oh, J.K., Mulvagh, S.L., and Wijdicks, E.F.M. (2006). Mechanisms in neurogenic stress cardiomyopathy after aneurysmal subarachnoid hemorrhage. Neurocritical Care 5 (3): 243–249.

95. Samuels, M.A. (2007). The brain–heart connection. Circulation 116 (1): 77–84.

96. James, P.A., Oparil, S., Carter, B.L. et al. (2014). 2014 Evidence-Based Guideline for the Management of High Blood Pressure in Adults Report From the Panel Members Appointed to the Eighth Joint National Committee (JNC 8). Journal of the American Medical Association 311 (5): 507–520.

97. Culebras, A. (2005). Sleep apnea and stroke. Reviews in Neurologic Disease 2 (1): 13–19.

98. Martinez-Garcia, M.A., Galiano-Blancart, R., Roman-Sanchez, P. et al. (2005). Continuous positive airway pressure treatment in sleep apnea prevents new vascular events after ischemic stroke. Chest 128 (4): 2123–2139.

99. Alexandrov, A.V., Sharma, V.K., Lao, A.Y. et al. (2007). Reversed robin hood syndrome in acute ischemic stroke patients. Stroke 38 (11): 3045–3048.

100. Bernhardt, J., Dewey, H., Thrift, A. et al. (2008). A very early rehabilitation trial for stroke (AVERT): phase II safety and feasibility. Stroke 39 (2): 390–396.

101. AVERT Trial Collaboration Group (2015). Efficacy and safety of very early mobilisation within 24 h of stroke onset (AVERT): a randomised controlled trial. The Lancet 386 (9988): 46–55.

102. Fraser, D.W., Moody, A.R., Morgan, P.S. et al. (2002). Diagnosis of lower-limb deep venous thrombosis: a prospective blinded study of magnetic resonance direct thrombus imaging. Annals of Internal Medicine 136 (2): 89–98.

103. Gregory, P.C. and Kuhlemeier, K.V. (2003). Prevalence of venous thromboembolism in acute hemorrhagic and thromboembolic stroke. American Journal of Physical Medicine and Rehabilitation 82 (5): 364.

104. Sherman, D.G., Albers, G.W., Bladin, C. et al. (2007). The efficacy and safety of enoxaparin versus unfractionated heparin for the prevention of venous thromboembolism after acute ischaemic stroke (PREVAIL study): an open-label randomised comparison. The Lancet 369 (9570): 1347–1355.

105. Geerts, W.H., Pineo, G.F., Heit, J.A. et al. (2004). Prevention of venous thromboembolism. Chest 126 (3): 338S–400S.

106. Kamphuisen, P.W., Agnelli, G., and Sebastianelli, M. (2005). Prevention of venous thromboembolism after acute ischemic stroke. Journal of Thrombosis and Haemostasis 3 (6): 1187–1194.

107. Geeganage, C.M., Sprigg, N., Bath, M.W., and Bath, P.M.W. (2013). Balance of symptomatic pulmonary embolism and symptomatic intracerebral hemorrhage with low-dose anticoagulation in secent ischemic stroke: a systematic review and meta-analysis of randomized controlled trials. Journal of Stroke and Cerebrovascular Diseases 22 (7): 1018–1027.

108. Paciaroni, M., Agnelli, G., Venti, M. et al. (2011). Efficacy and safety of anticoagulants in the prevention of venous thromboembolism in patients with acute cerebral hemorrhage: a meta-analysis of controlled studies. Journal of Thrombosis and Haemostasis 9 (5): 893–898.

109. The CLOTS Trials Collaboration (2009). Effectiveness of thigh-length graduated compression stockings to reduce the risk of deep vein thrombosis after stroke (CLOTS trial 1): a multicentre, randomised controlled trial. The Lancet 373 (9679): 1958–1965.

110. Adams, H.P. Jr., del Zoppo, G., Alberts, M.J. et al. (2007). Guidelines for the early management of adults with ischemic stroke: a guideline from the American Heart Association/American Stroke Association Stroke Council, Clinical Cardiology Council, Cardiovascular Radiology and Intervention Council, and the Atherosclerotic Peripheral Vascular Disease and Quality of Care Outcomes in Research Interdisciplinary Working Groups: the American Academy of Neurology affirms the value of this guideline as an educational tool for neurologists. Stroke 38 (5): 1655–1711.

111. Australian Commission on Safety and Quality in Health Care (2015). Acute Stroke Clinical Care Standard. Sydney: Australian Commission on Safety and Quality in Health Care.

CHAPTER 5

Nutritional Aspects of Stroke Care

Lin Perry[1] and Elizabeth Boaden[2]

[1] University of Technology Sydney and the Northern Hospitals Network, South Eastern Sydney Local Health District, Sydney, NSW, Australia
[2] School of Nursing, University of Central Lancashire, Preston, UK

KEY POINTS

- Good nutrition is essential for recovery and rehabilitation; malnourished patients fare worse, stay in hospital longer, experience more complications, and are more likely to die.
- Eating is a source of pleasure and an intrinsic part of social lives and quality of life.
- Dysphagia affects between one-third and one-half of all stroke patients. Early recognition and management is becoming widely accepted and addressed within routine care.
- Impairments that affect eating are dealt with in therapy programmes, but are seldom related to eating or practised at mealtimes as a carry-over of therapy.
- Recovery can be maximised through holistic assessment and with therapy focusing on the ability to eat and what is consumed.

This chapter maps to criteria within the following sections of the Stroke-Specific Education Framework (SSEF):

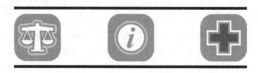

Stroke Nursing, Second Edition. Edited by Jane Williams, Lin Perry, and Caroline Watkins.
© 2020 John Wiley & Sons Ltd. Published 2020 by John Wiley & Sons Ltd.

INTERVIEWER   Since you mention food, is this a good point to ask how you are managing to eat, and what you're eating?

S1 (72-years-old male stroke survivor)   Oh, Diana will answer that.

S2 (survivor's wife)   We haven't used the PEG [percutaneous endoscopic gastrostomy] for a while because gradually over the weeks he's been eating a lot better, ordinary food, within reason. We're very fond of stewed apples –

S1   Egg and bacon, macaroni cheese – all sorts of things.

S2   Egg and chips, chicken livers, he's very fond of.

I   This doesn't sound very much like puree! Or even soft!

S2   No, he doesn't have puree now. We've given that up.

S1   Given that up completely!

S2   He eats pretty well ordinary food.

S1   I had pork steak –

S2   Pork chop.

S1   Pork chop! And pizza – I had pizza for my tea the other day! But I'm enjoying my food now.

(6 months post-stroke, London, UK)

5.1 Introduction

This chapter discusses food, nutrition, and malnutrition following stroke; nutrition as a risk factor and healthy eating to decrease the likelihood of stroke recurrence are discussed in Chapter 3.

Nutritional status is central to health and disease. Malnutrition is caused by not eating or absorbing enough essential components, such as vitamins, minerals, energy, and protein. Overnutrition is reflected in excessive, unbalanced, or disproportionate intake, such as too much carbohydrate or fats [2]. Key characteristics of malnutrition have been identified as:

- poor appetite, not eating enough; and
- muscle wasting and weight loss in the context of general health deterioration [3].

The signs, symptoms, and effects of malnutrition are many, and vary from subtle to florid (Table 5.1). However, measurements of these and related features during acute illness are difficult, because they are confused by the features of disease. Attempts to disentangle these factors and make comparisons across studies are hampered by the range and variety of different criteria for malnutrition [5]. Nonetheless, nutritional screening and assessment are critical first steps towards ensuring adequate dietary intake.

Malnutrition has been linked with increased risk of death or dependency post-stroke, so nutritional screening and assessment followed by action to overcome problems are essential elements of stroke care [6–10]. Food and eating are also fundamental to our social lives, contribute to well-being, have a substantial influence on quality of life, and are essential to consider as part of rehabilitation after stroke [11].

TABLE 5.1 **Consequences of malnutrition [4]**

Malnutrition affects every part of the body, increases vulnerability to illness, prolongs hospital stay, and increases the risk of complications and death.

Immune system

- Reduces ability to fight infection

Muscles

- Inactivity, leads to reduced ability to work, shop, cook, and self-care, may increase risk of pressure ulcers and blood clots, increases risk of falls
- Reduced ability to cough increases risks of chest infections and pneumonia
- Heart failure

Impaired wound-healing

Kidneys

- Inability to regulate salt and fluid can lead to overhydration or dehydration

Brain

- Malnutrition causes apathy, depression, introversion, self-neglect, and deterioration in social interactions

Reproduction

- Malnutrition reduces fertility
- During pregnancy, can predispose to problems with diabetes, heart disease, and stroke in the baby in later life

Impaired temperature regulation

- May lead to hypothermia

Consequences of malnutrition in children and adolescents

- Growth failure and stunting
- Delayed sexual development
- Reduced muscle mass and strength
- Impaired intellectual development
- Rickets
- Increased lifetime risk of osteoporosis

Consequences of specific micronutrient deficiencies

Many, but the commonest include:

- Iron deficiency → anaemia
- Zinc deficiency → skin rashes, decreased ability to fight infection
- Vitamin B12 deficiency → anaemia and problems with nerves
- Vitamin D deficiency → rickets in children, osteomalacia in adults
- Vitamin C deficiency → scurvy
- Vitamin A deficiency → night blindness

5.2 Do Stroke Patients Experience Nutritional Problems Pre-Stroke?

5.2.1 Nutrition and Malnutrition

It is vital that we eat in order to meet our bodies' requirements for energy, protein, fats, and other nutrients, so as to maintain health and activity. Nationally and internationally, estimated average requirements and recommended daily nutritional intakes have been established for optimal health, taking account of age and sex [12]. Calculations such as the Harris Benedict equation can adjust for activity and stress [13]. People can often cope short-term with eating poorly, especially if they were previously well-nourished. However, if poor eating continues, particularly in illness or disease, then outcomes are generally poor. Food and eating are also intricately linked with psychosocial well-being and community life [14], so anything that impairs eating is likely to cause much wider social disruption.

Older people tend to have greater risk of malnutrition when they become ill due to the pre-existing physiological and social changes that are associated with normal ageing [15]. With stroke incidence increasing with age, a substantial proportion of stroke patients are affected by age-related nutritional changes. These include:

- alterations in the gastrointestinal system – fewer taste buds, loss of teeth (with or without dentures), reduced gastric acid secretion, and decreased gastrointestinal peristalsis;
- altered awareness of hunger, enjoyment in eating, and satiety – sense of fullness [16];
- social factors – those bereaved or living alone may be less motivated to cook or eat well;
- limited choices due to practical issues such as dependence on others for shopping or meals; and
- psychological factors such as depression, which can affect appetite and eating habits.

Any or all of these factors may contribute to reduced dietary intake in terms of both quality and quantity. Studies of community-living older people have revealed insufficient energy intake in almost 25% of women and 22–29% of men [17], whilst across Europe dietary deficiencies have been found in 24% of men and 47% of women [18]. High levels of nutritional risk and dietary inadequacies have been shown in residential care settings, and in almost 10% of selected general practice patients [19, 20]. It is likely that some – perhaps many – stroke patients are undernourished before their first stroke.

For those who have experienced a previous stroke, the situation is compounded by the new stroke. In a cohort of stroke patients 6 months post-stroke, 66% had some degree of disablement that affected eating [21]. Earlier studies found 51% not cooking, 40–55% not shopping, 23% incapable of making a hot drink, and 39% dependent for eating [22, 23].

5.2.2 Nutritional Status on Admission to Hospital

Nutritional screening and assessment of stroke patients on admission to hospital has revealed substantial nutritional problems in many, predating the stroke. Comparison between studies is difficult because of the lack of an agreed clinical 'gold-standard' assessment for 'nutritional risk' or malnutrition [24]. However, there is general agreement that no single criterion is adequate and a combination of assessments is preferred. In the United Kingdom and internationally, the Malnutrition Universal Screening Tool [25] is often the screening tool of choice [26]; however, whilst described with stroke patients during rehabilitation [27], to date there has been no systematic study of its use with stroke patients. Table 5.2 shows assessments and findings from stroke patients. Further explanations of approaches to measuring nutrition (anthropometric, biochemical, clinical judgement) are discussed later in this chapter. Altogether, these studies identify up to one-third, and commonly around one in five, of all patients as malnourished and up to two-thirds as 'at risk' within the early days of hospital admission. Many patients show nutritional deterioration in hospital, in part at least due to the effects of both their stroke and post-stroke care [32, 34].

5.3 How Does Stroke Affect Dietary Intake?

5.3.1 Effects of Acute Illness

Strokes, particularly ischaemic events, are now recognised as a form of acute brain injury, in which an inflammatory component contributes to the pathological process (see Chapter 2). Acute injury is associated with a metabolic response. The initial period of acute stress lasts around 24 hours, but the subsequent anabolic (rebuilding) phase is much longer and involves increased nutritional requirements [35]. However, studies of acute stroke patients have not conclusively shown what this means in terms of dietary requirements. For some stroke patients, basal (resting) metabolic rates (BMRs) are increased [36–38], whilst for others either no significant difference is seen in BMR [39–41] or, longer-term, reduced requirements are indicated [42]. These studies used the Penn State (body size, temperature, and minute ventilation) and Harris Benedict (age, weight, and height) equations to estimate BMR and compared this with actual energy expenditure using indirect calorimetry in stroke patients 6–90 days after admission and long-term.

Despite inconclusive evidence of increased BMR, the energy 'cost' associated with physical activity may be affected by stroke-related disablement. On the one hand, activity-related energy expenditure may be less than estimated if disabilities restrict the type and duration of daily activities. On the other, the energy 'cost' of physical activity may be higher because of muscle inefficiency; stroke patients have to work relatively harder to complete actions. A study of 13 middle-aged stroke patients and 13 age- and sex-matched controls [43] measured oxygen uptake and reported significantly greater energy cost for stroke patients walking a

| | | TABLE 5.2 | Timing, assessments, and identified nutritional status of stroke patients |

Source	Timing	Assessments	Numbers (%) malnourished/ 'at risk'
Axelsson et al. [28]	Within 4 d of admission	2 or more under reference limits: weight TSF MAMC albumin, prealbumin, transferrin	16 (16)
Unosson et al. [29]	Within 48 h of admission	1 abnormal value in each category Anthropometric: weight index/MAC/TSF Blood tests: albumin/transthyretin/alpha$_1$-antitrypsin Skin tests: delayed hypersensitivity with 3 antigens	4 (8)
Dávalos et al. [6]	At 7 d from admission	Albumin $<35\,\text{g}\,\text{l}^{-1}$ or TSF or MAMC <10th centile	17 (16)
Choi-Kwon et al. [30]	Within 1 wk of admission	1 biochemical + 2 anthropometric measurements: <80% reference values of lean body mass or TSF at 3 sites BMI $<20\,\text{kg}\,\text{m}^{-2}$ lymphocytes $<1500\,\text{mm}^{-3}$ haemoglobin $<12\,\text{g}\,\text{dl}^{-1}$ albumin $<35\,\text{g}\,\text{l}^{-1}$	30 (34)
Gariballa and Sinclair [15]	Within 48 h of admission	TSF <5th centile MAC <5th centile BMI $<20\,\text{kg}\,\text{m}^{-2}$ albumin $<35\,\text{g}\,\text{l}^{-1}$	46 (23) 4 (2) 62 (31) 38 (19)
Westergren et al. [31]	After admission to rehab (median 6 d post-admission)	Modified SGA	20 (12) 32 (20) 'at risk'
Davis et al. [7]	Within 24 h of stroke	SGA	30 (16)
FOOD Trial Collaboration [9]	Within 7 d	Clinician judgement	279 (9)
Nip [32]	Within 2 wk of admission	MNA	7 (7) 66 (66) 'at risk'
Martineau et al. [33]	Within 48 h of admission to hospital	Patient-generated SGA	14 (19.2)

TSF, triceps skinfold; MAMC, mid-arm muscle circumference; MAC, mid-arm circumference; SGA, Subjective Global Assessment; MNA, Mini Nutritional Assessment.

much shorter distance compared to controls. Studies comparing various energy-predictive equations have yet to establish the best method to fine-tune calculation of energy requirements for individual stroke patients. Recommended dietary intakes for stroke patients therefore remain in line with national age- and sex-matched guidance, allowing for activity and metabolic stress [12].

5.3.2   Stroke-Related Eating Disabilities

Stroke produces a wide range of problems that can affect the ability to eat and increase the risk of malnutrition. Reliance upon assistance to eat increases the risk of inadequate intake and development of complications [29, 44, 45]. Even minor difficulties in people who eat independently may result in inadequate dietary intake [46]. Patients can be distressed by eating in public if their functional limitations mean that the way they eat does not match cultural expectations of well-mannered behaviour. They may limit what they eat and refuse to eat in company; this affects not just the stroke survivor, but their carer, families, and wider social networks [21, 47–49].

Eating disabilities include the inability to maintain head control and upright posture; loss of upper limb motor control and sensation; problems chewing and swallowing; and communication, visual, perceptual, and attention deficits. Table 5.3 lists the eating disabilities demonstrated by a cohort of patients admitted

TABLE 5.3   Eating disabilities of a cohort of acute stroke patients admitted to a South London hospital [34]

Eating disabilities at hospital	3–5 d after admission to hospital	Number	Percentage
Posture control	No functional impairment (0)[a]	325	56
	Mild impairment (1)	130	22
	Moderate impairment (2)	89	15
	Severe impairment (3)	43	7
Median (25, 75 centile) scores[b]		0 (0, 1)	
Arm movement	No functional impairment (0)	159	27
	Mild impairment (1)	209	35
	Moderate (2)	86	15
	Severe (3)	133	23
Median (25, 75 centile) scores[b]		1 (0, 2)	
Lip closure	No functional impairment (0)	449	76
	Partial impairment (1)	109	19
	Severe impairment (2)	29	5
Median (25, 75 centile) scores[b]		0 (0, 0)	

(continued)

TABLE 5.3	Eating disabilities of a cohort of acute stroke patients admitted to a South London hospital [34] *(continued)*		
Eating disabilities at hospital	**3–5 d after admission to hospital**	**Number**	**Percentage**
Chewing	No functional impairment (0)	369	63
	Partial impairment (1)	172	29
	Severe impairment (2)	46	8
Median (25, 75 centile) scores[b]		0 (0, 1)	
Swallowing	No functional impairment (0)	341	58
	Partial – can't tolerate 1 of 3 textures (1)	66	11
	Severe – can't tolerate 2 of 3 textures (2)	64	11
	Aspiration/high risk; nil orally (3)	116	20
Median (25, 75 centile) scores[b]		0 (0, 2)	
Communication	No functional impairment (0)	276	47
	Partial impairment (1)	149	25
	Severe impairment (2)	162	28
Median (25, 75 centile) scores[b]		1 (0, 2)	
Attention and praxis	No functional impairment (0)	417	71
	Partial impairment (1)	130	22
	Severe impairment (2)	39	7
Median (25, 75 centile) scores[b]		0 (0, 1)	
Visual field/perceptual loss/neglect	No functional impairment (0)	428	73
	Partial impairment (1)	132	23
	Severe impairment (2)	25	4
Median (25, 75 centile) scores[b]		0 (0, 1)	

n = 670 stroke patients, of whom 587 (586 for attention and praxis; 585 for visual fields) were able to be assessed.
[a] Eating Disabilities Assessment Scale [50].
[b] Scale point scores.

to a London hospital with acute stroke [34], whilst Case Study 5.1 describes what they meant for one of these patients. As well as physical problems, depression, which is common after stroke, may also influence dietary intake. Many stroke patients need help to eat. Of the London cohort of 670 stroke patients, in the early days after admission less than half (46.5%) ate independently, 4% were judged to

Case Study

Case 5.1   Evelyn

Evelyn is an 82-year-old woman admitted to hospital with an ischaemic stroke. She is not tall, but is a large woman. She has had a right hip replacement following a bad fall last year. She lives next door to her daughter, Jenny. On admission, she has a dense left hemiplegia and left visual inattention. She answers questions appropriately, although attention is required to understand her. Dysphagia is identified, and she is placed nil orally with intravenous hydration commenced. However, her chewing and swallow function is not the only eating-related problem: she is not able to keep herself upright (the safest position for eating); her left hand has minimal movement and all activities are one-handed; she neglects part of her left spatial field and needs prompting with a plate of food; and her speech makes communicating hunger, thirst, and food preferences an effort. She has a history of depression and says she feels a burden to her family.

require supervision, 26% needed assistance, 12.5% were fed, and 11% were tube fed [34]. Similarly, Westergren reported that 52.5% stroke patients needed help to eat on admission to rehabilitation [31].

5.3.2.1   Chewing and Dysphagia   Dysphagia is defined as 'eating and drinking disorders which may occur in the oral, pharyngeal, and oesophageal stages of deglutition' [51]. Dysphagia is important because it can cause aspiration pneumonia, malnutrition, dehydration, weight loss, and airway obstruction. It can lead to reduced stamina, increased complications, increased likelihood of pressure injury/ulcers, poorer physical recovery, reduced wound healing, and increased risk of anxiety or depression, infections, and, ultimately, death [52–54]. Predictive scores have demonstrated the significant contribution of dysphagia to risk of aspiration pneumonia, with tripled mortality rates following stroke [55, 56]. Fear of choking can also result in anxiety and a self-imposed restriction on what is eaten.

In the first 24 hours post-stroke, between 30 and 40% of conscious and assessable individuals have been observed with dysphagia. However, higher numbers have been reported as at risk of aspiration in the acute phases of stroke, from 67% when screened during the first 72 hours to 43% within 7 days [57]. Recovery rates have been reported at 73% within 7 days, with 11–19% retaining long-term (more than 6 months) swallowing difficulties [21, 58]. This is not a static condition, however, and both deterioration and recovery are seen. This means it is important to train carers and hospital staff to identify when swallowing difficulties arise or relapse, and to ensure they understand and are able to manage these difficulties [59].

Figure 5.1 outlines the anatomy of the head and neck, showing the main structures involved in swallowing, an activity that requires coordination of six cranial nerves and 26 pairs of muscles. Swallowing requires muscle function (to ensure stability), neuromuscular coordination, sensory and gastrointestinal function, normal heart and breathing control, and intact autonomic nervous system (to deliver overall coordination) [51]. Any or all of these can be disrupted

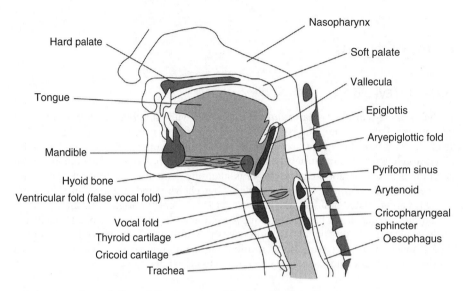

FIGURE 5.1 Lateral view of the anatomy of the head and neck.

by stroke at any or every stage of the swallowing process. For ease of analysis, the swallowing process may be divided into pre-oral, oral preparatory, oral transit, pharyngeal, and oesophageal stages.

5.3.2.1.1 Pre-Oral Stage Stroke may affect an individual's multisensory awareness of food and drink prior to its placement in the mouth. Cognitively affected individuals may fail to recognise food and drink by sight, smell, or sound. Sensory awareness of food and drink innervates memory centres via the limbic system. Inability to detect or process sensory attributes of food and drink may disrupt an individual's perception of their likes and dislikes, potentially leading to food refusal. Lack of cognitive awareness of food and drink may result in inability to grade the degree of lip and jaw opening and failure to approximate the vocal cords, which is usually a pre-emptive airway-protective response to liquids being brought to the mouth. Environmental influences, behavioural issues, and the mealtime assistant's behaviour affect positioning and muscle tone and may have a marked effect on oral stability and swallow physiology. Individuals with hemiparesis may find it difficult to feed themselves food and drink – reported as an independent predictor of poor patient outcome and death [60].

5.3.2.1.2 Oral Preparatory Stage Muscles of facial expression may be affected by stroke, with unilateral lip paresis allowing escape of fluids from the mouth. Poor oral control may result in:

- food and drink spilling prematurely into the pharynx and being aspirated pre-swallow;
- nasal backflow;
- reduced rotary lateral chewing action; and
- dysfunction in the sequential tongue elevation needed to move the food bolus back into the pharynx.

Absent or loose teeth or dentures significantly hinder chewing, limiting the sensory feedback from nerves in the teeth that govern differential chewing patterns in response to food type. Problems with teeth and dentures are common amongst elderly people, and often result in their opting for softer diets, often with consequently reduced nutritional quality [61]. Saliva produced from sublingual, submandibular, and parotid glands lubricates the food, and amylase enzymes begin the digestive process. Reduced saliva availability, resulting, for example, from dehydration, may lead to teeth demineralisation, loss of mucosal protection, and changes in the pH balance in the mouth. There may be difficulty forming and moving a food bolus, and subsequent digestion and gastric microbial control may be affected. Of concern is the reported colonisation in the mouths of over one-third of acute stroke patients with aerobic Gram-negative bacilli, which, if aspirated with saliva, may cause a chest infection [62]. Similarly, food and fluid residues in the mouth caused by reduced muscle tone in the cheeks or lips may allow aerobic bacteria to multiply.

Stroke patients can have difficulty clearing food from their mouths and may 'pocket' residues. If not removed after every meal, these can harbour bacterial growth, leading to bad breath and a bad taste in the mouth, which may deter eating. This may risk developing aspiration pneumonia if this material enters the lungs [63]. Stroke patients may also experience environmental, physical, or cognitive disturbances, which affect their ability to maintain their oral care. Medically compromised patients tend to harbour more oral aerobic and anaerobic Gram-negative bacilli compared to healthy people, and these have the potential to cause systemic infections [64]. See Chapter 6 for oral care.

Food and drink characteristics are ascertained by the anterior two-thirds of the tongue by touch (CN V) and taste (CN V11). Discrimination of flavour is unique to each individual, because of the numbers of taste buds and the memories they evoke. With advancing age, taste buds, taste, oral sensitivity, and muscle tone reduce. Sensory mechanisms in the mouth are less able to distinguish bolus characteristics (i.e. food consistency, viscosity, elasticity, volume, temperature, and mass), which may subsequently affect the timing and movement of upper oesophageal sphincter (UOS) opening. The oral preparatory stage concludes when a prepared bolus is placed on the tongue as a prerequisite to oral transit.

5.3.2.1.3 Oral Transit Stage Inability to create good lip seal, cheek tone, or soft palate elevation may result in drooling and reduce ability to generate the negative pressure necessary to move food backwards through the mouth and throat. Prior to oral transit, the vocal cords approximate in adduction (move together), which signals the onset of swallow apnoea (cessation of respiration). Sequential, differential anterior to posterior elevation of the tongue tip against the palate moves the bolus over a lowered tongue to the tongue base. Oral transit takes approximately 1 second, but this may be prolonged in older people with age-related changes in tongue motor function. Similarly, there is a greater propensity for the swallow to be triggered farther down the pharynx, at the lateral borders or even at the level of the pyriform sinus.

5.3.2.1.4 Pharyngeal Stage Valvular and pressure changes move the bolus across the pharynx to the oesophagus; therefore, swallowing is not considered a reflex activity but a neuromuscular, patterned, sequenced response [65]. The tongue base moves anteriorly to increase pharyngeal space for the bolus.

The presence of the bolus in the pharynx precipitates partial true vocal cord adduction in order to preclude pre-swallow aspiration. Usually, a swallow apnoea of 0.3–2.5 seconds occurs prior to the onset or termination of the oral transit stage and follows the initiation of an expiratory breath. However, the timing varies between and within individuals, as in approximately 10–20% of swallows, inspiration occurs prior to the swallow. Abnormal inspiratory breathing patterns observed in stroke patients post-swallow may serve to suck pharyngeal residue into the airway [66]. Incoordination and unilateral or bilateral paresis of the soft palate and the superior pharyngeal constrictor muscle (CN IX, X, XII) will allow backflow of the bolus into the nasal cavity, decrease the negative pressure required for movement of the bolus through the pharynx, generate longer pharyngeal transit times, and perhaps precipitate food and fluid residue in the valleculae and pyriform sinus, which can be readily aspirated post-swallow (Figure 5.2).

Three mechanisms protect the airway: adduction of the true and false vocal folds and approximation of the arytenoids – with an introverted epiglottis. This sequence of events serves to eject any part of the bolus that may have penetrated the laryngeal vestibule. An increase in the amplitude and duration of pharyngeal contraction behind the bolus together with a delay in pharyngeal transit may occur in response to an increase in bolus viscosity in older people.

Increased risk of aspiration occurs with delayed or absent superior and anterior hyoid movement, with limited movement of the thyroid and cricoid cartilages causing incoordination of UOS opening. Disorganised sensory information in the oral cavity will disrupt UOS opening, which usually occurs within 0.10 seconds of airway closure [65]. Resumption of expiration as the hyo-laryngeal structures lower facilitates removal of residue or any penetrated

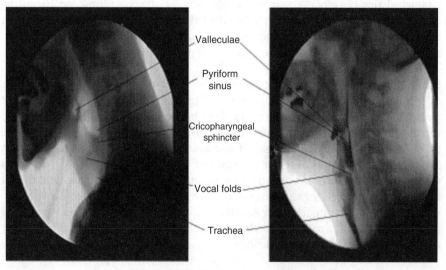

FIGURE 5.2 Lateral view of the pharynx: comparison of pre- and post-swallow aspiration of bolus into the trachea with residue in the valleculae and pyriform sinus. Anonymised X-ray images.

material in the laryngeal vestibule or hypopharynx post-swallow. There is an increase in respiratory rate post-swallow due to swallow apnoea. Normal respiratory rate is then resumed.

5.3.2.1.5   Oesophageal Stage   The oesophagus is under tonic closure at rest in order to limit air entering the stomach and reduce the potential for reflux of gastric acid to the pharynx. Oesophageal distension by the bolus triggers coordinated involuntary sequential waves of peristaltic contraction along the 18–25 cm-long tube by striated, striated and smooth, then smooth oesophageal muscle fibres. Descending inhibition (contraction above and relaxation below the bolus) allows variable oesophageal transit times of 2–3 seconds for liquids and 8–20 seconds for solids. Lubrication provided from the oesophageal mucosa facilitates bolus movement and provides mucosal protection. A secondary then tertiary peristaltic wave is initiated in response to bolus dysmotility. Oesophageal bolus transit promotes variations in neuronal activity, blood supply, and lymphatic drainage [67]. The lower oesophageal sphincter relaxes, demonstrating variable opening to allow passage of different-sized boluses into the stomach, then tonically closes to prevent acid reflux. Age influences the incidence of smooth muscle in the oesophagus, giving rise to an increase in the incidence of hiatus hernia and subsequent increase in the risk of aspiration pneumonitis secondary to refluxed material [68].

5.3.2.2   Posture and Head Control   Any disturbance of posture and sitting balance poses challenges for eating. The safest eating position is upright, with support as appropriate. Early assessments found almost 46% of patients with postural instability (Table 5.3) [34]. See Chapter 8 for posture and positioning.

5.3.2.3   Upper Limb Impairment   In the early weeks following stroke, the main motor impairments around the shoulder and upper limb are: weakness, lack of active range of movement, and reduced selective movement and dexterity (see Chapter 8). Overall, 77.4%, 79.0%, and 35.0% of patients have been reported with upper limb impairment, function, and limb ataxia, respectively, within 48 hours of admission [69, 70]. Observations of a select group of patients eating at up to 14 days post-stroke revealed 57% unable to manipulate cutlery or transfer food from plate to mouth, and arm movement impairment predicted reduced energy and protein intake [47, 50].

5.3.2.4   Problems with Cognition and Communication   Stroke causes a variety of communication problems, such as problems of expression (dysphasia, dyspraxia, dysarthria), problems understanding the emotional tone of speech, and lack of verbal comprehension, all ranging from subtle deficit to incomprehension (see Chapter 7). Reported incidence varies widely, from 18 to 74% of patients [71, 72]. At 48 hours after admission, communication deficits were found in 43%, with 59% dysarthric [69]. These data are derived predominantly from subjective judgement, which contributes to the widely varying findings.

Inability to communicate food preferences and requirements was identified in 48% of patients taking oral diet at 8–10 days post-stroke and has been
shown to be one of the factors that differentiate those with low dietary protein
intakes [50].

5.3.2.5 Visual and Perceptual Deficits
A wide range of visual, percep-
tual, and attention deficits have been reported following stroke, including visual
field deficits (hemianopias), apraxia, agnosia, and neglect (inattention). Reported
incidence varies widely, probably due to differing methods of assessment with
varying sensitivity, differing patient populations, and the timing of assessment
after stroke onset. At 48 hours after admission, visual or sensory inattention was
found in 38% of patients, and hemianopia in 46% [69]. Detection of meal components features in tests for visuospatial neglect [73]. Apraxia may directly affect the
ability to eat [74], and as both neglect and apraxia negatively influence rehabilitation of activities of daily living, they may indirectly influence eating and nutritional status [75, 76].

5.3.2.6 Smell and Taste
Smell and taste both contribute to the sensa-
tion of 'taste'; complaints of altered taste commonly arise from problems with
smell. Taste disturbance has been reported in stroke patients, with symptoms
including increased thresholds, reduced intensity of taste, loss of pleasant associations, conversion of some neutral sensations to unpleasant ones, development
of smell and taste intolerance, food aversion, and marked weight loss (see Case
Study 5.2) [77–80] . Case studies have reported taste disturbance in patients with
lesions at a variety of locations, including pontine, midbrain, thalamic, internal
capsule, insular haemorrhage and infarction, and unilateral cortical infarction
[77–80]. In one consecutive cohort of people admitted with stroke, 31 of 102
(30.5%) had reduced taste, most of whom had frontal lobe lesions. Of those with
abnormal taste, 6 of 21 (28.6%) also experienced impaired smell, compared to 4 of
33 (12.1%) with normal taste [78].

Case Study

Case 5.2 **Bill**

Bill, a bricklayer, was already having a rough time before his stroke. He admits to something
of a drinking habit, and says his wife left him, taking their two daughters, because of it. Bill
wasn't managing too well by himself before the stroke. He eventually recovered well from
his small internal capsule haemorrhage, and his main problem now is that everything he
eats tastes of burnt rubber. Even at 3 months post–stroke, the altered taste persists, and has
taken away any pleasure in food.

Bill is aware how important it is that he eats properly. His stay in hospital with his stroke
was prolonged by slow recovery and a chest infection, and he accepts that the dietitian
thinks he was malnourished when he was admitted. But he says he finds it hard to get excited
about meals that taste of old car tyres.

Taste dysfunction post-stroke is poorly studied, and there is little evidence of what might help [81].

5.3.2.7   Psychosocial Effects

5.3.2.7.1   Mood Disorder and Appetite   Post-stroke depression is common in the acute stages and for some years afterwards, reported to affect an estimated 31% of patients (95% confidence interval (CI) 28–35%) in the early stages, 25% (95% CI 16–33%) at between 1 and 5 years, and 23% (95% CI 14–31%) at 5 years [82].

Links have been demonstrated between nutrition and mood state, and a vicious cycle may become established, as what people eat may affect their mood, and depressed mood may be linked with altered food intake. Complex interrelationships are suggested. The most significant study of the effects of dietary intake in relation to mood entailed a 24-week period of semi-starvation for 32 young healthy male volunteers. A sustained intake of around 1470 kcal/day resulted in progressively increased tiredness, irritability, apathy, moodiness, depression and apprehension, with decreased ambition, concentration, self-discipline, and loss of mental alertness and drive to activity [83]. Depressed mood post-stroke has been consistently linked with poorer outcomes (e.g. with the ability to carry out activities of daily living, social function, and mortality) [84].

Altered appetite and weight changes have been identified as core symptoms of depression, although the relationship in stroke patients is obscured by the effects of acute illness and stroke-related eating disability. Work with participants with disordered eating and weight cycling ('yo-yo' dieting) has suggested that alterations to fatty acid intake (as a consequence of dietary restriction or manipulation) may be key contributors to mood disturbance [85, 86]. This may be relevant to stroke patients who experience sustained poor dietary intakes (see Case Study 5.3).

Exploring the relationship between mood state and nutritional status in hospitalised stroke patients, researchers failed to demonstrate a direct association between the two when using the General Health Questionnaire and Mini-Nutritional

Case Study

| Case 5.3 | John

John lost his wife when he was 62 years old. Now 88 years of age, both he and his daughter Jane say they are surprised he is still alive. Once a fit man weighing 70 kg and walking 2 miles to work and back every day, he slowly diminished from the time of his wife's death. Jane visits regularly, and takes him shopping every week to stock his fridge, but says she throws a lot out untouched. John says he just has no appetite. Losing his wife 'knocked the stuffing out of him'. Whilst he still worked, he ate lunch with his mates, but once he retired, his world shrank and he would go weeks seeing only Jane. Eating became a chore. Jane nags him (he says), and takes him out to make sure he gets a cooked lunch once a week. Now weighing 47 kg, John has been admitted with ischaemic stroke and right-sided weakness. Eating is even more of a chore today, and it is a challenge to find ways to encourage him to finish his meals.

Assessment. However, nutritional scores were significantly related to those for appetite, hunger, taste, and smell, which were linked to mood scores [32]. Comparing dietary intakes of those identified as depressed with those identified as not depressed, the former consistently consumed less energy and protein. During the first 2 weeks of admission, depressed participants consumed mean (standard deviation, SD) 1227 (711) kcal energy and 46.7 (20) g protein per day, compared to (still low) values of 1440 (677) kcal and 56 (20.2) g for non-depressed participants; this pattern was sustained, with depressed participants eating 299 kcal less energy and 16.8 g less protein per day than those not depressed in the week before discharge [32]. This effect continued, with links between appetite, mood state, and dietary intake still evident at 6 months post-stroke [11].

Altered body image may also have an effect on mood state, and hence dietary intake. Stroke effects such as uncontrolled drooling and facial palsy have obvious potential to affect the way people feel about themselves. However, even relatively subtle signs or symptoms (e.g. loss of sensation or tactile recognition in an upper limb, leading to reduced manual dexterity and clumsy eating) can have negative effects.

5.3.3   Impact of Dietary Provision and Hospital Meals

5.3.3.1   Nil by Mouth   Many stroke patients experience an initial period when they are maintained 'nil by mouth' in hospital whilst screening and assessment of swallowing function is arranged. It is generally well recognised that some form of fluid administration must be provided (by nasogastric, subcutaneous, or intravenous routes if oral administration is not judged safe) within a fairly short time period. Whilst it is also expedient that patients remain with nil orally until swallowing function can be screened and, if necessary, a full swallowing assessment conducted, the additional risks incurred by prolonged periods without nutrition are well recognised (see Table 5.1) and can be avoided or minimised by timely assessment and initiation of nutritional intake by an appropriate route (see Section 5.4.3).

5.3.3.2   Hospital Food   Dietary provision in hospital may influence what patients eat, because they are directly dependent on what catering services provide and indirectly affected by the eating environment. Numerous investigations have flagged the deficiencies of both [87]. A focus on hospital food in the United Kingdom resulted in the implementation of national standards [88]. It is worth noting that whilst many patients are wholly dependent upon hospital meals, 31% and 17% of one cohort of stroke patients consumed additional food and drinks not provided by the hospital. For the 5% prescribed supplements, these met an estimated 25–40% of daily energy and protein requirements [32].

Modified-consistency diets may single an individual out as requiring 'special' food. This can bring attention to them as different, cause embarrassment, and have a socially isolating effect. Even within the family, such diets may be perceived as burdensome, by both the patient and the family.

Altogether, stroke patients are known to experience pre-existing malnutrition that may be compounded by metabolic consequences of acute illness, with physical, psychological, social, and emotional stroke effects posing barriers to eating and adequate dietary intake. Whilst an integrated programme of eating rehabilitation focused on dysphagia amongst chronic stroke survivors has been described [89], components are more often addressed separately and may not be explicitly linked to eating.

5.4   How Can Stroke Patients Be Helped to Maintain Adequate Dietary Intake?

Nutritional support is essentially a multidisciplinary activity; many professional and lay people contribute to ensuring adequate and acceptable dietary provision and intake for stroke patients, and multidisciplinary initiatives are required to improve care and patient outcomes [21, 90]. Professional roles tend to vary across locations; hence, this section focuses on what can and should be done, rather than who might do it.

5.4.1   Screening and Assessment

Screening is the process used to identify those with an established problem or who have evidence of being 'at risk' of a particular problem, such as malnutrition or dysphagia. Once identified, these individuals can undergo clinical assessment to identify the nature, source, and extent of the problem.

5.4.1.1   Nutritional Screening
Nutritional screening is part of routine initial assessment, undertaken as soon as the patient's condition allows, ideally within the first 24 hours of admission or first contact. No single measurement is adequate, and many composite screening tools have been developed. Conclusive evidence of the effectiveness of nutritional screening in improving the quality of patient care or outcomes is lacking [91], but many screening tools lack demonstrated validity (ability to differentiate those with nutritional problems from those without) and all have limitations, especially when used with acutely ill patients. Clinical examination is important, but whilst malnutrition produces a range of clinical signs, these tend to be subtle and non-specific until malnutrition is advanced. Reliance upon clinical signs for nutritional screening may not be effective; use of screening tools with demonstrated validity and reliability (e.g. the Malnutrition Universal Screening Tool) is recommended by the National Institute for Health and Care Excellence (NICE) [92].

Weight is commonly used. A component of many screening tools, it may be compared to percentile weight tables, ideal weight tables, and previous or usual weight. Sequential weights can be recorded to track progress and response to nutrition support. However, weight has limitations as a nutritional index, particularly for stroke patients. Dehydration and shifting fluid balance, differing scales, clothing, and time of day may all cause changes that do not reflect nutritional state. Weighing scales in institutions require – but do not always receive – regular maintenance and calibration. Perry noted that only 48% of stroke patients were weighed at any point during admission, rising somewhat to 56.5% following a nutritional support project [34]. Weighing a patient with limited mobility is a labour-intensive process, and equipment may not be available to weigh immobile patients.

Weight measurement cannot differentiate muscle from fat and does not take account of overall bodily size unless height is used to calculate body mass index (BMI). The most common BMI equation is Quetelet's Index: weight (kg) divided by height (m^2). A cut-off value of $18.5\,\mathrm{kg\,m^{-2}}$ is often regarded as suggestive of malnutrition, or less than $20\,\mathrm{kg\,m^{-2}}$ if accompanied by recent weight loss. However, this is the subject of considerable debate, and in older people the criterion may be higher (e.g. $<23\,\mathrm{kg\,m^{-2}}$ [93]). Height may be difficult to measure in hospital patients, and may be misleading in older people. Knee height, ulnar length, and demi-span may be measured instead, and different calculations or tables applied [48]. The approaches taken to nutritional screening for the patient Evelyn are described in Case Study 5.4.

Other anthropometric measures, such as arm circumference and skinfold measurements, are seldom used in acute clinical practice; biochemical tests are affected by acute illness and are unreliable as nutritional indicators. Albumin has a long half-life and is a particularly poor nutritional index, although it may indicate prognosis. Recent dietary intake can be a useful pointer towards nutritional status. UK and European clinical guidelines are available to help healthcare staff identify patients who are malnourished or at risk of malnutrition [92, 94].

Many stroke patients experience nutritional deterioration during the course of treatment and rehabilitation; monitoring is therefore important, encompassing such aspects as nutritional intake, weight, gastrointestinal function, and general clinical condition [92]. As a minimum, weekly weighing has been advocated, with additional activities such as keeping food record charts recommended according to individual nutritional status.

5.4.1.2 Dysphagia Screening
Up to 67% of patients experience dysphagia in the first 3 days of stroke; 50% aspirate, one-third of whom develop

Case Study

Case 5.4 Evelyn (Cont.)

Evelyn is initially not easy to transfer, as she has left hemiplegia and a fairly recent right hip replacement. However, using hoist scales, she is weighed as 70 kg, and her knee height is measured at 47.5 cm, producing a height of 152 cm and a BMI of 30 (MUST score = 0). Asked whether her weight has changed recently, she denies this, but her notes for her hip replacement record her weight as 76 kg. She has therefore lost almost 8% of her body weight within the past 6 months (MUST score = 1). Evelyn was eating normally (according to both her and Jenny) up to the point of admission, but as she has severe dysphagia, is not taking anything orally, and it can be predicted this will take some days, at least, to resolve, she scores 2 for acute disease effect, giving her a total score of 3. This puts her in the 'high risk' category, despite her borderline obesity.

pneumonia [95]. It is therefore essential that all patients have their swallowing function screened as early as possible. An Australian cluster randomised trial found stroke patients allocated to an intervention that included swallow screening were significantly less likely to be dead or dependent at 90 days, with a number needed to treat of 6.4 [96].

Dysphagia screening is a pass-or-fail procedure used to identify an individual with any indication of swallowing dysfunction who may need a full dysphagia assessment. A clinical swallowing assessment is a behavioural assessment of swallowing function that entails cranial nerve testing and evaluation of swallowing using food and liquids of various textures and consistencies. An instrumental dysphagia assessment using, for example, videofluoroscopy or functional endoscopic evaluation of swallowing (FEES) aims to identify the specific swallowing impairment and the effects of compensatory strategies such as a chin tuck or the use of thickened liquids [97].

The last 3 decades have seen a proliferation of research into swallowing, important factors for identifying dysphagia and risk of aspiration (e.g. abnormal volitional cough, abnormal gag reflex, dysphonia, dysarthria, cough, and voice change after swallow) and their predictive abilities [57], and the feasibility of swallowing screening conducted by nurses [98]. What is needed for valid and reliable dysphagia screening is tool(s) of adequate sensitivity, specificity, and predictive strength to accurately detect risk of dysphagia when administered by frontline clinicians at the earliest contact with acute stroke patients: within 4 hours of admission in the United Kingdom [99] and as soon as possible (at least within 24 hours of admission) in Australia [100]. Such a tool must be valid: it should gauge dysphagia and aspiration risk, suitability for oral feeding, and need for further assessment. It must be reliable: various people should be able to administer the test with similar results (inter-rater reliability), and a single person should get similar results with repeat administration (intra-rater reliability). It must be sensitive and specific to the risk of dysphagia: it should differentiate those with and those without dysphagia (most available tests focus on high sensitivity, because of the concern over the increased morbidity and mortality associated with dysphagia). It should be quick and easy to determine: the likelihood of dysphagia/aspiration, whether swallowing assessment is required, and whether oral feeding is safe. The time parameter for initial screening should be stated, with serial screening implemented if full assessment cannot be achieved in a timely manner or there is neurological decline. Ideally, it should be established what professional group(s) delivers screening, and what training is required.

Other than its intrinsic merits, contextual factors influence selection of a screening tool: the organisational structure (size of hospital and stroke unit), volume of patient flow, and composition of healthcare personnel (nursing staffing, 24-hour availability of specialised personnel and radiology services). See Table 5.4 for examples of current tools.

5.4.2 Preventing Pneumonia

Patients cared for in stroke units are significantly less likely to experience pneumonia [34, 112]. There is probably a raft of reasons for this: timely dysphagia screening, earlier initiation and more appropriate use of modified consistency and texture diet and fluids/enteral feeding, and early mobilisation [34, 95, 96, 113, 114].

TABLE 5.4	Characteristics of commonly used validated swallow screening tools	
Tool	**Characteristics**	**Used by:**
'Any 2' [101]	Acute stroke; swallowing and non-swallowing items. Administer all items, screening positive if any 2 items are present	SLT
3 oz Water Swallow Test [102, 103]	Screening for all patients regardless of diagnosis; single water swallow assessment item	Not stated (SLT in publications)
Acute Stroke Swallow Screening [104]	Also called Barnes Jewish Hospital Stroke Dysphagia Screen. Acute stroke patients; non-swallowing and swallowing items; 10 min training. Discontinue if any item is positive	RN
Bedside Swallowing Assessment [58, 105–107]	Acute stroke; swallowing and non-swallowing items. Discontinue if any item is positive	Dr & SLT
Emergency Physician Dysphagia Screening [108]	Acute stroke; swallowing and non-swallowing items; training = brief explanation. Discontinue if any item is present	Emergency physicians
Gugging Swallow Screen [109]	Acute stroke; swallowing and non-swallowing items; swallowing involves multiple volumes and viscosities. Discontinue if any item is present	RN, SLT
Modified Mann Assessment of Swallowing Ability [110]	Acute stroke; non-swallowing items only	Stroke neurologists
Standardised Swallowing Assessment [57, 98]	Swallowing and non-swallowing items. Discontinue if any item is positive	RN, SLT, junior Drs
Toronto Bedside Swallowing Screening Test [111]	Stroke: acute and rehab; swallowing and non-swallowing items; 4 h training; up to 10 min to administer. Discontinue if any item is positive	RN

Source: Modified from Donovan et al. [97].

Selective oral decontamination has been suggested to lower oropharyngeal colonisation with pathogenic Gram-negative bacteria [115]. Prophylaxis against vomiting and regurgitation may also be helpful, particularly for tube-fed patients, using the antiemetic agent metoclopramide [116], as stroke is associated with lower oesophageal sphincter dysfunction, gastroparesis, increased gastric residual volumes, and reflux [117]. Prophylactic antibiotics may significantly reduce post-stroke infection generally, but not pneumonia, without affecting mortality [118–120].

Although a key source of ongoing morbidity and mortality post-stroke, dysphagia management to prevent or reduce the incidence of pneumonia remains a neglected area of research and clinical care [121].

5.4.2.1   Oral Hygiene   Good oral hygiene is essential in maintaining a healthy mouth, teeth, and gums, providing patient comfort, and enabling patients to eat a full range of foods. The multiple effects of stroke can make it difficult for patients to manage their oral care and teeth cleaning independently; especially in the acute stage, many need help. The flora of the oral cavity are altered by the stroke itself [115], by oropharyngeal food residues and dental plaque, by antibiotics, and by candida infections. Saliva production and consistency may change, and the oral cavity may become dry with poor oral closure and positioning. Poor oral care and dental hygiene cause discomfort, reduce quality of life, and pose an increased risk for pneumonia. See Chapter 6 for oral care.

5.4.3   Timing of Initiation of Nutritional Support

There is no clear evidence to identify a 'safe' maximum period of starvation or nutritional depletion, and individual circumstances, degree of nutritional risk, and actual dietary intake guide individual decisions. However, the clear association between malnutrition and increased mortality in stroke patients should be borne in mind, as should the significant reduction in complications seen with fewer numbers of days spent with nil orally [21, 122]. However, systematic review failed to find any significant difference in death and dependency for early compared to late initiation of feeding [123].

Ethical dilemmas may be posed in relation to decision-making around initiation of tube feeding for severely impaired, acutely unwell stroke patients. Difficulties arise from not knowing the prognosis, not knowing values and preferences, and not being able to elicit them. Families may or may not be able to indicate the patient's perspective, and may have different views themselves (see Case Study 5.5

Case Study

Case 5.5   Margaret

Margaret is 92 years old and has been living with her daughter Frances, son-in-law Martin, and young adult grandchildren since she had a below-knee amputation following a road traffic accident some years ago. On admission, she has a dense hemiplegia, is incontinent, and her speech is only intelligible with effort. She also has severe dysphagia, and is placed nil orally with subcutaneous hydration. Her swallow function is reassessed daily, but by 5 days shows no sign of improvement.

Repeat attempts to place a nasogastric tube (NGT) fail. Margaret tells the nurses that she is too tired to do anything, and switches between saying she wants to eat and get better, and saying she can't cope anymore and just wants to die.

Frances is desperate for her to make progress and come home; Martin is very anxious about whether Frances will cope with her mother, who is more dependent than before the stroke. Gastroscopy shows a large sliding hiatus hernia, and a gastrostomy is successfully placed after a longer-than-usual procedure. Recovery is slow and complicated by poor tolerance of feeding and leakage from the gastrostomy insertion site. Eventually, admission to nursing home care is arranged, once Frances finally agrees that return home is unrealistic.

for an example). Provision of nourishment is a fundamental and very emotive topic [14]; excellent communication between and amongst families and health-care professionals is essential. UK guidance flags artificial nutrition support as a medical intervention, decisions concerning which need to consider likely benefit, risks, and harms. Where there is real concern that such an intervention may be futile, it is clearly important that this is discussed and understood by all concerned [124]. The UK Mental Capacity Act [125] provides guidance on establishing whether and to what extent someone can contribute to decisions about their care, and when Lasting Power of Attorney can be used or a deputy appointed.

5.4.4 Managing Eating Disabilities

As eating-related disabilities are experienced across the spectrum from acute to long-term care, management strategies may need to span similar time frames.

5.4.4.1 Chewing Difficulties
The risk of stroke is increased in people with both significant periodontal disease and no natural teeth [126]. With increasing age, the mouth changes shape and dentures no longer fit the gums, compounding difficulties in mastication. Dentures are only one-sixth as effective as teeth when chewing [127], and although digestion has been shown to be independent of chewing, edentulous patients consumed less calcium, protein, niacin, and vitamin C compared to individuals with intact dentition [128–130].

Poor jaw closure requires facilitated jaw support (manual assistance); if the tongue cannot move the bolus across the midline on to the teeth, the food bolus needs to be placed on the non-damaged side of the tongue in the short term, and tongue lateralisation exercises are required in the long term. External pressure to the cheek in patients with unilateral facial weakness increases the negative intraoral pressure required for swallowing, prevents food falling between teeth and cheek, and assists the tongue in forming food into a cohesive bolus. It may also help to avoid food of mixed textures that are difficult to chew, and to serve several smaller meals to allow the person to rest between meals.

5.4.4.2 Restorative and Compensatory Strategies for Dysphagia Management
Restorative (direct) therapy aims to change dysfunctional swallowing physiology (Table 5.5), including behavioural changes (such as swallowing exercises and environmental modifications), acupuncture, drug therapy, neuromuscular and pharyngeal electrical stimulation, thermal and tactile stimulation, transcranial direct current, and magnetic stimulation. Research evidence is limited; to date, only behavioural interventions and acupuncture have been shown to reduce dysphagia. Transcutaneous electrical stimulation may have value as an adjuvant therapy alongside behavioural therapies [131].

Where the swallow is weak with poor laryngeal elevation, Mendelssohn's manoeuvre entails deliberately prolonging laryngeal elevation during mid-swallow, aiming to increase the proportion of bolus going into the oesophagus and decrease pharyngeal residues. The patient is taught to feel his or her larynx

TABLE 5.5 Compensatory strategies and restorative behavioural therapies for dysphagia

Stage of swallow	Swallow disorder	Compensatory strategy	Restorative/rehabilitative exercises/therapy
Pre-oral	Lack of cognitive or sensory awareness	Provide cues on food characteristics	Ensure dentures and spectacles are fitting
Oral preparatory	Poor lip seal	Supported lip and jaw closure	Lip exercises
	Poor cheek tone	Intraoral prosthesis, cheek hold technique (apply pressure to weak side), tilt head towards unaffected side	Cheek tone exercises
	Poor sensation in oral cavity	Increase bolus taste, volume, density, temperature, carbonated drinks	Sensory awareness programme
	Poor tongue movement	Modify consistency of bolus, pace rate of bolus presentation, avoid mixed consistencies, remove residue from oral cavity post-swallow	Tongue lateralisation exercises
	Poor chewing/jaw closure	Jaw support, diet modification	Chewing exercises
Oral transit	Poor tongue movement/oral transit	Head back posture	
Pharyngeal	Delayed swallow	Adapted cutlery and crockery to assist in self-feeding, chin tuck posture, increase bolus taste, volume, density, temperature, carbonated drinks	Proprioceptive neuromuscular facilitation (PNF) to the fauceal arches
	Reduced base-of-tongue movement	Chin tuck, clearing swallows, effortful swallow, decrease bolus size, increase bolus consistency	Tongue hold technique, gargle and yawn exercises, supersupraglottic swallow
	Unilateral pharyngeal paresis	Head rotation to damaged side, head tilt to unaffected side, back or side lying, clearing swallows, liquid wash down	

(continued)

TABLE 5.5 Compensatory strategies and restorative behavioural therapies for dysphagia (*continued*)

Stage of swallow	Swallow disorder	Compensatory strategy	Restorative/rehabilitative exercises/therapy
	Unilateral tongue and pharyngeal paresis	Head tilt to unaffected side, clearing swallows	
	Reduced laryngeal closure	Chin tuck, head rotation to damaged side, supraglottic swallow, supersupraglottic swallow, alter bolus consistency	Supraglottic swallow, supersupraglottic swallow, breath hold manoeuvre, push–pull voicing
	Reduced laryngeal elevation	Chin tuck and lie on side/back, supersupraglottic swallow, Mendelssohn's manoeuvre, clearing swallows	Falsetto voicing, Mendelssohn's manoeuvre, shaker technique, chin tuck against resistance
	Crico-pharyngeal dysfunction/reduced anterior movement of hyo-laryngeal structure	Head rotation, avoid mixed consistencies	Shaker technique, chin tuck against resistance,
Oesophageal	Oesophageal dysmotility	Effortful swallow	
	Fatigue	Nutritional supplements, decrease meal size, increase frequency of meals	

rising during the swallow, and at its highest point, to hold it in that position for several seconds. A double swallow may improve clearance of food remaining in the pharynx. Supraglottic swallowing is intended to maximise closure of the laryngeal inlet. Breath is held before swallowing, with the aim of adducting the vocal cords and protecting the airway, although videonasoendoscopy has shown that breath-holding does not always result in the vocal cords coming together. The patient swallows twice and immediately afterwards coughs to expel anything that has penetrated the laryngeal vestibule. Exercises specific to individual impairments (e.g. of tongue, lips, and facial muscles) are frequently recommended [53]. However, evaluation of these techniques is limited.

Compensatory postures and strategies eliminate or reduce the volume of material aspirated into the airway. These were initially designed for use with patients with oropharyngeal cancer, and they require that patients are able to understand and cooperate with instructions. Compensatory postures do not necessarily match with principles of normal neurological movement patterns, and, whilst effective in the short term in ensuring that respiration and nutrition are not compromised, they should not be regarded as long-term management without considering how to promote normal tone, reflexes, and sensory integration and prevent abnormal patterns of movement and reflexes from becoming established [53]. Such strategies aim to compensate for specific impairments (Table 5.5). For example, head and neck may be deliberately positioned. With the chin down ('chin tuck'), the epiglottis shifts backwards and may narrow the laryngeal entrance and increase airway protection. This may be helpful if the pharyngeal phase is delayed, but it does not eliminate aspiration in all patients. Where there is unilateral pharyngeal paralysis, lateral head rotation may open the UOS and direct the bolus away from the paralysed side. Excluding the flaccid oesophageal sidewall, which otherwise weakens pharyngeal pressure gradients, allows remaining peristaltic contractions to achieve faster, more complete bolus transit. Described in research but seldom used in clinical practice, palatal prostheses reshape the oral cavity to address individual problems in bolus manipulation and triggering of swallowing [53].

5.4.4.3   Texture Modification and Fluid Consistencies   As swallow physiology is dependent on consistencies consumed, modification of food, liquid, and medication can be utilised therapeutically. Modifying taste, temperature, texture, viscosity, and volume can affect bolus preparation and swallow performance [132–134]. Thicker fluids and modified-consistency diets compensate for deficits in swallow physiology and improve efficient transit through the mouth and pharynx, thereby improving the safety of the swallow. Thin liquids lose cohesion very rapidly, so if a delay exists, naturally thicker or artificially thickened drinks are indicated to improve swallow efficiency [127]. However, decisions regarding thickener need to be client-specific, dictated by the length of delay. Prescription of thickened fluids is not without potential problems: patients often do not like them and may decline to drink them and thus become dehydrated [135]. Longer-term adherence to thickener use is poor, but education programmes for patients and carers have been linked with more consistent use and thus improved patient safety [136]. Offering free fluids without thickener may not increase patients' risk of developing aspiration pneumonia [137].

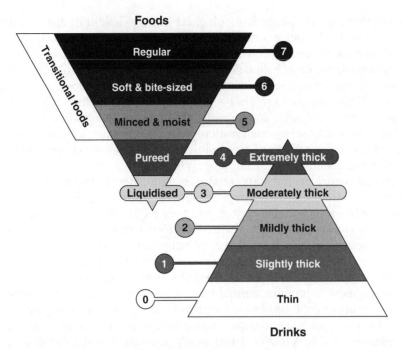

FIGURE 5.3 The International Dysphagia Diet Standardisation Initiative framework for texture-modified foods and thickened fluids [138, 139].

Historically, there have been a number of different classifications of modified-texture foods and fluids, using descriptors and terminologies that vary between locations (e.g. terms such as 'nectar', familiar in the United States, are seldom used in the United Kingdom) – as does interpretation of the same terms (e.g. the consistency understood by 'custard'). There is now an international consensus taxonomy of descriptors (Figure 5.3), which is being increasingly adopted. This comprises eight levels, with three (levels 3 and 4) applicable to both fluid consistencies and food textures. Table 5.6 details these levels.

Liquidising food increases the volume without increasing calories. It is important that food, however prepared, should look colourful and appetising, which can be achieved by blending different foods separately, using food moulds and garnishes. Most community meal schemes are able to supply modified-texture meals, although menu choice may be limited.

5.4.4.4 Nutritional Supplementation

Foods and drinks can be fortified to add extra calories by using full-fat products, sugars, and milk. Increasing the number of meals and introducing snacks between meals to approximately six per day will also increase nutritional intake. Supplements, available on prescription or over the counter, may augment normal intake or provided complete nutritional intake in themselves. Nutritional supplementation has not demonstrated significant difference in case fatality, death, or dependency, but can significantly increase energy (MD 430.18 kcal/day; 95% CI 141.61–718.75; P = 0.003) and protein intake and reduce pressure ulcers (OR 0.56; 95% CI

TABLE 5.6	Descriptors of consistency and texture modification of fluids and foods [139]
Consistency/texture	**Description of fluid consistency/food texture**
0 Thin fluid	Fast flow; flows like water through any teat or straw
1 Slightly thick	Thicker than water; requires more effort than thin fluid to get through a teat or straw
2 Mildly thick	Pours off a spoon quickly, but slower than thin drinks; sippable; effort required to drink through a standard straw
3 Liquidised/ Moderately thick	Can be drunk from cup; effort required to suck through standard or wide-bore straw; cannot be piped, moulded, layered on a plate; cannot be eaten with a fork, can be eaten with a spoon; no oral processing or chewing required, can be swallowed directly; smooth texture with no 'bits'; prongs of a fork do not leave a pattern; spreads out if spilled on a flat surface
4 Extremely thick/Pureed	Usually eaten with a spoon (or fork); cannot be drunk from a cup or straw; does not require chewing; can be piped, moulded, layered; very slow movement under gravity but cannot be poured; holds shape on a plate; no lumps; liquid does not separate from solids; prongs of a fork leave a pattern and food retains the indentation of the fork; sample sits in a mound above the fork; a small amount may flow through to form a tail below the fork, but it does not flow continuously; may spread out slowly or slump and spread out slightly on a plate
5 Minced and moist	Can be eaten with a fork or spoon, or with chopsticks if the individual has very good hand control; can be scooped and shaped on a plate; soft and moist with no separate thin liquid; small lumps within the food are easy to squash with a tongue; when pressed with a fork, particles are easily separated and come through the prongs; can be easily mashed with little pressure from a fork; holds shape on a spoon; may spread or slump very slowly on a plate
6 Soft & bite-sized	Can be eaten with a fork, spoon, or chopsticks; can be easily mashed with pressure on a fork, spoon, or chopsticks; chewing but not biting required before swallowing; soft, tender, and moist throughout, with no separate thin liquid; a fork on its side can be used to separate or break up into smaller pieces; when a sample is pressed by the base of a fork, the sample squashes and changes shape and will not return to its original shape when pressure is removed
7 Regular	Normal, everyday, age-appropriate foods; includes stringy, fibrous, hard, tough, crispy, crunchy, pips, seeds, husks, bone

0.32–0.96; P = 0.03) [123]. In line with general nutritional recommendations, supplement use should be targeted at those with demonstrated need [140], taking into consideration patient preference, adherence, and the potential for 'taste fatigue', as well as availability.

5.4.4.5 **Enteral Nutrition** Enteral feeding may be used to provide

nutritional support for patients with a functioning gastrointestinal tract who are unable to eat orally; dysphagia as a result of stroke is one of the most common reasons for enteral tube feeding worldwide [141]. Recent years have seen dramatic increases in the numbers maintained on home enteral nutrition; the United Kingdom saw a 42.8% increase over a 10-year period [141], although more recent figures have declined [142]. Enteral tube feeding may also be used, less commonly, to augment inadequate oral intake; in long-term management, it may be appropriate to have complementary routes of intake, with quality of life being the focus [143].

An NGT is normally a short-term solution (up to around 28 days) for individuals with nutritional difficulties. Potential complications include oesophagitis, ulceration (most commonly nasal or gastric), inadvertent removal and tube displacement, blockage, and poor patient compliance [123]. Particular considerations are methods of checking accurate placement; pH testing of gastric aspirate is preferred, with chest X-ray where this is not possible [92]. Auscultation and many other previously common approaches have not demonstrated acceptable levels of accuracy [144]. Management of intubated but confused patients also poses problems, with cultural, national, and personal differences of opinion about the ethics of restraint, whether via sedation, bed clothes, tying hands to bed rails, or mittens. A device known as a bridle is increasingly used to minimise tube displacement amongst select patient groups [145]. Nasojejunal (NJ) tubes are uncommon but may be used for patients with abnormal gastric function where there is a greater risk of aspiration due to reflux.

Gastrostomies are a longer-term solution but patient selection is important owing to the impact on quality of life. They can be placed surgically, via endoscopy (percutaneous endoscopic gastrostomy, PEG), or radiographically (RIG). For patients with abnormal gastric function, percutaneous endoscopic jejunostomy (PEJ) tubes are the preferred option, although reflux may not be abolished [146]. Gastrostomies with balloon retention devices are useful for some patients, as they allow for rapid replacement by appropriately trained staff. Symptoms associated with this route of feeding include diarrhoea, vomiting, site infection and leakage, infection and hypergranulation at the stoma site, and 'buried bumper' (where the gastric retaining device migrates into the gastric or abdominal wall). Blocked tubes are not uncommon but can be minimised by good management and patient and carer education [147].

No significant difference has been found between PEG and NGT feeding for case fatality or the composite outcome of death or dependency, but PEG has been linked with fewer treatment failures (OR 0.09; 95% CI 0.01–0.51; P = 0.007), lower gastrointestinal bleeding (OR 0.25; 95% CI 0.09–0.69; P = 0.007), and higher feed delivery (MD 22.00; 95% CI 16.15–27.85; P < 0.001) and albumin concentration (MD 4.92 g l^{-1}; 95% CI 0.19–9.65; P = 0.04). Comparing bridle to conventional NGT securement, there was no difference in case fatality, death, or dependency, but feed delivery was higher with bridles [123].

Feed can be delivered either as a continuous infusion or as a bolus. UK nutrition guidelines are supportive of either approach, taking into account patient preference, convenience, and drug administration. For patients in ICU, however, continuous feeding over 16–24 hours daily is recommended [92].

Parenteral nutrition (PN) is a means of supplying full nutritional support intravenously for individuals who have a non-functioning gastrointestinal tract. It is rarely required in the stroke population.

In many areas, local standards for PEG management are available, and the British Association for Parenteral and Enteral Nutrition (BAPEN) sets standards for home enteral tube feeding [148] which include contact with a support group, such as Patients on Intravenous & Nasogastric Nutrition Therapy (PINNT). Various systems of long-term support or back-up are provided, entailing, for example, hospital outreach, community nursing, and/or support services contracted from commercial companies. For all patients with neurological damage who have nothing orally, oral stimulation programmes are essential in order to prevent hypersensitive oral defensive patterns becoming established, which may make oral hygiene routines difficult to maintain.

5.4.4.6   Smell and Taste
Amongst groups of older adults, taste dysfunction has been linked with low body weight and energy intake, reduced appetite, and poorer immune function; dietary intervention with flavour-modified meals increased dietary intake and improved immunity and muscle function. Smell and taste are intimately linked with when and why people want to start and stop eating, the quantity and qualities of food eaten, and outcomes related to this [149–151]. It has not been established whether taste impairment in stroke patients affects dietary intake, or whether similar approaches to flavour modification for taste-impaired stroke patients might enhance nutritional intake. Currently, taste and smell dysfunction are seldom sought as part of neurological assessment of stroke patients, but questions could be included as part of nursing nutritional assessment, with a view to tailoring menu choices to sensory abilities and preferences.

5.4.4.7   Management of Other Eating-Related Disabilities
Posture and head control, upper limb impairment, cognitive, communication, and visual and perceptual deficits all impact on ability to recognise and communicate dietary wants and needs and to eat safely. Clearly, eating is a complex activity requiring integration of multiple skills. For many stroke patients, focusing on more than single actions affects performance; for example, Harley et al. [152] reported that the effort of just speaking could be sufficient to disturb postural control early after stroke. Rehabilitation interventions are normally related to the activities of daily living in which actions are applied. Rehabilitation interventions are available and used for eating-related deficits (see Chapters 7, 8, 10, and 14); the relevance of rehabilitation in relation to the ability to eat is recognised [153] but is seldom the specific focus. Meal times present rehabilitation opportunities, where patients may practise application of a range of skills worked on during therapy sessions.

Assistance with eating – skilled feeding – requires sensitive management. It should not attract attention to what is occurring, and when done well, has been described as a 'silent dance', in which the person fed sees their own actions reflected in those of their helper [154]. A wide range of assistive devices may be helpful (e.g. plate-guards, non-slip mats, adapted cutlery). Many can also be useful in relation to meal preparation. Reviewing patients at 3–5 years post-stroke,

Sorensen et al. [155] found a significant increase in the use of aids for cooking and eating, flagging either changing patterns of need or previous poor knowledge of what was available.

5.4.4.8 Mood Disorder and Appetite

Identification and treatment of mood disorder post-stroke is now widely accepted as an important component of standard stroke care. Pharmacological treatment of depression in stroke patients has demonstrated beneficial effects for symptoms but also increased adverse events, so decisions whether to treat depend on individual risk–benefit assessment [156]. Similarly, it is not known whether treatment of depression will relieve depression-related appetite suppression or carbohydrate craving. In high-risk situations such as cachexia, appetite stimulants such as prednisolone may be used: there is no evidence that such an approach may confer benefit for stroke patients.

5.4.4.9 The Eating Environment

Non-pharmacological means may enhance dietary intake. These include attention to the psychosocial dimension of eating by creating a pleasant, relaxed atmosphere in which food is eaten as a shared social experience. This is not easy in hospital wards, where people eat in isolation at their bedsides with ward activities going on around them, limited by set meal delivery and collection times. However, given recognition of its importance, and particularly with the help of family and friends, this may be addressed, ensuring meal systems meet individual food preferences and patients are able to choose what they eat. This is especially an issue for certain ethnic groups, for whom choice is often more limited, especially when combined with the need for texture modification. In hospital systems where patients experience transfers between wards, catering systems do not always keep track of patient movements in a timely fashion. Ensuring out-of-hours availability of palatable snacks is also important; given decreasing lengths of stay and increasing investigations, it is increasingly important that food is available not just at set meal times. Such an approach may not fit easily within systems that regard food as hotel services, targeted for cost-containment.

5.5 Conclusion

A considerable proportion of stroke patients demonstrate evidence of malnutrition or nutritional risk at admission to hospital; many will experience a wide range of eating-related disabilities that will prevent or deter them from eating for at least part of their recovery period. Depression, common at all stages post-stroke, is linked with appetite changes and, sometimes, reduced dietary intake; the sequence of this is unclear – whether depression causes or follows appetite changes. This is important, because malnutrition has been linked with increased complication rates, poorer rehabilitation outcomes, and more deaths amongst stroke patients. Eating is also an important component of quality of life, and nutritional status and ability to eat have long-term effects for stroke survivors, their families, and their social circles.

Nutritional screening and assessment is the essential first stage in identifying individual needs, goals, care plans, and programmes. However, whilst nutritional screening for all patients is widely advocated (unless a good case for exemption can be made), it does not always occur. In part, this may be attributed to the challenges posed by undertaking screening with immobile, possibly aphasic or cognitively impaired, acutely unwell patients. Nonetheless, without some form of screening and assessment, this important component of rehabilitation may be neglected or ineffectively addressed.

Many eating-related disabilities are already the subject of rehabilitation interventions, although meal times may be underutilised as opportunities to bring together and practise skills addressed during therapy sessions. Others, such as smell and taste dysfunction, remain underexplored. Decision-making in relation to provision of artificial nutrition support may pose challenges, and can require active involvement and collaboration between the whole team and the patient (insofar as this is possible), their family, and their carers. Decision-making for severely disabled patients presents particular difficulties, and may require engagement with family members with power of attorney and independent advocates.

Nutrition may be provided to patients through a range of means; care-planning and goal-setting need to be established collaboratively, monitored, and reviewed regularly. Methods to address long-term problems, continuing beyond hospital discharge, need to be discussed in relation to what is available within and through community resources. The need for ongoing review should be borne in mind. Education and training for patients and carers is important at all stages, but perhaps especially in relation to long-term management. Ultimately, patients may make decisions to take risks within their context of overall quality of life which healthcare professionals would not sanction, based on differing perceptions of the balance of benefit and risk.

I manage to do a bit of cooking but sometimes I can't, because I can't do it or because of safety reasons. My husband does all the shopping, when he comes in the evening. I go in the kitchen and I just help him, because I feel I want to be part of it. I manage some things, if there's no limited time for it I can do it. So it's OK to do those things, and I feel more myself, don't feel so hopeless.
(56-year-old female stroke survivor, 6 months post-stroke, London)

References

1. UK Stroke Forum Education & Training. About the SSEF. Available from: http://www. stroke-education.org.uk/about. [30 November 2018]
2. Keller, H.H. (1993). Malnutrition in institutionalized elderly: how and why? Journal of the American Geriatrics Society 41 (11): 1212–1218.
3. Chen, C.C.H., Schilling, L.S., and Lyder, C.H. (2001). A concept analysis of malnutrition in the elderly. Journal of Advanced Nursing. 36 (1): 131–142.
4. British Association for Parenteral and Enteral Nutrition (BAPEN). Introduction to Malnutrition. Available from: http://www.bapen.org.uk/malnutrition-undernutrition/ introduction-to-malnutrition?start=2 [30 November 2018]
5. Reilly, H. (1996). Nutrition in clinical management: malnutrition in our midst. Proceedings of the Nutrition Society 55: 841–853.
6. Dávalos, A., Ricart, W., Gonzalez-Huix, F. et al. (1996). Effect of malnutrition after acute stroke on clinical outcome. Stroke 27 (6): 1028–1032.

7. Davis, J.P., Wong, A.A., Schluter, P.J. et al. (2004). Impact of premorbid undernutrition on outcome in stroke patients. Stroke 35 (8): 1930–1934.

8. Finestone, H.M., Greene-Finestone, L.S., Wilson, E.S., and Teasell, R.W. (1996). Prolonged length of stay and reduced functional improvement rate in malnourished stroke rehabilitation patients. Archives of Physical Medicine and Rehabilitation 77 (4): 340–345.

9. FOOD Trial Collaboration (2003). Poor nutritional status on admission predicts poor outcomes after stroke: observational data from the FOOD trial. Stroke 34 (6): 1450–1456.

10. Zhang, J., Zhao, X.-Q., Wang, A. et al. (2015). Emerging malnutrition during hospitalisation independently predicts poor 3-month outcomes after acute stroke: data from a Chinese cohort. Asia Pacific Journal of Clinical Nutrition 24 (3): 379–386.

11. Perry, L. and Mclaren, S. (2004). An exploration of nutrition and eating disabilities in relation to quality of life at 6 months post-stroke. Health & Social Care in the Community 12 (4): 288–297.

12. British Nutrition Foundation. Nutrient Requirements. Available from: http://www.nutrition.org.uk/nutritionscience/nutrients-food-and-ingredients/nutrient-requirements.html [30 November 2018].

13. Harris Benedict Equation. BMI calculator Available from: http://www.bmi-calculator.net/bmr-calculator/harris-benedict-equation [30 November 2018].

14. Lupton, D. (1996). Food, the Body and the Self. London: Sage.

15. Gariballa, S. and Sinclair, A. (1998). Assessment and treatment of nutritional status in stroke patients. Postgraduate Medical Journal 74 (873): 395–399.

16. Duffy, V.B., Backstrand, J.R., and Ferris, A.M. (1995). Olfactory dysfunction and related nutritional risk in free-living, elderly women. Journal of the Academy of Nutrition and Dietetics 95 (8): 879–884.

17. Finch, S., Doyle, W., Lowe, C. et al. (1998). National Diet and Nutrition Survey: People Aged 65 Years and Over. London: The Stationary Office.

18. de Groot, C., Van Den Broek, T., and Van Staveren, W. (1999). Energy intake and micronutrient intake in elderly Europeans: seeking the minimum requirement in the SENECA study. Age and Ageing 28 (5): 469–474.

19. Edington, J., Kon, P., and Martyn, C. (1996). Prevalence of malnutrition in patients in general practice. Clinical Nutrition 15 (2): 60–63.

20. Vir, S.C. and Love, A. (1979). Nutritional status of institutionalized and noninstitutionalized aged in Belfast, Northern Ireland. American Journal of Clinical Nutrition 32 (9): 1934–1947.

21. Perry, L. and McLaren, S. (2003). Eating difficulties after stroke. Journal of Advanced Nursing 43 (4): 360–369.

22. Ebrahim, S., Barer, D., and Nouri, F. (1987). An audit of follow-up services for stroke patients after discharge from hospital. International Disability Studies 9 (3): 103–105.

23. Wilkinson, P.R., Wolfe, C.D., Warburton, F.G. et al. (1997). A long-term follow-up of stroke patients. Stroke 28 (3): 507–512.

24. Foley, N.C., Salter, K.L., Robertson, J. et al. (2009). Which reported estimate of the prevalence of malnutrition after stroke is valid? Stroke 40 (3): e66–e74.

25. British Association for Parenteral and Enteral Nutrition (BAPEN). Malnutrition Universal Screening Tool. Available from: http://www.bapen.org.uk/pdfs/must/must_full.pdf [30 November 2018].

26. Stratton, R.J., Hackston, A., Longmore, D. et al. (2004). Malnutrition in hospital outpatients and inpatients: prevalence, concurrent validity and ease of use of the 'malnutrition universal screening tool' ('MUST') for adults. British Journal of Nutrition 92 (5): 799–808.

27. Aadal, L., Mortensen, J., and Nielsen, J.F. (2015). Weight reduction after severe brain injury: a challenge during the rehabilitation course. Journal of Neuroscience Nursing 47 (2): 85–90.

28. Axelsson, L.T., Chung, T.C., Dobrogosz, W.J., and Lindgren, S.E. (1989). Production of a broad spectrum antimicrobial substance by *Lactobacillus reuteri*. Microbial Ecology in Health and Disease 2 (2): 131–136.

29. Unosson, M., Ek, A., Bjurulf, P. et al. (1994). Feeding dependence and nutritional status after acute stroke. Stroke 25 (2): 366–371.

30. Choi-Kwon, S., Yang, Y.H., Kim, E.K. et al. (1998). Nutritional status in acute stroke: undernutrition versus overnutrition in different stroke subtypes. Acta Neurologica Scandinavica 98 (3): 187–192.

31. Westergren, A., Karlsson, S., Andersson, P. et al. (2001). Eating difficulties, need for assisted eating, nutritional status and pressure ulcers in patients admitted for stroke rehabilitation. Journal of Clinical Nursing 10 (2): 257–269.

32. Nip, W. (2007). Mood and Food: An Investigation of Mood State and Nutritional Status After Stroke. London: University of London.

33. Martineau, J., Bauer, J.D., Isenring, E., and Cohen, S. (2005). Malnutrition determined by the patient-generated subjective global assessment is associated with poor outcomes in acute stroke patients. Clinical Nutrition 24 (6): 1073–1077.

34. Perry, L. (2002). Eating after an Stroke: Natural History and Investigation of an Evidence-Based Intervention. London: University of London.

35. Broom, J. (1993). Sepsis and trauma. In: Human Nutrition and Dietetics, 9e (ed. J.S. Garrow and W.P.T. James), 456–463. Edinburgh: Churchill Livingstone.

36. Chalela, J.A., Haymore, J., Schellinger, P.D. et al. (2004). Acute stroke patients are being underfed. Neurocritical Care 1 (3): 331–334.

37. Touho, H., Karasawa, J., Shishido, H. et al. (1990). Measurement of energy expenditure in acute stage of cerebrovascular diseases. Neurologia Medico-Chirurgica 30 (7): 451–455.

38. Frankenfield, D.C. and Ashcraft, C.M. (2012). Description and prediction of resting metabolic rate after stroke and traumatic brain injury. Nutrition 28 (9): 906–911.

39. Esper, D.H., Coplin, W.M., and Carhuapoma, J.R. (2006). Energy expenditure in patients with nontraumatic intracranial hemorrhage. Journal of Parenteral and Enteral Nutrition 30 (2): 71–75.

40. Finestone, H.M., Greene-Finestone, L.S., Foley, N.C., and Woodbury, M.G. (2003). Measuring longitudinally the metabolic demands of stroke patients: resting energy expenditure is not elevated. Stroke 34 (2): 502–507.

41. Weekes, E. and Elia, M. (1992). Resting energy expenditure and body composition following cerebro-vascular accident. Clinical Nutrition 11 (1): 18–22.

42. Leone, A. and Pencharz, P.B. (2010). Resting energy expenditure in stroke patients who are dependent on tube feeding: a pilot study. Clinical Nutrition 29 (3): 370–372.

43. Platts, M.M., Rafferty, D., and Paul, L. (2006). Metabolic cost of overground gait in younger stroke patients and healthy controls. Medicine and Science in Sports and Exercise 38 (6): 1041–1046.

44. Kayser-Jones, J. and Schell, E. (1997). The effect of staffing on the quality of care at mealtime. Nursing Outlook 45 (2): 64–72.

45. Siebens, H., Trupe, E., Siebens, A. et al. (1986). Correlates and consequences of eating dependency in institutionalized elderly. Journal of the American Geriatrics Society 34 (3): 192–198.

46. Aquilani, R., Galli, M., Guarnaschelli, C. et al. (1999). Prevalence of malnutrition and inadequate food intake in self-feeding rehabilitation patients with stroke. Europa Medicophysica 35 (2): 75–81.

47. Jacobsson, C., Axelsson, K., Österlind, P.O., and Norberg, A. (2000). How people with stroke and healthy older people experience the eating process. Journal of Clinical Nursing 9 (2): 255–264.

48. Perry, L. and McLaren, S. (2003). Nutritional support in acute stroke: the impact of evidence-based guidelines. Clinical Nutrition 22 (3): 283–293.

49. Sidenvall, B., Fjellström, C., and Ek, A.-C. (1996). Cultural perspectives of meals expressed by patients in geriatric care. International Journal of Nursing Studies 33 (2): 212–222.

50. McLaren, S. and Dickerson, J. (2000). Measurement of eating disability in an acute stroke population. Clinical Effectiveness in Nursing 4 (3): 109–120.

51. Royal College of Speech and Language Therapy (2006). Communicating Quality 3: RCSLT's Guidance on Best Practice in Service Organisation and Provision. London: Royal College of Speech and Language Therapy.

52. Kuhlemeier, K., Rieve, J., Kirby, N., and Siebens, A. (1989). Clinical correlates of dysphagia in stroke patients. Archives of Physical Medicine and Rehabilitation 70: 56.

53. Logemann, J. (1998). Evaluation and Treatment of Swallowing Disorders, 2e. Austin: Pro Ed.

54. Sala, R., Munto, M., Preciado, I. et al. (1998). Swallowing changes in cerebrovascular accidents: incidence, natural history, and repercussions on the nutritional status, morbidity, and mortality. Revista de Neurologia 27 (159): 759–766.

55. Hoffmann, S., Malzahn, U., Harms, H. et al. (2012). Development of a clinical score (A2DS2) to predict pneumonia in acute ischemic stroke. Stroke 43 (10): 2617–2623.

56. Zhang, X., Yu, S., Wei, L. et al. (2016). The A2DS2 score as a predictor of pneumonia and in-hospital death after acute ischemic stroke in Chinese populations. PLoS One 11 (3): 1–9.

57. Perry, L. and Love, C.P. (2001). Screening for dysphagia and aspiration in acute stroke: a systematic review. Dysphagia 16 (1): 7–18.

58. Smithard, D., O'Neill, P., Park, C. et al. (1996). Complications and outcome after acute stroke: does dysphagia matter? Stroke 27 (7): 1200–1204.

59. Boaden, E., Davies, S., Storey, L., and Watkins, C. (2006). Inter Professional Dysphagia Framework. Preston: University of Central Lancashire.

60. Langmore, S.E., Terpenning, M.S., Schork, A. et al. (1998). Predictors of aspiration pneumonia: how important is dysphagia? Dysphagia 13 (2): 69–81.

61. Choi, Y., Park, D., and Kim, Y. (2014). Relationship between prosthodontic status and nutritional intake in the elderly in Korea: National Health and Nutrition Examination Survey (NHANES IV). International Journal of Dental Hygiene 12 (4): 285–290.

62. Millns, B., Gosney, M., Jack, C. et al. (2003). Acute stroke predisposes to oral Gram-negative bacilli – a cause of aspiration pneumonia? Gerontology 49 (3): 173–176.

63. Yoneyama, T., Yoshida, M., Ohrui, T. et al. (2002). Oral care reduces pneumonia in older patients in nursing homes. Journal of the American Geriatrics Society 50 (3): 430–433.

64. Lam, O., McGrath, C., Bandara, H. et al. (2012). Oral health promotion interventions on oral reservoirs of *Staphylococcus aureus*: a systematic review. Oral Diseases 18 (3): 244–254.

65. Hiiemae, K.M. and Palmer, J. (1999). Food transport and bolus formation during complete feeding sequences on foods of different initial consistency. Dysphagia 14 (1): 31–42.

66. Pitts, T., Morris, K., Lindsey, B. et al. (2012). Co-ordination of cough and swallow in vivo and in silico. Experimental Physiology 97 (4): 469–473.

67. Newman, R.D. and Nightingale, J.M. (2012). Videofluoroscopy: A Multidisciplinary Team Approach. Abingdon: Plural Publishing.

68. Marik, P.E. (2001). Aspiration pneumonitis and aspiration pneumonia. New England Journal of Medicine 344 (9): 665–671.

69. Brott, T., Adams, H., Olinger, C. et al. (1989). Measurements of acute cerebral infarction: a clinical examination scale. Stroke 20 (7): 864–870.

70. Lawrence, E.S., Coshall, C., Dundas, R. et al. (2001). Estimates of the prevalence of acute stroke impairments and disability in a multiethnic population. Stroke 32 (6): 1279–1284.

71. Kalra, L., Smith, D., and Crome, P. (1993). Stroke in patients aged over 75 years: outcome and predictors. Postgraduate Medical Journal 69 (807): 33–36.

72. Taub, N., Wolfe, C., Richardson, E., and Burney, P. (1994). Predicting the disability of first-time stroke sufferers at 1 year. 12-month follow-up of a population-based cohort in Southeast England. Stroke 25 (2): 352–357.

73. Stone, S., Wilson, B., Wroot, A. et al. (1991). The assessment of visuo-spatial neglect after acute stroke. Journal of Neurology, Neurosurgery & Psychiatry 54 (4): 345–350.

74. Foundas, A.L., Macauley, B.L., Raymer, A.M. et al. (1995). Ecological implications of limb apraxia: evidence from mealtime behavior. Journal of the International Neuropsychological Society 1 (1): 62–66.

75. Hochstenbach, J. and Mulder, T. (1999). Neuropsychology and the relearning of motor skills following stroke. International Journal of Rehabilitation Research 22 (1): 11–19.

76. Kalra, L., Perez, I., Gupta, S., and Wittink, M. (1997). The influence of visual neglect on stroke rehabilitation. Stroke 28 (7): 1386–1391.

77. Finsterer, J., Stöllberger, C., and Kopsa, W. (2004). Weight reduction due to stroke-induced dysgeusia. European Neurology 51 (1): 47–49.

78. Heckmann, J.G., Stössel, C., Lang, C.J. et al. (2005). Taste disorders in acute stroke: a prospective observational study on taste disorders in 102 stroke patients. Stroke 36 (8): 1690–1694.

79. Kim, J.S. and Choi, S. (2002). Altered food preference after cortical infarction: Korean style. Cerebrovascular Diseases 13 (3): 187–191.

80. Pritchard, T.C., Macaluso, D.A., and Eslinger, P.J. (1999). Taste perception in patients with insular cortex lesions. Behavioral Neuroscience 113 (4): 663.

81. Kumbargere Nagraj, S., Naresh, S., Srinivas, K. et al. (2014). Interventions for the management of taste disturbances. Cochrane Database of Systematic Reviews 11 (Art. No.: CD010470). https://doi.org/10.1002/14651858.CD010470.pub2.

82. Hackett, M.L. and Pickles, K. (2014). Part I: frequency of depression after stroke: an updated systematic review and meta-analysis of observational studies. International Journal of Stroke 9 (8): 1017–1025.

83. Brozek, J. (1985). Malnutrition and Human Behavior. New York: Van Nostrand Reinhold.

84. Gillen, R., Tennen, H., McKee, T.E. et al. (2001). Depressive symptoms and history of depression predict rehabilitation efficiency in stroke patients. Archives of Physical Medicine and Rehabilitation 82 (12): 1645–1649.

85. Bruinsma, K.A. and Taren, D.L. (2000). Dieting, essential fatty acid intake, and depression. Nutrition Reviews 58 (4): 98–108.

86. Chen, Z., Sea, M., Kwan, K. et al. (1997). Depletion of linoleate induced by weight cycling is independent of extent of calorie restriction. American Journal of Physiology-Regulatory, Integrative and Comparative Physiology 272 (1): R43–R50.

87. Age Concern (2006). Hungry to Be Heard: The Scandal of Malnourished Older People in Hospital. London: Age Concern England.

88. Department of Health (2004). Standards for Better Health. London: Department of Health.

89. Jacobsson, C., Axelsson, K., Norberg, A. et al. (1997). Outcomes of individualized interventions in patients with severe eating difficulties. Clinical Nursing Research 6 (1): 25–44.

90. Gandolfi, M., Smania, N., Bisoffi, G. et al. (2014). Improving post-stroke dysphagia outcomes through a standardized and multidisciplinary protocol: an exploratory cohort study. Dysphagia 29 (6): 704–712.

91. Omidvari, A.H., Vali, Y., Murray, S.M. et al. (2013). Nutritional screening for improving professional practice for patient outcomes in hospital and primary care settings. Cochrane Database of Systematic Reviews 6 (Art. No.: CD005539) https://doi.org/10.1002/14651858.CD010470.pub2.

92. National Institute for Health and Care Excellence (NICE) (2006). Nutrition Support in Adults: Oral Nutrition Support, Enteral Tube Feeding and Parenteral Nutrition. London: National Institute for Health and Clinical Excellence.

93. Beck, A. and Ovesen, L. (1998). At which body mass index and degree of weight loss should hospitalized elderly patients be considered at nutritional risk? Clinical Nutrition 17 (5): 195–198.

94. Council of Europe Committee of Ministers. Resolution ResAP(2003)3 on Food and Nutritional Care in Hospitals. Strasbourg: Council of Europe Committee of Ministers; 2003.

95. Hinchey, J.A., Shephard, T., Furie, K. et al. (2005). Formal dysphagia screening protocols prevent pneumonia. Stroke 36 (9): 1972–1976.

96. Middleton, S., McElduff, P., Ward, J. et al. (2011). Implementation of evidence-based treatment protocols to manage fever, hyperglycaemia, and swallowing dysfunction in acute stroke (QASC): a cluster randomised controlled trial. The Lancet 378 (9804): 1699–1706.

97. Donovan, N.J., Daniels, S.K., Edmiaston, J. et al. (2013). Dysphagia screening: state of the art. Invitational conference proceeding from the state-of-the-art nursing symposium. Stroke 44 (4): e24–e31.

98. Perry, L. (2001). Screening swallowing function of patients with acute stroke. Part one: Identification, implementation and initial evaluation of a screening tool for use by nurses. Journal of Clinical Nursing 10 (4): 463–473.

99. Scottish Intercollegiate Guidelines Network. Management of patients with stroke: identification and management of dysphagia, a national clinical guideline. No. 119. Edinburgh: SIGN; 2010. Available from: https://www.sign.ac.uk/assets/sign119.pdf [30 November 2018].

100. Stroke Foundation (2017). Clinical Guidelines for Stroke Management. Melbourne: Stroke Foundation.

101. Daniels, S.K., McAdam, C.P., Brailey, K., and Foundas, A.L. (1997). Clinical assessment of swallowing and prediction of dysphagia severity. American Journal of Speech-Language Pathology 6 (4): 17–24.

102. DePippo, K.L., Holas, M.A., and Reding, M.J. (1992). Validation of the 3-oz water swallow test for aspiration following stroke. Archives of Neurology 49 (12): 1259–1261.

103. Suiter, D.M. and Leder, S.B. (2008). Clinical utility of the 3-ounce water swallow test. Dysphagia 23 (3): 244–250.

104. Edmiaston, J., Connor, L.T., Loehr, L., and Nassief, A. (2010). Validation of a dysphagia screening tool in acute stroke patients. American Journal of Critical Care 19 (4): 357–364.

105. Smithard, D.G., O'Neill, P.A., England, R.E. et al. (1997). The natural history of dysphagia following a stroke. Dysphagia 12 (4): 188–193.

106. Smithard, D.G., O'Neill, P.A., Park, C. et al. (1998). Can bedside assessment reliably exclude aspiration following acute stroke? Age and Ageing 27 (2): 99–106.

107. Ramsey, D.J., Smithard, D.G., and Kalra, L. (2003). Early assessments of dysphagia and aspiration risk in acute stroke patients. Stroke 34 (5): 1252–1257.

108. Turner-Lawrence, D.E., Peebles, M., Price, M.F. et al. (2009). A feasibility study of the sensitivity of emergency physician dysphagia screening in acute stroke patients. Annals of Emergency Medicine 54 (3): 344–348.

109. Trapl, M., Enderle, P., Nowotny, M. et al. (2007). Dysphagia bedside screening for acute-stroke patients: the Gugging Swallowing Screen. Stroke 38 (11): 2948–2952.

110. Antonios, N., Carnaby-Mann, G., Crary, M. et al. (2010). Analysis of a physician tool for evaluating dysphagia on an inpatient stroke unit: the modified mann assessment of swallowing ability. Journal of Stroke and Cerebrovascular Diseases 19 (1): 49–57.

111. Martino, R., Silver, F., Teasell, R. et al. (2009). The Toronto Bedside Swallowing Screening Test (TOR-BSST): development and validation of a dysphagia screening tool for patients with stroke. Stroke 40 (2): 555–561.

112. Govan, L., Langhorne, P., and Weir, C.J. (2007). Does the prevention of complications explain the survival benefit of organized inpatient (stroke unit) care? Further analysis of a systematic review. Stroke 38 (9): 2536–2540.

113. Cuesy, P.G., Sotomayor, P.L., and Piña, J.O.T. (2010). Reduction in the incidence of poststroke nosocomial pneumonia by using the 'turn-mob' program. Journal of Stroke and Cerebrovascular Diseases 19 (1): 23–28.

114. Titsworth, W.L., Abram, J., Fullerton, A. et al. (2013). Prospective quality initiative to maximize dysphagia screening reduces hospital-acquired pneumonia prevalence in patients with stroke. Stroke 44 (11): 3154–3160.

115. Gosney, M., Martin, M., and Wright, A. (2006). The role of selective decontamination of the digestive tract in acute stroke. Age and Ageing 35 (1): 42–47.

116. Warusevitane, A., Karunatilake, D., Sim, J. et al. (2015). Safety and effect of metoclopramide to prevent pneumonia in patients with stroke fed via nasogastric tubes trial. Stroke 46 (2): 454–460.

117. Gomes, G.F., Pisani, J.C., Macedo, E.D., and Campos, A.C. (2003). The nasogastric feeding tube as a risk factor for aspiration and aspiration pneumonia. Current Opinion in Clinical Nutrition & Metabolic Care 6 (3): 327–333.

118. Westendorp, W.F., Vermeij, J.-D., Vermeij, F. et al. (2012). Antibiotic therapy for preventing infections in patients with acute stroke. Cochrane Database of Systematic Reviews 1 (Art. No.: CD008530). https://doi.org/10.1002/14651858.CD008530.pub2.

119. Westendorp, W.F., Vermeij, J.-D., Zock, E. et al. (2015). The Preventive Antibiotics in Stroke Study (PASS): a pragmatic randomised open-label masked endpoint clinical trial. The Lancet 385 (9977): 1519–1526.

120. Kalra, L., Irshad, S., Hodsoll, J. et al. (2015). Prophylactic antibiotics after acute stroke for reducing pneumonia in patients with dysphagia (STROKE-INF): a prospective, cluster-randomised, open-label, masked endpoint, controlled clinical trial. The Lancet 386 (10006): 1835–1844.

121. Cohen, D.L., Roffe, C., Beavan, J. et al. (2016). Post-stroke dysphagia: a review and design considerations for future trials. International Journal of Stroke 11 (4): 399–411.

122. Dennis, M., Lewis, S., Cranswick, G., and Forbes, J. FOOD Trial Collaboration.(2006). FOOD: a multicentre randomised trial evaluating feeding policies in patients admitted to hospital with a recent stroke. Health Technology Assessment 10 (2): 1–120.

123. Geeganage, C., Beavan, J., Ellender, S., and Bath, P.M.W. (2012). Interventions for dysphagia and nutritional support in acute and subacute stroke. Cochrane Database of Systematic Reviews 10 (Art. No.: CD000323). https://doi.org/10.1002/14651858. CD000323.pub2.

124. Lennard-Jones, J.E. (1998). Ethical and Legal Aspects of Clinical Hydration and Nutritional Support. Maidenhead: British Association for Parenteral and Enteral Nutrition.

125. Department of Health (2005). Mental Health Capacity Act. London: Her Majesty's Stationery Office.

126. Elter, J., Offenbacher, S., Toole, J., and Beck, J. (2003). Relationship of periodontal disease and edentulism to stroke/TIA. Journal of Dental Research 82 (12): 998–1001.

127. Marks, L. and Rainbow, D. (2003). Working with Dysphagia. Oxon: Speechmark Publishing.

128. Farrell, J.H. (1956). The effect of mastication on the digestion of food. British Dental Journal 100: 149–155.

129. Krall, E., Hayes, C., and Garcia, R. (1998). How dentition status and masticatory function affect nutrient intake. Journal of the American Dental Association 129 (9): 1261–1269.

130. Sheiham, A., Steele, J., Marcenes, W. et al. (2001). The relationship among dental status, nutrient intake, and nutritional status in older people. Journal of Dental Research 80 (2): 408–413.

131. Chen, Y.-W., Chang, K.-H., Chen, H.-C. et al. (2016). The effects of surface neuromuscular electrical stimulation on post-stroke dysphagia: a systemic review and meta-analysis. Clinical Rehabilitation 30 (1): 24–35.

132. Bisch, E.M., Logemann, J.A., Rademaker, A.W. et al. (1994). Pharyngeal effects of bolus volume, viscosity, and temperature in patients with dysphagia resulting from neurologic impairment and in normal subjects. Journal of Speech and Hearing Research 37 (5): 1041–1049.

133. Logemann, J.A., Pauloski, B.R., Colangelo, L. et al. (1995). Effects of a sour bolus on oropharyngeal swallowing measures in patients with neurogenic dysphagia. Journal of Speech, Language, and Hearing Research 38 (3): 556–563.

134. Rosenbek, J.C., Roecker, E.B., Wood, J.L., and Robbins, J. (1996). Thermal application reduces the duration of stage transition in dysphagia after stroke. Dysphagia 11 (4): 225–233.

135. Whelan, K. (2001). Inadequate fluid intakes in dysphagic acute stroke. Clinical Nutrition 20 (5): 423–428.

136. Rosenvinge, S.K. and Starke, I.D. (2005). Improving care for patients with dysphagia. Age and Ageing 34 (6): 587–593.

137. Garon, B.R., Engle, M., and Ormiston, C. (1997). A randomized control study to determine the effects of unlimited oral intake of water in patients with identified aspiration. Journal of Neurologic Rehabilitation 11 (3): 139–148.

138. Cichero, J.A., Lam, P., Steele, C.M. et al. (2017). Development of international terminology and definitions for texture-modified foods and thickened fluids used in dysphagia management: the IDDSI framework. Dysphagia 32 (2): 293–314.

139. International Dysphagia Diet Standardization Initiative Complete. IDDSI Framework 2016. Available from: https://iddsi.org/framework/ [30 November 2018]

140. Dennis, M.S., Lewis, S.C., and Warlow, C. (2005). Routine oral nutritional supplementation for stroke patients in hospital (FOOD): a multicentre randomised controlled trial. The Lancet 365 (9461): 755–763.

141. Ojo, O. (2015). The challenges of home enteral tube feeding: a global perspective. Nutrients 7 (4): 2524–2538.

142. British Association for Parenteral and Enteral Nutrition (BAPEN). BANS Reports. Available from: https://www.bapen.org.uk/resources-and-education/publications-and-reports/bans [30 November 2018]

143. Rabeneck, L., McCullough, L.B., and Wray, N.P. (1997). Ethically justified, clinically comprehensive guidelines for percutaneous endoscopic gastrostomy tube placement. The Lancet 349 (9050): 496–498.

144. Metheny, N., Wehrle, M.A., Wiersema, L., and Clark, J. (1998). Testing feeding tube placement: auscultation vs. pH method. American Journal of Nursing 98 (5): 37–42.

145. Williams, J. (2005). Using an alternative fixing device for nasogastric tubes. Nursing Times 101 (35): 26–27.

146. Lien, H.-C., Chang, C.-S., and Chen, G.-H. (2000). Can percutaneous endoscopic jejunostomy prevent gastroesophageal reflux in patients with preexisting esophagitis? American Journal of Gastroenterology 95 (12): 3439.

147. Colagiovanni, L. (2000). Preventing and clearing blocked feeding tubes. Nursing Times 96 (17 Suppl.): 3–4.

148. Elia M. The Malnutrition Advisory Group consensus guidelines for the detection and management of malnutrition in the community. Available from: https://onlinelibrary.wiley.com/doi/full/10.1046/j.1467-3010.2001.00111.x [30 November 2018].

149. de Jong, N., Mulder, I., de Graaf, C., and van Staveren, W.A. (1999). Impaired sensory functioning in elders: the relation with its potential determinants and nutritional intake. Journals of Gerontology Series A: Biomedical Sciences and Medical Sciences 54 (8): B324–B331.

150. Schiffman, S. and Graham, B. (2000). Taste and smell perception affect appetite and immunity in the elderly. European Journal of Clinical Nutrition 54 (S3): S54–S63.

151. Schiffman, S.S. and Warwick, Z.S. (1993). Effect of flavor enhancement of foods for the elderly on nutritional status: food intake, biochemical indices, and anthropometric measures. Physiology & Behavior 53 (2): 395–402.

152. Harley, C., Boyd, J., Cockburn, J. et al. (2006). Disruption of sitting balance after stroke: influence of spoken output. Journal of Neurology, Neurosurgery & Psychiatry 77 (5): 674–676.

153. Koltin, S.E. and Rosen, H.S. (1996). Hemiplegia and feeding: an occupational therapy approach to upper extremity management. Topics in Stroke Rehabilitation 3 (3): 69–86.

154. Martinsen, B., Harder, I., and Biering-Sorensen, F. (2008). The meaning of assisted feeding for people living with spinal cord injury: a phenomenological study. Journal of Advanced Nursing 62 (5): 533–540.

155. Sorensen, H.V., Lendal, S., Schultz-Larsen, K., and Uhrskov, T. (2003). Stroke rehabilitation: assistive technology devices and environmental modifications following primary rehabilitation in hospital – a therapeutic perspective. Assistive Technology 15 (1): 39–48.

156. Hackett, M.L., Anderson, C.S., House, A., and Halteh, C. (2008). Interventions for preventing depression after stroke. Cochrane Database of Systematic Reviews 3 (Art. No.: CD003689). https://doi.org/10.1002/14651858.CD003689.pub3.

CHAPTER 6

Oral Care After Stroke

Mary Lyons

Liverpool School of Tropical Medicine, Liverpool, UK

University of Central Lancashire, Preston, UK

KEY POINTS

- Poor oral hygiene may be linked with an increased risk of aspiration pneumonia – a leading cause of mortality post-stroke.
- Oral care is often done poorly and delegated to the least qualified members of the care team.
- Nursing staff receive little training and guidelines are based on weak evidence, and lack detail about how best to provide oral care.
- Evidence is lacking whether good oral care can reduce the risk of aspiration pneumonia or mortality.
- Clinically relevant, effective, feasible, evidence-based oral care interventions capable of improving patient outcomes in stroke care are urgently needed.

This chapter maps to criteria within the following sections of the Stroke-Specific Education Framework (SSEF):

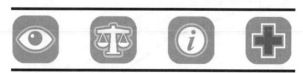

And you know you're wanting to go and give him a kiss to reassure him and give him a love, but ... at the same time kind of thinking hmm no, no. And it's awful because it's your dad and you shouldn't have to feel like that.

Stroke Nursing, Second Edition. Edited by Jane Williams, Lin Perry, and Caroline Watkins.
© 2020 John Wiley & Sons Ltd. Published 2020 by John Wiley & Sons Ltd.

6.1 Introduction

Poor oral care can have serious mental, physical and social consequences, and adversely affect quality of life after a stroke [2–4]. Poor oral hygiene may increase the risk of developing aspiration pneumonia [5, 6], which causes the highest attributable mortality of all medical complications following a stroke; its prevention is therefore of great importance [7, 8]. Evidence is weak but suggests that good oral hygiene and plaque control may reduce the risk of aspiration pneumonia [9–14].

Several common problems occurring after a stroke increase the risk of pneumonia. Dysphagia and loss of oro-motor and sensory function can affect up to 78% of patients who have recently had a stroke (see Chapter 5), causing stasis of saliva and food in the oral cavity [15–18]. Reduced tongue pressure and altered lateral movements are common and can result in food pooling in the sulci of the oral cavity, leading to stomatitis and problems with dentures [19, 20]. Higher-than-normal pathogenic bacterial and yeast counts have been recorded in the oral cavity of patients during the acute phase of stroke [10, 21, 22].

Stroke is common in the elderly [23] and improvements in diet and dental care mean that there is an increasing trend for people to retain their own natural teeth as they age [24]. Figure 6.1 shows the proportion of people with 21 or more natural teeth increasing in all age groups over recent decades. This has implications for dental care, as very few elderly people have excellent oral health; most have periodontal disease and fillings, with implants becoming more common [25]. A significant proportion of the expected increase in the cost of dental care in the European Union, from €54 billion in 2000 to €93 billion in 2020, comes from the provision of oral care for the growing number of dependent older people – including those who have had a stroke [26, 27].

The trend towards better dental health is further indicated by the fall in the proportion of people who are edentulous (i.e. have no natural teeth). Figure 6.2 shows how the risk of being edentulous in all age groups reduced in England

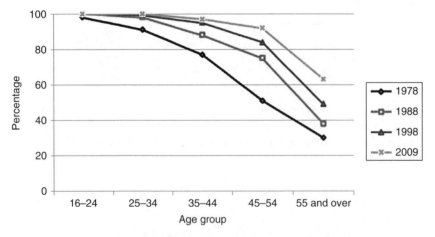

FIGURE 6.1 Trends in the percentage of adults with 21 or more natural teeth by age, England 1978–2009. *Source: [24]. Copyright © 2016, Re-used with the permission of the NHS Health and Social Care Information Centre, also known as NHS Digital. All rights reserved.*

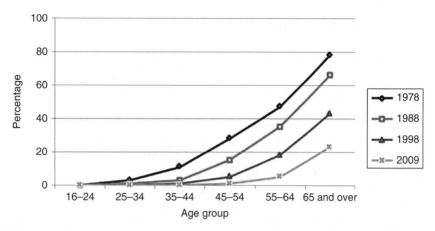

FIGURE 6.2   Trends in percentage edentate by age, England 1978–2009. *Source: [24].*
Copyright © 2016, Re-used with the permission of the NHS Health and Social Care
Information Centre, also known as NHS Digital. All rights reserved.

between 1978 and 2009. It can be more difficult to maintain oral hygiene in
those with partial dentition than in the edentulous, who tend to be better on this
score [28].

6.2   Oral Assessment

A prompt oral assessment facilitates the development of an oral care plan based
on individual stroke patient's needs. Poor oral hygiene is a risk factor for stroke,
and together with neglect of oral care is common in stroke patients [13, 29]. A
recent systematic review of oral health amongst patients with stroke found that
they had poorer oral health across a range of parameters (tooth loss, dental caries,
and periodontal status) than healthy controls [29]. Although a cause-and-effect
relationship cannot be presumed, a growing body of work suggests an association
between the inflammatory processes associated with periodontal disease and
increased risk of stroke [30–33].

An oral assessment can also identify potential problems that could affect
recovery and would benefit from referral for specialist dental or speech and language therapy input [34]. Few evidence-based oral assessment tools or guidelines
exist; those that do are rarely used, and none have been specifically developed
or validated with stroke patients [35, 36]. Available oral assessment protocols
score features such as saliva, soft tissues, and odour; some also include dental
plaque, oral function, swallowing, voice quality, and hard tissue assessment. For
example, the BRUSHED assessment (Bleeding, Redness, Ulceration, Saliva, Halitosis, External factors, Debris) is a useful mnemonic designed to prompt nurses to
assess these important oral health signs and symptoms [37]. The holistic and reliable oral assessment tool (THROAT) was originally developed to assess oral health
in elderly hospitalised patients, but has been used with acute stroke patients [38].
Nurses are well placed to conduct an initial oral assessment and can be trained to
identify patients who may need referral to a dental specialist [39].

Management and Care

Regular oral care is important for the maintenance of healthy teeth and gums, and promotes comfort [2]. Hospitalisation, reduced food and drink intake, increased exposure to antibiotics, and dependency are some of the factors that can reduce stroke patients' ability to maintain oral hygiene effectively [35, 40]. Until safe swallowing is established, stroke patients are not given oral fluids [34]. Dehydration is common, and is exacerbated by oxygen therapy, mouth breathing, and the side-effects of medications; xerostomia can quickly develop, increasing the risk of oral infections, root surface caries, and discomfort [41, 42].

Dependent stroke patients rely on nurses for oral care, but this can be particularly challenging in dysphagic patients, who may be unable to prevent toothpaste or rinsing fluids from entering their airway. Oral care is often given low priority by nurses and delegated to the least qualified member of the care team [43]. A number of national guidelines refer to oral care following a stroke, and discuss the lack of evidence to support detailed guidance [44–49]. For example, Section 4.11 of the English Clinical Guideline for Stroke [34] refers to the need to brush teeth with toothpaste or chlorhexidine gel and mentions the possibility of using an electric toothbrush. It also advises that patients with dentures should have them cleaned and put in during the day, and flags the need for staff training. The Guidelines for the Oral Healthcare of Stroke Survivors [50] are more comprehensive, but focus on dental healthcare. Section 3.2 says that oral health should form part of the early stroke unit assessment and that continual monitoring of oral health is needed until independence is resumed. Section 4.2 suggests that an oral hygiene care plan should be developed based on specific protocols taken from the British Society for Disability and Oral Health Guidelines [51]. Key points are that brushing the teeth of a dysphagic stroke patient should be done using aspiration and a small amount of toothpaste and that dehydration-related xerostomia, a common problem, can be managed using sugar-free chewing gum, which stimulates salivary flow [52]. Saliva substitutes in the form of mouth rinses, sprays, and gels may be helpful, but their effect can be short-lived [53]. When there is no risk of dysphagia, the guidelines recommend encouraging oral fluids.

There is currently neither evidence nor consensus guidance for best practice in the assessment, equipment, procedure, or frequency of oral care for dysphagic and other stroke patients. No guidelines contain information or advice on how best to reduce the risk of choking when delivering oral care for this group. Despite some degree of shared understanding about what good oral care might include, practice in different locations varies widely, and staff report feeling insufficiently trained to deliver oral care effectively [35, 54–56].

As the stroke patient moves from the acute to the recovery stage, oral care priorities change, but still still need to focus on maintaining simple preventative care measures. Basic oral care should be combined with early diagnosis and referral for the management of dental pathology so that dentition, natural or prosthetic, can be maintained. Lack of appropriate training and failure to prioritise oral care within the stroke care pathway has the biggest impact on the patients with greatest need, who are at high risk of complications [12]. A Cochrane review of staff-led interventions for improving oral hygiene following a stroke concluded that provision of training in oral care interventions can improve staff knowledge and attitudes, the cleanliness of patients' dentures, and perhaps the incidence of pneumonia [2]. However, the evidence was weak, and improvements in the cleanliness of patients' teeth were not observed. Whilst there is little high-quality evidence, several oral hygiene interventions appear to be feasible and well-tolerated in early-stage studies [57–63]. Antiseptic agents such as chlorhexidine appear to reduce oropharyngeal carriage of bacteria, but in many studies the impact of antiseptic agents could not be distinguished from the adjunctive mechanical oral hygiene measures, and no significant decrease in risk of pneumonia was apparent [14, 59, 64].

6.4 Patient and Carer Perspective

Stroke patients often experience oral discomfort and pain, oral infections (especially oral candidiasis), and difficulties in denture-wearing [3, 4, 40, 58]. Normal daily activities that affect oral hygiene, such as eating, drinking and tooth-brushing, can be severely disrupted [65]. Over time, lack of adequate oral care will lead to progression of dental caries and periodontal disease, which can result in tooth loss and pain. This impacts patients' ability to eat and their quality of life, and may complicate ongoing medical management [66, 67]. Case Study 6.1 highlights some common oral care issues. Table 6.1 summarises findings from studies exploring stroke patients', carers', and professionals' experience of oral care [2, 69, 70].

Case Study

Case 6.1 Bert

Following his stroke, 78-year-old Bert has a severe right-sided weakness, expressive and receptive dysphasia, and dysphagia. Initially treated in an acute stroke unit, he is later moved to a rehabilitation ward. He has poor sitting balance and limited right-sided movement. Bert takes nothing orally, receives nutrition through a percutaneous endoscopic gastrostomy (PEG) tube, and is dependent on the nurses for his care.

Bert's daughter Jenny is his principal advocate. Jenny says that prior to the stroke, Bert took great pride in his appearance. He regularly visited the dentist and was vigilant about his oral care. In the initial period after his stroke, Bert was diagnosed with pneumonia and was given antibiotics and oxygen therapy. During this time, he tended to breathe through his mouth and developed oral candidiasis with cold sores on his lips. Jenny talks about him having 'Yellow filmy stuff on his teeth'. The state of Bert's mouth and teeth affects Jenny's relationship with her father and makes her want to keep her distance.

Jenny notices inconsistencies in the way the nurses clean her father's mouth. Sometimes they use pink sponges, sometimes swabs or cotton-wool balls. She remarks that the pink sponges are not very effective in removing the yellow film but may help keep the mouth moist. In the rehabilitation ward, the nurses use toothbrushes which can be attached to a suction machine and toothpaste, which results in a big improvement in her father's oral health. Bert clearly appreciates the oral care he receives, and Jenny comments that leaving someone's mouth in an unhygienic state must be uncomfortable.

Jenny says that she would be more than willing to help with oral care, but doesn't know how to, and is afraid of making her father choke. She feels that if carers such as herself were given training, they could provide oral care when they visited their relatives. Jenny judges that delivering oral care is an intimate procedure that provides nurses an opportunity to interact with their patients.

TABLE 6.1	Stroke patients', carers', and professionals' experience of oral care

- Oral care is perceived as important by patients, carers, and professionals [68].
- Patients feel anxious and distressed about their appearance and worry about their lack of control over saliva or that they may have halitosis [3, 68].
- Lack of care is common and is a cause of distress for patients and their families [68].
- Nurses make assumptions about patients' ability to attend to their own oral care, and patients find it difficult to ask for what they need [54, 68].
- Relatives and friends express empathy but feel powerless to intervene and provide oral care [54, 68].
- Basic materials needed to provide good oral care are often unavailable in stroke units [56].
- There is uncertainty and fear amongst nurses and carers about the best way to provide oral care for stroke patients, especially when dysphagia is present [35, 54].

6.5   Conclusion

Lack of knowledge and understanding about oral care and inadequate research to inform best practice in acute stroke care, rehabilitation, and nursing home settings are hampering best practice. Evidence on the impact of oral care on risk of pneumonia in the acute stroke setting is lacking [57]. Nurses feel inadequately trained to provide oral care, especially when dysphagia or other problems are present, and it tends to be given low priority [54]. There is an urgent need for evidence and guidance on nursing care standards to overcome the barriers to good oral health care experienced by stroke patients.

Acknowledgements

Lyons M, Smith CEB, Brady M, Brocklehurst P, Dickinson H, Hamdy S, Higham S, Langhorne P, Lightbody L, McCracken G, Medina-Lara A, Sproson L, Walls A, and Watkins C. Oral care after stroke: where are we now? *European Stroke Journal* 2018. 10.1177/2396987318775206

References

1. Stroke Specific Education Framework. Available from: http://www.stroke-education.org.uk/framework [30 November 2018].
2. Brady, M.C., Furlanetto, D., Hunter, R. et al. (2006). Staff-led interventions for improving oral hygiene in patients following stroke (updated 2011). Cochrane Database of Systematic Reviews 4 (Art. No.: CD003864). https://doi.org/10.1002/14651858.CD003864.pub2.

3. Schimmel, M., Leemann, B., Christou, P. et al. (2011). Oral health-related quality of life in hospitalised stroke patients. Gerodontology 28 (1): 3–11.

4. Locker, D., Clarke, M., and Payne, B. (2000). Self-perceived oral health status, psychological well-being, and life satisfaction in an older adult population. Journal of Dental Research 79 (4): 970–975.

5. Scannapieco, F.A., Bush, R.B., and Paju, S. (2003). Associations between periodontal disease and risk for nosocomial bacterial pneumonia and chronic obstructive pulmonary disease. A systematic review. Annals of Periodontology 8 (1): 54–69.

6. Terpenning, M.S., Taylor, G.W., Lopatin, D.E. et al. (2001). Aspiration pneumonia: dental and oral risk factors in an older veteran population. Journal of the American Geriatrics Society 49 (5): 557–563.

7. Langhorne, P., Stott, D.J., Robertson, L. et al. (2000). Medical complications after stroke: a multicenter study. Stroke 31 (6): 1223–1229.

8. Katzan, I.L., Cebul, R.D., Husak, S.H. et al. (2003). The effect of pneumonia on mortality among patients hospitalized for acute stroke. Neurology 60 (4): 620–625.

9. Sjögren, P., Nilsson, E., Forsell, M. et al. (2008). A systematic review of the preventive effect of oral hygiene on pneumonia and respiratory tract infection in elderly people in hospitals and nursing homes: effect estimates and methodological quality of randomized controlled trials. Journal of the American Geriatrics Society 56 (11): 2124–2130.

10. Chipps, E., Gatens, C., Genter, L. et al. (2014). Pilot study of an oral care protocol on poststroke survivors. Rehabilitation Nursing 39 (6): 294–304.

11. Yoneyama, T., Yoshida, M., Ohrui, T. et al. (2002). Oral care reduces pneumonia in older patients in nursing homes. Journal of the American Geriatrics Society 50 (3): 430–433.

12. Wagner, C., Marchina, S., Deveau, J.A. et al. (2016). Risk of stroke-associated pneumonia and oral hygiene. Cerebrovascular Diseases 41 (1–2): 35–39.

13. Kuo, Y.W., Yen, M., Fetzer, S. et al. (2015). Effect of family caregiver oral care training on stroke survivor oral and respiratory health in Taiwan: a randomised controlled trial. Community Dental Health 32 (3): 137–142.

14. Juthani-Mehta, M., Van Ness, P.H., McGloin, J. et al. (2015). A cluster-randomized controlled trial of a multicomponent intervention protocol for pneumonia prevention among nursing home elders. Clinical Infectious Diseases 60 (6): 849–857.

15. Singh, S. and Hamdy, S. (2006). Dysphagia in stroke patients. Postgraduate Medical Journal 82 (968): 383–391.

16. Martino, R., Foley, N., Bhogal, S. et al. (2005). Dysphagia after stroke: incidence, diagnosis, and pulmonary complications. Stroke 36 (12): 2756–2763.

17. Teismann, I.K., Steinstraeter, O., Stoeckigt, K. et al. (2007). Functional oropharyngeal sensory disruption interferes with the cortical control of swallowing. BMC Neuroscience 8 (1): 62.

18. Sorensen, R.T., Rasmussen, R.S., Overgaard, K. et al. (2013). Dysphagia screening and intensified oral hygiene reduce pneumonia after stroke. Journal of Neuroscience Nursing 45 (3): 139–146.

19. Hori, K., Ono, T., Iwata, H. et al. (2005). Tongue pressure against hard palate during swallowing in post-stroke patients. Gerodontology 22 (4): 227–233.

20. Kim, I.S. and Han, T.R. (2005). Influence of mastication and salivation on swallowing in stroke patients. Archives of Physical Medicine and Rehabilitation 86 (10): 1986–1990.

21. Zhu, H.W., McMillan, A.S., McGrath, C. et al. (2008). Oral carriage of yeasts and coliforms in stroke sufferers: a prospective longitudinal study. Oral Diseases 14 (1): 60–66.

22. Millns, B., Gosney, M., Jack, C. et al. (2003). Acute stroke predisposes to oral gram-negative bacilli – a cause of aspiration pneumonia? Gerontology 49 (3): 173–176.

23. Feigin, V.L., Forouzanfar, M.H., Krishnamurthi, R. et al. (2014). Global and regional burden of stroke during 1990–2010: findings from the Global Burden of Disease Study 2010. The Lancet 383 (9913): 245–254.

24. Office for National Statistics Social Survey Division Information Centre for Health and Social Care. Adult Dental Health Survey 2009. 2nd Edition, 2012. Available from: https://beta.ukdataservice.ac.uk/datacatalogue/doi/?id=6884#!#2 [30 November 2018].

25. Derks, J. and Tomasi, C. (2015). Peri-implant health and disease. A systematic review of current epidemiology. Journal of Clinical Periodontol 42 (Suppl. 16): S158–S171.

26. Glick, M., Monteiro da Silva, O., Seeberger, G.K. et al. (2012). FDI vision 2020: shaping the future of oral health. International Dental Journal 62 (6): 278–291.

27. Widström, E., Eaton, K., and Vanobbergen, J. (2004). Oral healthcare systems in the extended European Union, partim: [Oral Health care system in] Belgium. Oral Health and Preventive Dentistry 2 (3): 155–194.

28. Zuluaga, D.J.M., Ferreira, J., Montoya, J.A.G., and Willumsen, T. (2012). Oral health in institutionalised elderly people in Oslo, Norway and its relationship with dependence and cognitive impairment. Gerodontology 29 (2): e420–e426.

29. Dai, R., Lam, O.L., Lo, E.C. et al. (2015). A systematic review and meta-analysis of clinical, microbiological, and behavioural aspects of oral health among patients with stroke. Journal of Dentistry 43 (2): 171–180.

30. Dorfer, C.E., Becher, H., Ziegler, C.M. et al. (2004). The association of gingivitis and periodontitis with ischemic stroke. Journal of Clinical Periodontology 31 (5): 396–401.

31. Slowik, J., Wnuk, M.A., Grzech, K. et al. (2010). Periodontitis affects neurological deficit in acute stroke. Journal of the Neurological Sciences 297 (1–2): 82–84.

32. Sellars, C., Bowie, L., Bagg, J. et al. (2007). Risk factors for chest infection in acute stroke. A Prospective Cohort Study 38 (8): 2284–2291.

33. Azarpazhooh, A. and Leake, J.L. (2006). Systematic review of the association between respiratory diseases and oral health. Journal of Periodontology 77 (9): 1465–1482.

34. Intercollegiate Stroke Working Party (2016). National Clinical Guideline for Stroke, 5e. London: Royal College of Physicians.

35. Kwok, C., McIntyre, A., Janzen, S. et al. (2015). Oral care post stroke: a scoping review. Journal of Oral Rehabilitation 42 (1): 65–74.

36. Abidia, R.F. (2007). Oral care in the intensive care unit: a review. Journal of Contemporary Dental Practice 8 (1): 76–82.

37. Hayes, J. and Jones, C. (1995). A collaborative approach to oral care during critical illness. Dental Health 34: 6–10.

38. McKenzie, K. (2015). Feasibility and Criterion Validity of the Holistic and Reliable Oral Assessment Tool (THROAT) in Acute Dysphagic Stroke Patients. Manchester: University of Manchester.

39. Jones, H. (2005). Oral care in intensive care units: a literature review. Special Care in Dentistry 25 (1): 6–11.

40. Hunter, R.V., Clarkson, J.E., Fraser, H.W., and MacWalter, R.S. (2006). A preliminary investigation into tooth care, dental attendance and oral health related quality of life in adult stroke survivors in Tayside, Scotland. Gerodontology 23 (3): 140–148.

41. Kerr, G.D., Sellars, C., Bowie, L. et al. (2009). Xerostomia after acute stroke. Cerebrovascular Diseases 28 (6): 624–626.

42. Bahouth, M.N., Bahrainwala, Z., Hillis, A.E., and Gottesman, R.F. (2016). Dehydration status is associated with more severe hemispatial neglect after stroke. The Neurologist 21 (6): 101–105.

43. Costello, T. and Coyne, I. (2008). Nurses' knowledge of mouth care practices. British Journal of Nursing 17 (4): 264–268.

44. Casaubon, L.K., Boulanger, J.M., Glasser, E. et al. (2016). Canadian stroke best practice recommendations: acute inpatient stroke care guidelines, update 2015. International Journal of Stroke 11 (2): 239–252.

45. Boddice, G., Brauer, S., Gustafsson, L. et al. (2010). Clinical Guidelines for Stroke Management. Melbourne: Australian Government National Health and Medical Research Council.

46. Management of stroke rehabilitation working group (2010). VA/DOD clinical practice guideline for the management of stroke rehabilitation. Journal of Rehabilitation Research and Development 47 (9): 1–43.

47. Scottish Intercollegiate Guidelines Network. Management of patients with stroke: identification and management of dysphagia, a national clinical guideline. No. 119. Edinburgh: SIGN; 2010. Available from: https://www.sign.ac.uk/assets/sign119.pdf [30 November 2018].

48. Raghunathan, S., Freeman, A., and Bhowmick, B. (2009). Mouth care after stroke. Gerimed: Midlife Beyond 39: 582–586.

49. Griffiths, J. and Lewis, D. (2002). Guidelines for the oral care of patients who are dependent, dysphagic or critically ill. Journal of Disability and Oral Health 3 (1): 30–33.

50. British Society of Gerodontology (2010). Guidelines for the Oral Healthcare of Stroke Survivors. London: British Society of Gerodontology.

51. Griffiths, J., Jones, V., Leeman, I. et al. (2000). Guidelines for the Development of Local Standards of Oral Health Care for Dysphagic, Critically and Terminally Ill Patients. London: British Society for Disability and Oral Health.

52. Davies, A.N. (2000). A comparison of artificial saliva and chewing gum in the management of xerostomia in patients with advanced cancer. Palliative Medicine 14 (3): 197–203.

53. Bots, C.P., Brand, H.S., Veerman, E.C. et al. (2005). Chewing gum and a saliva substitute alleviate thirst and xerostomia in patients on haemodialysis. Nephrology Dialysis Transplantation 20 (3): 578–584.

54. Horne, M., McCracken, G., Walls, A. et al. (2015). Organisation, practice and experiences of mouth hygiene in stroke unit care: a mixed-methods study. Journal of Clinical Nursing 24 (5–6): 728–738.

55. Willumsen, T., Karlsen, L., Næss, R., and Bjørntvedt, S. (2012). Are the barriers to good oral hygiene in nursing homes within the nurses or the patients? Gerodontology 29 (2): e748–e755.

56. Talbot, A., Brady, M., Furlanetto, D.L.C. et al. (2005). Oral care and stroke units. Gerodontology 22 (2): 77–83.

57. Brady, M.C., Stott, D.J., Norrie, J. et al. (2011). Developing and evaluating the implementation of a complex intervention: using mixed methods to inform the design of a randomised controlled trial of an oral healthcare intervention after stroke. Trials 12: 168.

58. Kim, E.K., Jang, S.H., Choi, Y.H. et al. (2014). Effect of an oral hygienic care program for stroke patients in the intensive care unit. Yonsei Medical Journal 55 (1): 240–246.

59. Lam, O.L.T., McMillan, A.S., Samaranayake, L.P. et al. (2013). Effect of oral hygiene interventions on opportunistic pathogens in patients after stroke. American Journal of Infection Control 41 (2): 149–154.

60. Lam, O.L., McMillan, A.S., Samaranayake, L.P. et al. (2013). Randomized clinical trial of oral health promotion interventions among patients following stroke. Archives of Physical Medicine and Rehabilitation 94 (3): 435–443.

61. Seguin, P., Laviolle, B., Dahyot-Fizelier, C. et al. (2014). Effect of oropharyngeal povidone-iodine preventive oral care on ventilator-associated pneumonia in severely brain-injured or cerebral hemorrhage patients: a multicenter, randomized controlled trial. Critical Care Medicine 42 (1): 1–8.

62. Smith, C.J., Horne, M., McCracken, G. et al. (2017). Development and feasibility testing of an oral hygiene intervention for stroke unit care. Gerodontology 34 (1): 110–120.

63. Fields, L.B. (2008). Oral care intervention to reduce incidence of ventilator-associated pneumonia in the neurologic intensive care unit. Journal of Neuroscience Nursing 40 (5): 291–298.

64. Lam, O.L., McMillan, A.S., Li, L.S., and McGrath, C. (2016). Oral health and post-discharge complications in stroke survivors. Journal of Oral Rehabilitation 43 (3): 238–240.

65. Terezakis, E., Needleman, I., Kumar, N. et al. (2011). The impact of hospitalization on oral health: a systematic review. Journal of Clinical Periodontology 38 (7): 628–636.

66. Weening-Verbree, L., Huisman-de Waal, G., van Dusseldorp, L. et al. (2013). Oral health care in older people in long term care facilities: a systematic review of implementation strategies. International Journal of Nursing Studies 50 (4): 569–582.

67. Karki, A.J., Monaghan, N., and Morgan, M. (2015). Oral health status of older people living in care homes in Wales. British Dental Journal 219 (7): 331–334.

68. Dickinson, H. (2016). Improving the Evidence Base for Oral Assessment in Stroke Patients. Preston: University of Central Lancashire.

69. Wårdh, I., Hallberg, L.R.M., Berggren, U. et al. (2000). Oral health care – a low priority in nursing. Scandinavian Journal of Caring Sciences 14 (2): 137–142.

70. Adams, R. (1996). Qualified nurses lack adequate knowledge related to oral health, resulting in inadequate oral care of patients on medical wards. Journal of Advanced Nursing 24 (3): 552–560.

CHAPTER 7

Communication

Jane Marshall[1], Katerina Hilari[2], Madeline Cruice[3], and Kirsty Harrison[3]

[1]Division of Language and Communication Science, School of Health Sciences, City, University of London, London, UK

[2]Acquired Communication Disorders, School of Health Sciences, City, University of London, London, UK

[3]School of Health Sciences, City, University of London, London, UK

KEY POINTS

- Communication difficulties are common and varied post-stroke.
- Not all difficulties are immediately obvious, particularly those affecting the understanding of speech or writing.
- It is important to understand the range of problems that individuals experience, and to make best use of remaining communication abilities.
- Particular care should be taken when evaluating communication in people from language minority groups and those with more than one language, ensuring a full delineation of all issues.
- Communication difficulties significantly affect quality of life, causing distress and frustration for families, friends, staff, and stroke survivors.
- Staff should be able to support patients in expressing their basic needs and in participating in higher-level activities requiring communication, including discussing their condition, making treatment and care decisions, and interacting with family and friends.

This chapter maps to criteria within the following sections of the Stroke-Specific Education Framework (SSEF):

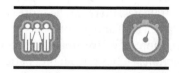

Stroke Nursing, Second Edition. Edited by Jane Williams, Lin Perry, and Caroline Watkins.
© 2020 John Wiley & Sons Ltd. Published 2020 by John Wiley & Sons Ltd.

They were talking to me and sometimes I didn't even know ... they'd say something but by the end of the sentence they was saying I didn't know what it was because I'm still thinking of the first little bit ... I really wanted to get into people's conversations but I couldn't ... and I would look at them

('Jenny') [2]

7.1 Introduction

Communication is important for all stroke care. This chapter describes communication impairments caused by stroke, and suggests strategies that nurses and others in the stroke team can use to facilitate communication. The particular needs of people from language minority groups are flagged. The role of speech and language therapists (SLTs; also termed speech (and language) pathologists) is described for the rehabilitation of communication. We consider psychosocial factors and the impact of communication difficulties on quality of life.

7.1.1 Communication in the Acute Stroke Care Context

A variety of factors can make communication in hospital difficult for any patient, such as anxiety, pain, sleep deprivation, and lack of privacy. For those post-stroke, such problems are often compounded by speech and language impairments. Graham, who was unable to speak after his stroke, gives this example:

[I] attracted the nurses attention in hospital by throwing things at their office, as [I] was unable to call them ... [they] thought I was delirious [3]

For David, the problems were worsened by the insensitivity and lack of awareness of one member of staff. He recounts an incident on the ward during lunch:

We were there one day, on lunchtime, can't remember now, and this woman came along and said, pushed in front of me, quite without manners, and said, 'Whadya want?' in a rude tone, and I said 'Can you hang on a minute, Mary's not able to read', and she said 'Well, she won't get anything again' and I went spare. I said 'Don't you realise she can't read or speak'. [4]

Sadly, David's experience was not exceptional. Some healthcare providers in hospital stroke units are not aware of patients' communication impairments, with negative consequences for patient care [5]. If staff are aware, and are skilled in using communication strategies, there can be more successful interactions [6]. Good communication between staff and patients has many advantages, including more accurate diagnoses, more effective treatment, better patient compliance, and higher patient satisfaction [7]. It is crucial that patients can make their needs known to staff and participate in decision-making about care. Whilst SLTs have a role in creating a positive communication environment, it is the responsibility of all the stroke team. Perhaps most importantly, staff need to ensure that their communication behaviours do not add to the barriers faced by stroke patients. This chapter will suggest techniques and strategies to reduce communication barriers, particularly when nursing patients who have post-stroke communication problems.

7.2 Aphasia

Aphasia is an acquired language disorder arising from brain injury, with stroke being the most common cause. A third of acute stroke patients have aphasia [8, 9], a quarter of whom have persistent symptoms [10]. Aphasia affects all aspects of language (i.e. speaking, listening, reading, and writing), and can even impair non-verbal modalities like gestures [11]. It mostly occurs in people with left-hemisphere damage, as the left brain plays the primary role in processing language. Following are some examples of how people with aphasia define it:

> *'It's taken my voice'*
> *'My brain is just buzzing about and me lips is a different kettle of fish'*
> *'It was just as if my brain was a cake and a piece was cut out'*
> *'I know the right word, but the wrong word comes out' [2]*

Loss of speech is the most obvious sign of aphasia, affecting content, not just pronunciation. For some people, the loss is total. Others, like Karl in Case Study 7.1, can produce isolated words or phrases. Repetitive utterances are also common; unfortunately, these are often swear words and cannot be inhibited [12].

Case Study

Case 7.1 Karl

Karl is a 49-year-old car salesman. He was admitted a week ago following a left middle cerebral artery stroke. This caused a right-sided hemiplegia and severe aphasia.

Karl grew up in India and spoke Hindi and English fluently pre-stroke. Now he can only say one phrase, 'I've got it', and occasional single words, such as 'arm' and 'coffee'. Ward staff are unsure whether these words are accurate. For example, Karl was pointing to his leg when he said 'arm'. His wife has tried speaking to him in Hindi, but says that he was unable to reply.

Karl is cooperative with the nurses and follows instructions. For example, if a nurse wants to check his blood pressure (BP), he holds out his arm. Karl is also resourceful. On one occasion, a student nurse wanted to take him for a bath. He said 'No', which surprised the nurse. Then Karl found his calendar of appointments and indicated that he was expecting his physiotherapy.

Karl sometimes becomes very agitated and distressed. These episodes have recently become more frequent. Karl is due to be discharged in a few days.

7.2.1 Fluent and Non-fluent Aphasia

Aphasia is often described as fluent or non-fluent. Karl has non-fluent aphasia, since his speech is hesitant and fragmented. This is also termed Broca's aphasia, after the nineteenth-century neurologist who first described it. People with Broca's cannot produce grammatical sentences. For example, they might say, 'Saturday ... shops' instead of, 'On Saturday I went shopping'. Usually, there are problems with word-finding, and often apraxia (see later). Broca's aphasia typically arises from lesions to the left frontal lobe.

In fluent aphasia, the quantity and rate of speech is typically unchanged. However, speech is difficult to understand because of multiple errors. Here are two extracts of fluent aphasic speech:

> *I was quite ... erm ... that's why I can't get weyerdkeep makes me very erm here up here makes him all ... all setoytaid but these come and I can't it might be because I had another minsing. [13]*

> *She has lugyburger ... she has radio ... she has pigyburger pigyburger and uh blop ... I guess there shoes and a spade ... then if they were ... but this bow is good. [14]*

As illustrated by these examples, people with fluent aphasia often produce non-words (neologisms). These can be very repetitive and formed from similar sounds. Puzzlingly, some people with fluent aphasia seem unaware their speech is disordered [15, 16]. Thus, they are surprised and even angry when care staff fail to understand them, and may refuse rehabilitation. Such speakers are sometimes described as having Jargon aphasia or Wernicke's aphasia (again after a nineteenth-century scientist). They typically have more posterior lesions than those with Broca's aphasia.

7.2.2 Comprehension Problems with Aphasia

Aphasia problems extend beyond speech; there can also be comprehension difficulties [17]. These may be subtle, only affecting the understanding of complex language, or profound, where even single words are affected. Typically, comprehension difficulties are most evident in Wernicke's aphasia, although there are exceptions to this.

Comprehension impairments are difficult to detect. Karl seemed to understand speech. He followed instructions and, when asked if he wanted a bath, responded appropriately. However, he may have gathered clues from the environment, helping him understand what was being said. For example, the student nurse may have (helpfully) pointed to the bathroom when asking about the bath. We must test comprehension when no clues are available before drawing firm conclusions.

7.2.3 Reading and Writing with Aphasia

Reading and writing are usually impaired in aphasia. Being unable to read in the acute care environment can be particularly disorientating for patients. For example, they may be unable to read basic signs ('Toilet', 'Dining Room', 'Call Bell'), recognise their name, or select menu-card options. Some individuals can read single words, but not text [18]. As a result, they struggle with correspondence and other forms of written information, and may no longer read for pleasure. Writing varies across individuals. Some are unable to write, whilst others achieve occasional words or sentences. Importantly, we often see dissociations between writing and speech, such as someone with no meaningful speech who can write a few words (and vice versa). As with speech, people with aphasia often make errors in writing; they might write 'mother' when they meant 'wife', or make a spelling error, such as 'wite'. Many people with aphasia have to write with their non-preferred hand, because they have a right hemiplegia. This adds to their difficulties, making writing slow and effortful. Writing problems can be very distressing, and have a negative impact on self-esteem.

7.2.4 Recovery from Aphasia

About 40% of people with aphasia in acute stroke experience language recovery [19]; some studies suggest recovery rates may be even higher [20]. Factors predicting recovery are unclear. For example, some studies find an effect of age [9, 21], whilst others do not [22]. Less disputed is the relationship between initial severity and recovery; people with severe stroke symptoms or low initial scores on language tests typically have the poorest outcomes [20, 21, 23–26]. Despite this, most people with aphasia improve somewhat, providing there are no further neurological events. Progress is most rapid early post-stroke, but may continue throughout the first year and even beyond. Recovery is assisted by speech and language therapy, particularly when treatment is provided intensively [27].

7.2.5 Identifying Aphasia

The SLT plays the key role in diagnosing aphasia. However, most patients are referred to SLTs by nurses, doctors, and other rehabilitation staff. Nurses play a crucial role in early detection of aphasia [28], and they must be aware of its signs (see Table 7.1). For some patients, there are obvious communication problems, but it may not be obvious that they are due to aphasia. For example, relatives may hint at dementia pre-stroke. Here, an SLT referral should still be made so they can clarify the diagnosis. Aphasia can be difficult to identify in patients who speak little or no English. Again, a referral should be made, with a language assessment being conducted through an interpreter or bilingual coworker (see later).

The SLT will be able to confirm if aphasia is present, often using a screening test. This may be a quick-to-administer language measure, such as the Frenchay Aphasia Screening Test [29]. The Inpatient Functional Communication Interview (IFCI) [30] may be used to assess communication needs in hospital. The therapist will also be interested in nurses' observations about the patient's communication, as nurses typically spend more time with patients than therapists, observing more communication exchanges [28]. Indeed, the IFCI includes a Staff Questionnaire asking nurses (or others) to indicate how patients communicate on the ward.

The current UK National Institute for Health and Care Excellence (NICE) guidelines for stroke rehabilitation in adults (CG 162) recommend that all stroke patients be screened for communication difficulties within 72 hours of onset, and that all stroke rehabilitation services devise a standardised screening protocol [31].

TABLE 7.1 **Signs of aphasia**

Modality	Possible signs
Speech	Limited output with long pauses
	Obvious word-finding difficulties
	Word selection or production errors, such as calling a carrot a 'potato' or a 'karrik'
	Fluent but incomprehensible speech that may contain non-words
	Grammatical errors or a lack of grammar
Comprehension	Failure to follow instructions
	Errors in following instructions, such as looking down when asked to look up
	Helped by repetition, simplified speech, pointing, and gesture
Reading and writing	Refusal of books and newspapers, or opting only for texts with pictures
	Failure to complete a menu card or makes obviously incorrect selections
	Inability to clarify information when given a pen and paper
	Distress when asked to write
	Obvious discrepancy between pre-morbid writing and current abilities
	Word selection or spelling errors in writing; only parts of words achieved

7.2.6 Strategies to Use When Nursing Patients with Aphasia

Communication problems from aphasia make nursing difficult. However, there are a number of helpful strategies that can be employed, with Karl's use of his calendar being a good example.

7.2.6.1 Careful Language Choice

Everyone should think carefully about the language they use. Most people with aphasia struggle to comprehend long or complex sentences and most understand concrete words better than abstract ones. Concrete words are things that can be seen and touched, such as 'pillow' and 'trolley'. Abstract words are concepts that cannot be experienced by the senses, such as 'idea' and 'diagnosis'. Therefore, short, simple speech, constructed mainly from concrete words, is easier for patients to comprehend. Many people with aphasia are helped by slowed speech, although it is important that

TABLE 7.2   **Adapting language for the patient with aphasia**

Message	Aphasia-friendly version
After I have taken your blood pressure, I need to give you your cardiac medication.	I am going to take your blood pressure [the nurse shows the patient the equipment and carries out the test]. Now I need to give you your pills [the nurse shows the patient the medication]. They are for your heart [the nurse gestures to his or her own heart].
After you have been discharged tomorrow, you will receive correspondence from us about your review appointment.	Tomorrow, you are going home. The doctor will write to you. She will ask you to come back to the hospital so we can find out how you are getting on.

this does not sound patronising. Table 7.2 gives examples of how to make speech 'aphasia-friendly'.

7.2.6.2 Using Clues   Clues about what is being said can accompany speech. So, if a nurse wants to tell a male patient with aphasia that they are going to give him an injection, it is a good idea to show him the syringe, or make a simple gesture. Many people with aphasia find written words and pictures helpful. So, if the patient is being taken for a scan, it is a good idea to show him the written sign and a picture of the equipment. It can be difficult to know whether a patient with aphasia has understood. Sometimes, they may repeat what you say, but without comprehension. Therefore, important information should be conveyed several times, with the support of pictures, written words, and symbols.

7.2.6.3 Other Strategies   Other strategies can help people with aphasia to get their message across. First, give them plenty of time and do not be afraid of silences. Remind them to use alternatives to speech. For example, if the patient has a pain, they can be asked to point to where it hurts. Some people with aphasia make very effective use of *gesture or drawing*, either spontaneously or in response to therapy [32, 33]. It is worth exploring whether writing is better than speech, such as by giving them a pen and paper when they are trying to convey something. If the patient is able to produce some speech, remember that it may contain errors: important information should be checked for accuracy. This is an example of a nurse doing this:

NURSE   Do you take any pills or medicine?
PATIENT   Yes ... Er, espro
NURSE   Is that aspirin [writes 'aspirin']?
PATIENT   Yes
NURSE   How many do you take each day?
PATIENT   Er ... four

NURSE   [Writes '4' and holds up four fingers] You take four. Is that right?
PATIENT No ... Er, one
NURSE   [Writes '1' and holds up one finger] You take one. Is that right?
PATIENT Yes

Some people with aphasia are helped by *cues* when they are stuck for a word. For example, providing them with the first sound of a word or information about its meaning may help them to say it [34]. However, this is rather unnatural and only works if the nurse knows the target word. An alternative is to provide people who have aphasia with *props* to assist with communication. Karl had a written weekly calendar of his rehabilitation appointments by his bed. By using this, he could show the student nurse that it was not a good time for his bath. Other props include communication charts, with symbols for everyday basic needs, maps, family photographs, and pictures.

Using strategies is particularly important when essential information has to be communicated, such as that relating to medications and medical tests. The IFCI contains a helpful list of strategies for supporting a patient's understanding and helping them to respond [30], and the Stroke Association has a booklet about how to make information accessible to people with aphasia [35]. The SLT team should also be able to suggest specific ideas for individual patients. Nurses who work frequently with patients with aphasia might seek training about communication disorders and how to facilitate communication. There is evidence that training is effective [36].

7.3   Dysarthria and Apraxia of Speech

Roughly 42% of stroke patients experience dysarthria and 11% apraxia (sometimes termed 'dyspraxia') of speech [37]. Dysarthria and apraxia are impairments of speech production, rather than of language. So, assuming there are no other deficits, the patient will be able to read, write, and comprehend what other people say. Their own speech, however, will be difficult, if not impossible, to understand.

In dysarthria, neurological control of the muscles involved in speech is disrupted. These are the muscles of: the chest, used for breathing; the larynx, used for voice production; and the face, tongue, lips, and throat, used for articulation (making different speech sounds). Different types of dysarthria reflect the site of neurological damage and the cerebral hemispheres affected (e.g. for spastic dysarthria, damage is present in both hemispheres) (see Table 7.3). Unilateral upper motor neurone dysarthria is the most common type of dysarthria following a single stroke (see Case Study 7.2) [38]. Dysarthria can be caused by conditions other than stroke, such as Parkinson's disease and motor neurone disease.

To complicate matters, dysarthria and apraxia of speech can coexist. Similarly, dysarthria can also co-occur with dysphagia (eating and swallowing difficulties). Dysphagia and dysarthria are found together in 28% of patients, with both dysarthria and aphasia in 15% [37].

TABLE 7.3 **The seven different types of dysarthria**

Type of dysarthria	Signs and symptoms
Unilateral upper motor neuron	Unilateral lower facial weakness (below the eye), slow speech rate, quiet voice and intermittent speech sound errors
Spastic	Slow speech rate, with strained or strangled voice quality; monotone and effortful speech
Flaccid	Nasal-sounding speech, breathy voice, use of short phrases, audible breathing, and imprecise consonants; specific speech characteristics depend on which cranial nerves are damaged
Hypokinetic	Monotone and typically quiet speech; lots of inappropriate silences and increased or 'rushed' speech rate; reduced stress (or emphasis)
Hyperkinetic	Abnormal involuntary movements, which disturb the rhythm and rate of speech
Ataxic	Inaccurate articulation, excess and equal stress (affecting intonation and emphasis), and excessively loud speech
Mixed	Multiple types of dysarthria present at the same time, e.g. spastic-flaccid in motor neuron disease

Source: Adapted from Duffy [38].

Case Study

Case 7.2 Earl

Earl is a 67-year-old retired science teacher. He lives with his wife, and has 4 children and 12 grandchildren. Computed tomography (CT) confirms a left middle cerebral artery stroke. He has been in the acute stroke unit for 6 days. His swallowing difficulties are resolving, but he has a mild speech impairment and the nurses are finding it difficult to understand him during busy times on the ward. He speaks slowly and his articulation breaks down at times. The predominant feature of his speech is his quiet voice, which his wife says is a dramatic change from his strong voice pre-stroke. The SLT has assessed his communication and feels his symptoms demonstrate a unilateral upper motor neurone dysarthria.

7.3.1 The Role of the SLT in Managing Dysarthria

In acute stroke, the assessment and management of dysphagia is typically a greater priority than speech (see Chapter 5). Assessment of communication aims to determine the patient's level of intelligibility, or the degree to which speech can be understood, and why this is breaking down. A commonly used test is the Frenchay Dysarthria Assessment (FDA-2) [39]. This explores each aspect of speech, such as breathing, volume, pitch, and rate. It also examines movements of the tongue and lips and measures the patient's intelligibility with single words, sentences, and conversation. Such systematic assessment helps identify which aspects of speech are impaired or intact, and pinpoint aims for therapy.

As time progresses, the SLT will involve the patient and family in discussing their perception of the patient's speech. This is important, as therapy for dysarthria typically requires the patient to monitor and exert more control over their speech. Therapy may include speech exercises and training in compensatory strategies, such as slowed speech, gesture, and writing (for examples, see [40]). In some cases, particularly where there is no accompanying aphasia, communication may be supplemented with technological aids, such as electronic voice-output communication aids.

Patients with dysarthria post-stroke often have a good prognosis. Up to 40% of patients have normal speech at 6 months post-stroke, and most others have mild impairments [41].

7.3.2 Apraxia of Speech

Apraxia of speech disrupts the planning and sequencing of speech movements. Unlike dysarthria, the neuromuscular system is intact and the impairment results from faulty programming and speech planning. Difficulties arise whenever the person wants to say something, or is asked to talk. Surprisingly, automatic speech may still be possible; so they may be able to recite days of the week or count without difficulty. Apraxia of speech is marked by hesitant, imprecise speech, with inconsistent errors on the sounds of words. Often, there are signs of struggle during speech, as the person tries to control the movements of their tongue and lips. In severe cases, all speech is impossible. Although apraxia of speech may occur in isolation, it often coexists with aphasia. It typically arises from left-hemisphere damage. Both aphasia and apraxia of speech are more commonly associated with stroke than dysarthria [42].

7.3.3 Strategies to Use When Nursing a Patient with Dysarthria

Dysarthria makes it difficult for the patient to communicate their needs and concerns (see Table 7.4). Often, problems are worse with *fatigue*, so it is best to hold important conversations in the morning or after rest. They are also affected by *posture*, so it is important that the patient is in an upright sitting position. Talking during concurrent activities, especially eating, is no longer possible, so *distractions need to be removed*. It is important that communication is made as easy as possible, so, for example, ensure that the patient *can hear properly* and is wearing *correctly fitted dentures*. Depending on the nature of the damage, patients with dysarthria often have unimpaired language and cognition, so they can make good use of strategies such as *writing down key words*. They will also follow *spoken or written instructions*.

The problems of dysarthria can discourage communication and distort patterns of interaction. When nurses interact with patients with dysarthria, they often use task-orientated language, relating to aspects of care, but neglect more social

TABLE 7.4 Communication strategies for the patient with dysarthria

Tips for the patient

- Introduce your topic with a single word or short phrase before attempting more complete sentences.
- Speak slowly and loudly; pause frequently.
- Check with the listeners to make sure that they understand you.
- Try to limit conversations when you feel tired, as your speech will be more difficult to understand.
- Use other methods as well as speech, such as pointing, gesturing, and writing key words; if you get very frustrated, take a rest and try again later.

Tips for the nurse

- Try to speak to the patient in a quiet environment with no distractions.
- Make sure the patient is in a good sitting posture.
- If relevant, make sure the patient has their hearing aid and glasses.
- Pay attention to the patient and watch them as they talk.
- Be honest and let the patient know if you do not understand them; do not pretend to understand.
- Repeat the part of the message that you understood so that the patient does not have to repeat the entire thing.
- If you cannot understand the message after repeated attempts, ask yes/no questions or encourage the patient to write.

uses of communication, which are valued by patients [43]. The Royal College of Physicians Guidelines highlight the importance of *training* for carers of people with dysarthria and apraxia of speech post-stroke; nurses should liaise with the SLT to ascertain the best ways of communicating with a patient [44].

7.4 Right-Hemisphere Damage (RHD) Communication Deficit

Lesions causing right-hemisphere damage (RHD) produce a range of problems (see Chapter 9). These include left-side neglect, visual agnosia (inability to recognise objects), constructional apraxia (inability to assemble parts correctly to make a meaningful whole, e.g. inability to copy a two- or three-sided design), and disorientation in space. There may be anosognosia (a lack of awareness of illness or disability) and problems of attention, memory, organisation, and problem-solving. Occasionally, individuals display prosopagnosia (face-blindness). Some individuals lose the perception of sounds, making it difficult for them to appreciate music. Many of these problems have consequences for communication [45] and are distressing for the person and their family. Face-blindness, for example, can result in patients not recognising their spouse or children.

Between 50 and 78% of people with RHD show communication and social interaction difficulties, with 20% having a marked impairment [46, 47]. Problems include:

- Difficulties interpreting the context of a conversation or the speaker's intentions. These are called pragmatic difficulties. For example, a person with RHD might want to ask a passing nurse a question, whilst missing signs that the nurse is dealing with something else and is in a hurry. Pragmatic difficulties are often evident in non-verbal behaviours, such as reduced eye contact, reduced facial expression, and reduced use of gesture. There may also be difficulties with intonation and the marking of stress (emphasis) in speech. The patient's speech may sound flat, and they may be unable to interpret other people's intonation (e.g. to detect anger or amusement).

- Difficulties with non-literal uses of language. These include difficulties with jokes, metaphors, and inferences.

- Difficulties with conversation, such as verbosity (wordiness), poor turn-taking, and going off topic.

- Reading and writing deficits. People with RHD may struggle to follow the plot of a story and may misinterpret humour, irony, and metaphor. Their reading and writing may be affected by visuospatial impairments. For example, they may have left neglect dyslexia (failure to read information in the left visual field), causing misreading of the beginnings of words or sentences; there may also be comparable problems in writing, affecting the spelling of words.

Case Study 7.3 describes a person with RHD who displays some of these problems.

Case Study

| Case 7.3 | James

James is an 83-year-old retired judge. He lives with his wife, who has disabling visual and hearing problems, and is her main carer. James is admitted to hospital with left-sided weakness and slurred speech. A CT scan confirms a small area of haemorrhage in the right parietal lobe. He has left facial weakness, left neglect, absent reflexes and sensation on the left, and reduced power on the left.

James is referred to an SLT for his speech and swallowing problems. Sarah, his nurse, says he follows instructions and, although his speech is quiet and somewhat slurred (James has dysarthria), she can understand what he is saying. Sarah is puzzled because James' daughter has reported difficulties conversing with her father. Sarah cannot understand why this is, although she has noticed that James misses light-hearted comments and does not smile or engage much with the other patients. Betty, the person in the bed next to his, has complained that he ignores her and describes him as 'odd'. Once, she wanted to borrow James' newspaper. She hinted at this by saying, 'I wonder what's in the news today'. James completely missed her intention and simply said, 'I don't know', which upset her. Finally, James seems forgetful and excessively worried about things. He asks the same questions again and again (e.g. who is looking after his wife whilst he is in hospital).

In his initial assessment, the SLT notes that James has a flat facial expression and intonation. He talks a lot but has a tendency to take everything literally and veer off the topic of conversation.

7.4.1 Strategies to Use When Nursing a Person with RHD

Right-hemisphere communication deficits will affect communication on the ward and social interactions with staff and other patients. In addition, difficulties in laying down new memories will affect the patient's ability to cope with the changes caused by stroke. This may manifest in different ways. The patient might appear obsessively worried, for example, asking the same questions over and over again. Alternatively, awareness and memory disorders could make them seem indifferent to their problems and to the efforts of the stroke team. **Being aware of these difficulties** is essential to ensuring their well-being on the ward. Strategies that help with RHD cognitive and communication issues include *being literal and clear* (e.g. say, 'I am only joking' after a joke), keeping to a *regular routine*, and using *memory aids*. Table 7.5 summarises some ways to help.

7.5 Language Minorities

It is very important that aphasia and other communication impairments are not missed in stroke patients from language minority groups (for evidence that this can happen, see [48, 49]). For example, we should not assume that communication

TABLE 7.5	Strategies to help the patient with right-hemisphere damage (RHD)	
Modality	**Sign**	**Strategy**
Comprehension	Takes expressions like 'the physio will be up in a minute' literally and gets anxious when the physio is 'late'	Be literal, e.g. say, 'The physio will be up soon'
	Has difficulty drawing inferences	Be clear and check understanding.
		If appropriate, alert other patients to the nature of RHD communication difficulties
	Has difficulty recognising the speaker's intention	Make your intention obvious, e.g. if you are being funny, say, 'I am only joking'
Memory	Gets disorientated; asks the same questions again and again	Have a daily routine; discuss it e.g. at the beginning of the day and after lunch
	Forgets appointments	Have a diary of events and frequently remind the patient to use it
	Does not practise exercises	
Reading	Has difficulty reading menu card or TV guide due to left-side neglect	Have something of different texture and colour under reading material, and track the left edge with the finger before starting reading
		Write key words vertically

problems following stroke simply reflect limited pre-morbid English. Ideally, the patient should be assessed by an SLT from his or her language community. If this is not possible, the therapist will assess through interpreters or bilingual coworkers. It is important not to use family members and friends as interpreters, as this can disrupt family relationships and yield unreliable data [50]. Relatives can, however, provide invaluable insights about what happens when the patient tries to speak in their home language(s).

If the patient is bi- or multilingual, it is important that all their languages are assessed. In our example of aphasia (see Case Study 7.1), Karl's Hindi and English were both affected. Karl's case is typical, in that aphasia rarely leaves one language unscathed. However, the profile of impairments may vary, with one language being stronger than another (see examples in [51]). Typically, the language that was learnt earlier in life, or which is used most commonly by the individual, is most resistant to damage. Occasionally, however, a patient's second language is less impaired following stroke [52, 53]. Discrepancies like this call for careful assessment to uncover whatever language resources remain to the individual.

7.6 What Can SLTs Contribute in Acute Stroke Care?

The SLT has four main responsibilities:

- to assess the patient's communication and swallowing impairments and their impact on the patient's life;
- to support communication on the ward;
- to advise the patient, family members, and staff about communication and swallowing; and
- to provide intervention to reduce the communication and swallowing problems.

7.6.1 Assessment

By sharing their observations of patients, nurses can play a vital role in identifying those who need further assessment [28]. Detailed SLT assessment aims to find out the nature and severity of the communication impairment, its effect on communication activities, and the role played by environmental factors. Assessment may additionally explore broader issues such as social participation and quality of life [54], and provide a baseline against which recovery can be compared. Therapists draw upon the views of the patient and their family during assessment. For example, they will ask how they perceive difficulties and elicit their priorities for intervention [55]. Therapists will consult with nursing and rehabilitation staff to determine how the patient is communicating with them during daily activities (e.g. at mealtimes or ward rounds).

Therapists have a number of measures for exploring these issues, such as formal tests and interview protocols (for the patient and their family members). They will often record and analyse samples of the patient's language and carry out informal observation (e.g. to find out how the person responds to conversation or copes with situations on the ward with nurses and other rehabilitation staff). It is imperative to identify facilitators and barriers in the communication environment, including how supportive others' communication skills are and what use is made of resources such as communication aids, writing, drawing, and gesture [5].

7.6.2   Communication

Hospital patients have important communication needs. For example, they need to understand their medical diagnosis and its implications. They probably want to ask questions about their care and the procedures they are undergoing. At the most basic level, they need to be able to call for a nurse. These functions are hard if there are communication impairments post-stroke. Patients who experience difficulty in communicating their needs have more problems with low mood and depression, higher mortality rates, and worse functional outcomes [28]. Through observation and discussion with ward staff, the SLT can pinpoint the communication needs of each patient, and help them meet those needs during their hospital stay. This is likely to involve the implementation of strategies such as providing pictures or symbols in place of words for important signs. Often, the therapist will offer short training sessions for ward staff on how to make communication easier for stroke patients in general, and for certain patients in particular. Training should cover how to use tools and techniques for communicating with patients, and ideally support staff to make specific adjustments to their practices, such as devising local guidelines, amending menu cards, and making information accessible with pictographs [36, 56].

7.6.3   Advice

Members of the general public know very little about the communication impairments arising from stroke [57, 58]. Those affected, therefore, are likely to be similarly uninformed, at least when the stroke first happens. A recent systematic review indicated that stroke survivors and members of their family have a wide range of information needs [59]. These include the causes and nature of the stroke, prognosis, rehabilitation plans, services available after hospital, how to cope with communication impairments, and sources of emotional and psychosocial support [59]. Advice may be provided individually or through relatives' support groups and training programmes. Such provision makes a positive impact on family interactions [60].

7.6.4   Intervention

Results from assessment and observation, and discussions with the patient and their family, will help the therapist to determine treatment goals and select interventions. Therapy methods are diverse. They may include language exercises (focussing on speaking, understanding, reading, or writing), practice on functional communication tasks, conversation groups, and work on strategic compensation (e.g. gesture, drawing). Therapy frequently involves family members, friends, and staff, when available, to give them skills in communicating with the patient. Intensity of rehabilitation is important [27]. Clinical trials suggest that those receiving intensive aphasia therapy make greater gains in language and communication than those on usual care [61–63]. Guidelines advise at least 45 minutes of speech and language therapy per day for 5 days per week, providing this is tolerated by the patient [31]. Nurses have a role in enhancing therapeutic input for patients with communication impairments, using any techniques advocated by the SLT [28]. Case Study 7.4 provides an example of therapy.

Case Study

| Case 7.4 | Rachael |

Rachael is 75 years old. She has a left-hemisphere stroke causing severe aphasia and a right hemiplegia. Her speech is fluent but incomprehensible, with few recognisable words. Her writing is affected, although she can occasionally write part of a word. Rachael can understand spoken and written words, but not complex sentences. She is a retired academic who lives alone in a first-floor flat. She has two loyal friends who visit regularly.

Communication about Rachael's nursing and care needs results in frequent misunderstandings. For example, Rachael often refuses to be taken to physiotherapy, particularly if the therapist is unfamiliar. She also finds it very difficult to make requests (e.g. if she needs her glasses or the lavatory). The first communication aim, therefore, is to alleviate these difficulties. The SLT produces a chart of strategies to use when communicating with Rachael. This is discussed with Rachael and given to all staff and her friends. She also develops a simple booklet of Rachael's main rehabilitation and care needs. On one page is written 'physiotherapy', alongside a photo of the gym. Another shows words and symbols that can be used with nurses (e.g. if she is in pain). The SLT practises using the booklet with Rachael and the nurses.

The therapist also employs writing therapy. The aim is for Rachael to write 10 words that relate to her immediate needs, such as the names of clothing, her friends, and objects like 'toothbrush'. Rachael practises these words in tasks that progress from copying to copying after a delay, to filling in a missing letter, to writing the name from a picture. Once Rachael can make a recognisable attempt at these words, they are incorporated into communication activities. For example, the therapist might ask Rachael, 'Who is visiting this afternoon?' as a cue for her to write her friend's name. Therapy is stepped up by introducing new words.

It is clear that Rachael will have long-term mobility, daily living, and communication needs. It is important that this is discussed with Rachael and that she is fully involved in decisions about her future. Working with Rachael's friends, the SLT and occupational therapist (OT) institute a programme of consultation. They use photographs of Rachael's flat to identify the obstacles that she will face (e.g. the stairs). They also map out a typical day (with pictures) and think about the help that she will need (e.g. with dressing). The therapists then provide Rachael with labels and images of the different care options. For example, they outline how Rachael might be supported at home, using images of a stair-lift, visiting care staff, meals-on-wheels, bath hoist, and a panic button. They also show her brochures from local residential homes, with simplified information about fees. Rachael is able to use these images to indicate her preference, which is for residential care. This is followed up with a visit to a care home and a successful trial stay.

7.7 Psychological Issues and Quality of Life

7.7.1 Onset and Acute Care

The onset of stroke with a communication impairment is a crisis point in a person's life. To date, much of our evidence about this comes from people with aphasia. For example, they report feelings of shock, anger, frustration, anxiety, aggression, shame, guilt, grief, loss, and embarrassment [2, 64]. It is also important to recognise that stroke can isolate patients, as illustrated by Betty and James earlier in this chapter, and by Jean's comment here:

> When I had a stroke I found nobody talk to me and that other patients you know walk by the bed and look and um let's [never] say a word because they knew I couldn't speak.
> *(Jean, Personal Insights audiotape, Dysphasia Matters package [65])*

Family members may also be overwhelmed by negative feelings, and they need support and information in acute stroke [66]. Families want answers to questions such as, What is stroke?, What is aphasia?, What are the co-existing problems?, and Where can we get more information? A particular need is for honest but hopeful information about the prognosis. For example, one participant in a study by Avent et al. [66] stated:

> When I was talking to the therapist, I was like, I have heard all the bad. How about the positive?

It is essential to provide accessible information for people with aphasia and their families. The SLT can help by identifying leaflets that people with aphasia can read and understand. Useful resources are available from organisations such as the Stroke Association [35] and National Institute for Health Research (NIHR) on engaging with people with aphasia [67].

7.7.2 Discharge

Discharge from hospital, although eagerly anticipated, can be a time of particular stress for both the patient and their family. There is uncertainty about the future and worries about coping with mobility and communication problems at home. Further anxieties may focus on the availability of ongoing therapy and support services, and access to these post-discharge [2, 59]. Karl (Case Study 7.1) showed increasing distress as discharge approached. A big concern is safety, including communication safety. For example, it is essential that the patient has a method of summoning help in an emergency.

It is important to ensure that patients have accurate information and support strategies post-discharge, in order to assist communication [59, 66]. For example, the participants in Avent et al. [66] felt it was crucial to leave hospital with information about support groups and other community resources. It is critical that care plans are in place, and that these are effective; often, there are shortfalls in services:

> *You leave with this great package and are told you will be getting all this back-up. You think great ... then nothing materialises for six weeks. You get home and think great, physio is going to come and this person is going to come and nobody comes at all and then six weeks later they come. Once it happens it's alright, but when you first get home nothing, it's really awful. [68]*

Not all needs can be anticipated prior to discharge [69]. Services need to be flexible and responsive to a patient's 6-month or annual stroke review [31].

7.7.3 Long-term Effects

Communication disability has a long-term negative impact on recovery post-stroke [70]. It significantly affects quality of life, even when other variables, such as emotional state and social support, are factored out [71–73]. The long-term social consequences of stroke and aphasia often include loss of work and a consequent drop in income, a need to give up driving, restrictions in social life, and the falling away of friends [2, 74–76]. Fatigue is often a profound and persistent problem. Additionally, there may be lasting emotional effects, with a high incidence of depression in people with aphasia in the long term (62% [77]). These consequences are particularly concerning, as after stroke, poor social support is associated with worse recovery [78] and increased likelihood of a future adverse event such as a second stroke [79]; depression, too, is associated with worse rehabilitation outcomes, lower quality of life, and higher mortality [80].

These findings suggest that to improve quality of life, interventions need to focus not just on communication, but also on promoting emotional well-being, facilitating activities, and strengthening social networks and participation. Therapies to address these factors are emerging and report positive findings [81, 82].

Those with severe communication impairment and additional problems post-stroke may require nursing home care. A recent population-based study of people living in long-term care facilities in Canada (n = 66 193) compared the impact of 60 diseases and 15 conditions on caregiver-assessed preference-based quality of life. After adjusting for age, sex, and other diagnoses, aphasia exhibited the largest negative impact on quality of life, even over and beyond cancer and Alzheimer's disease [83]. It is therefore paramount to address the communication needs and support the psychosocial well-being of people with post-stroke communication problems in long-term care. SLTs play an important role in educating others on how to communicate effectively with people with aphasia and on how to establish a supportive communication environment in nursing homes [84].

The long-term picture for people with communication difficulties post-stroke is not all negative. Those with aphasia report developing new positive social interactions [85]. They also report that participation in activities, meaningful relationships, and a sense of autonomy and independence help them live successfully with their condition [86]. There are personal accounts in the literature of individuals with long-term aphasia who have achieved new and satisfying lives (see [87] and the Aphasia Now Web site: www.aphasianow.org). Positive experiences of care in the acute phase can be the first step towards attaining this goal.

7.8 Conclusion

Strokes can cause a range of communication impairments. In some cases, problems are confined to the pronunciation of words. In others, all aspects of language are affected, including understanding. These problems, in turn, affect recovery, rehabilitation, well-being, and quality of life, with consequences for the stroke survivor and their family and friends. Even when problems are severe, the picture is not all bleak. Most people experience some degree of spontaneous recovery, and effective therapies are available, as are a wide range of strategies to support communication. These include: using simplified language, supporting speech with pointing and gesture, and, above all, giving the person time to communicate. Family members and carers can also be helped. They need education and advice, for example about the nature of stroke and aphasia and how to maintain communication.

SLTs are key to supporting people with communication impairments post-stroke. It is vital that patients are referred if impairments are suspected, and all members of the multidisciplinary team (MDT) should understand the potential consequences of stroke for communication. Nurses, who have the most contact with acute stroke patients, make a particular difference to the quality of care. By using sensitive and thoughtful communication strategies in the early stages, a nurse can help to lay the foundations for successful stroke rehabilitation.

References

1. Stroke Specific Education Framework. Available from: http://www.stroke-education.org.uk/framework [30 November 2018].
2. Parr, S., Byng, S., and Gilpin, S. (1997). Talking About Aphasia: Living with Loss of Language After Stroke. Miton-Keynes: McGraw-Hill Education.
3. Jordan, L. and Kaiser, W. (1996). Aphasia: A Social Approach. London: Chapman Hall.
4. Cruice, M., Cocks, N., Lancashire, T. et al. (2011). You've Got to Realize When You Have a Stroke It's a Stroke for Life. In: The Impact of Communication Disability Across the Lifespan (ed. K. Hilari and N. Botting), 596. Guildford: J&R Press.
5. O'Halloran, R., Worrall, L., and Hickson, L. (2011). Environmental factors that influence communication between patients and their healthcare providers in acute hospital stroke units: an observational study. International Journal of Language & Communication Disorders 46 (1): 30–47.
6. O'Halloran, R., Hickson, L., and Worrall, L. (2008). Environmental factors that influence communication between people with communication disability and their healthcare providers in hospital: a review of the literature within the International Classification of Functioning, Disability and Health (ICF) framework. International Journal of Language & Communication Disorders 43 (6): 601–632.

7. McCooey, R., Toffolo, D., and Code, C. (2000). A socioenvironmental approach to functional communication in hospital in-patients. In: Neurogenic Communication Disorders: A Functional Approach (ed. L. Worrall and C. Frattali), 295–311. New York: Thieme.

8. Engelter, S.T., Gostynski, M., Papa, S. et al. (2006). Epidemiology of aphasia attributable to first ischemic stroke: incidence, severity, fluency, etiology, and thrombolysis. Stroke 37 (6): 1379–1384.

9. Laska, A., Hellblom, A., Murray, V. et al. (2001). Aphasia in acute stroke and relation to outcome. Journal of Internal Medicine 249 (5): 413–422.

10. Ali, M., Lyden, P., and Brady, M. (2015). Collaboration. V. Aphasia and dysarthria in acute stroke: recovery and functional outcome. International Journal of Stroke 10 (3): 400–406.

11. Hogrefe, K., Ziegler, W., Weidinger, N., and Goldenberg, G. (2012). Non-verbal communication in severe aphasia: influence of aphasia, apraxia, or semantic processing? Cortex 48 (8): 952–962.

12. Code, C. (1982). Neurolinguistic analysis of recurrent utterance in aphasia. Cortex 18 (1): 141–152.

13. Robson, J., Marshall, J., Pring, T., and Chiat, S. (1998). Phonological naming therapy in jargon aphasia: positive but paradoxical effects. Journal of the International Neuropsychological Society 4 (6): 675–686.

14. Bose, A. (2013). Phonological therapy in jargon aphasia: effects on naming and neologisms. International Journal of Language & Communication Disorders 48 (5): 582–595.

15. Marshall, J. (2006). Jargon aphasia: what have we learned? Aphasiology 20 (5): 387–410.

16. Sampson, M. and Faroqi-Shah, Y. (2011). Investigation of self-monitoring in fluent aphasia with jargon. Aphasiology 25 (4): 505–528.

17. Morris, J. and Franklin, S. (2017). Disorders of auditory comprehension. In: Aphasia and Related Neurogenic Communication Disorders, 2e (ed. I. Papathanasiou and P. Coppens), 151–168. Burlington: Jones & Bartlett Learning.

18. Meteyard, L., Bruce, C., Edmundson, A., and Oakhill, J. (2014). Profiling text comprehension impairments in aphasia. Aphasiology 29 (1): 1–28.

19. Inatomi, Y., Yonehara, T., Omiya, S. et al. (2008). Aphasia during the acute phase in ischemic stroke. Cerebrovascular Diseases 25 (4): 316–323.

20. Maas, M.B., Lev, M.H., Ay, H. et al. (2012). The prognosis for aphasia in stroke. Journal of Stroke and Cerebrovascular Diseases 21 (5): 350–357.

21. El Hachioui, H., Lingsma, H.F., van de Sandt-Koenderman, M.W. et al. (2013). Long-term prognosis of aphasia after stroke. Journal of Neurology, Neurosurgery, and Psychiatry 84 (3): 310–315.

22. Pedersen, P.M., Vinter, K., and Olsen, T.S. (2004). Aphasia after stroke: type, severity and prognosis. Cerebrovascular Diseases 17 (1): 35–43.

23. Basso, A. (1992). Prognostic factors in aphasia. Aphasiology 6 (4): 337–348.

24. de Riesthal, M. and Wertz, R. (2004). Prognosis for aphasia: relationship between selected biographical and behavioural variables and outcome and improvement. Aphasiology 18 (10): 899–915.

25. Lazar, R.M., Minzer, B., Antoniello, D. et al. (2010). Improvement in aphasia scores after stroke is well predicted by initial severity. Stroke 41 (7): 1485–1488.

26. Plowman, E., Hentz, B., and Ellis, C. (2012). Post-stroke aphasia prognosis: a review of patient-related and stroke-related factors. Journal of Evaluation in Clinical Practice 18 (3): 689–694.

27. Brady, M.C., Kelly, H., Godwin, J. et al. (2016). Speech and language therapy for aphasia following stroke. Cochrane Database of Systematic Reviews 6 (Art. No.: CD000425). https://doi.org/10.1002/14651858.CD000425.pub3.

28. Poslawsky, I.E., Schuurmans, M.J., Lindeman, E., and Hafsteinsdóttir, T.B. (2010). A systematic review of nursing rehabilitation of stroke patients with aphasia. Journal of Clinical Nursing 19 (1–2): 17–32.

29. Enderby, P., Wood, V., and Wade, D. (1987). Frenchay Aphasia Screening Test. Windsor: NFER-Nelson.
30. McCooey, R., Worrall, L., Toffolo, D. et al. (2004). Inpatient Functional Communication Interview. Norwich: Singular Publishing.
31. National Institute for Health and Care Excellence (NICE) (2013). Stroke Rehabilitation in Adults: Clinical Guideline (CG162). Manchester: National Institute for Health and Care Excellence.
32. Rose, M.L. (2006). The utility of arm and hand gestures in the treatment of aphasia. Advances in Speech Language Pathology 8 (2): 92–109.
33. Sacchett, C., Byng, S., Marshall, J., and Pound, C. (1999). Drawing together: evaluation of a therapy programme for severe aphasia. International Journal of Language and Communication Disorders 34 (3): 265–289.
34. Nickels, L. (1997). Spoken Word Production and its Breakdown in Aphasia. Hove: Psychology Press.
35. Stroke Association (2012). Accessible Information Guidelines. London: Stroke Association.
36. Jensen, L.R., Løvholt, A.P., Sørensen, I.R. et al. (2015). Implementation of supported conversation for communication between nursing staff and in-hospital patients with aphasia. Aphasiology 29 (1): 57–80.
37. Flowers, H.L., Silver, F.L., Fang, J. et al. (2013). The incidence, co-occurrence, and predictors of dysphagia, dysarthria, and aphasia after first-ever acute ischemic stroke. Journal of Communication Disorders 46 (3): 238–248.
38. Duffy, J.R. (2013). Motor Speech Disorders-E-Book: Substrates, Differential Diagnosis, and Management. St. Louis: Elsevier Health Sciences.
39. Enderby, P. and Palmer, R. (2008). Frenchay Dysarthria Assessment-2. Austin: Pro-Ed.
40. Mackenzie, C. and Lowit, A. (2007). Behavioural intervention effects in dysarthria following stroke: communication effectiveness, intelligibility and dysarthria impact. International Journal of Language & Communication Disorders 42 (2): 131–153.
41. Urban, P., Rolke, R., Wicht, S. et al. (2006). Left-hemispheric dominance for articulation: a prospective study on acute ischaemic dysarthria at different localizations. Brain 129 (3): 767–777.
42. Yorkston, K., Beukelman, D., Strand, E., and Hakel, M. (2010). Management of Motor Speech Disorders in Adults and Children. Austin: Pro-ED.
43. Gordon, C., Ellis-Hill, C., and Ashburn, A. (2009). The use of conversational analysis: nurse–patient interaction in communication disability after stroke. Journal of Advanced Nursing 65 (3): 544–553.
44. Royal College of Physicians (2016). National Clinical Guideline for Stroke, 5e. London: Royal College of Physicians.
45. Elman, R.J. (1999). Group treatment for patients with right hemisphere damage. In: Group Treatment of Neurogenic Communication Disorders: The Expert Clinician's Approach, 2e (ed. L.R. Cherney and A.S. Halper), 269–296. Boston: Butterworth-Heinemann.
46. Benton, E. and Bryan, K. (1996). Right cerebral hemisphere damage: incidence of language problems. International Journal of Rehabilitation Research 19 (1): 47–54.
47. Ferré, P., Clermont, M.F., Lajoie, C. et al. (2009). Identification de profils communicationnels parmi les individus cérébrolésés droits: profils transculturels. Neuropsicologia Latinoamericana 1 (1): 32–40.
48. Marshall, J., Atkinson, J., Thacker, A., and Woll, B. (2003). Is speech and language therapy meeting the needs of language minorities? The case of deaf people with neurological impairments. International Journal of Language & Communication Disorders 38 (1): 85–94.
49. Centeno, J.G. (2009). Issues and principles in service delivery to communicatively-impaired minority bilingual adults in neurorehabilitation. Seminars in Speech and Language 30 (3): 139–153.

50. Roberts, P. (2008). Issues in assessment and treatment for bilingual and culturally diverse patients. In: Language Intervention Strategies in Aphasia and Related Neurogenic Communication Disorders, 5e (ed. R. Chapey), 245–274. Baltimore: Lippincott Williams and Wilkins.
51. Fabbro, F. (1999). The Neurolinguistics of Bilingualism. Hove: Psychology Press.
52. García-Caballero, A., García-Lado, I., González-Hermida, J. et al. (2007). Paradoxical recovery in a bilingual patient with aphasia after right capsuloputaminal infarction. Journal of Neurology, Neurosurgery & Psychiatry 78 (1): 89–91.
53. Adrover-Roig, D., Galparsoro-Izagirre, N., Marcotte, K. et al. (2011). Impaired L1 and executive control after left basal ganglia damage in a bilingual Basque–Spanish person with aphasia. Clinical Linguistics & Phonetics 25 (6–7): 480–498.
54. Hilari, K., Byng, S., Lamping, D.L., and Smith, S.C. (2003). Stroke and Aphasia Quality of Life Scale-39 (SAQOL-39): evaluation of acceptability, reliability, and validity. Stroke 34 (8): 1944–1950.
55. Pound, C., Parr, S., Lindsay, J., and Woolf, C. (2000). Beyond Aphasia: Therapies for Living with Communication Disability. Bicester: Speechmark.
56. Simmons-Mackie, N.N., Kagan, A., O'Neill Christie, C. et al. (2007). Communicative access and decision making for people with aphasia: implementing sustainable healthcare systems change. Aphasiology 21 (1): 39–66.
57. Code, C., Mackie, N.S., Armstrong, E. et al. (2001). The public awareness of aphasia: an international survey. International Journal of Language and Communication Disorders 36 (S1): 1–6.
58. Elman, R.J., Ogar, J., and Elman, S.H. (2000). Aphasia: awareness, advocacy, and activism. Aphasiology 14 (5–6): 455–459.
59. Hilton, R., Leenhouts, S., Webster, J., and Morris, J. (2014). Information, support and training needs of relatives of people with aphasia: evidence from the literature. Aphasiology 28 (7): 797–822.
60. Turner, S. and Whitworth, A. (2006). Conversational partner training programmes in aphasia: a review of key themes and participants' roles. Aphasiology 20 (6): 483–510.
61. Breitenstein, C., Grewe, T., Flöel, A. et al. (2017). Intensive speech and language therapy in patients with chronic aphasia after stroke: a randomised, open-label, blinded-endpoint, controlled trial in a health-care setting. The Lancet 389 (10078): 1528–1538.
62. Godecke, E., Hird, K., Lalor, E.E. et al. (2012). Very early poststroke aphasia therapy: a pilot randomized controlled efficacy trial. International Journal of Stroke 7 (8): 635–644.
63. Godecke, E., Ciccone, N.A., Granger, A.S. et al. (2014). A comparison of aphasia therapy outcomes before and after a very early rehabilitation programme following stroke. International Journal of Language & Communication Disorders 49 (2): 149–161.
64. Lafond, D., Joanette, Y., Ponzio, J. et al. (1993). Living with Aphasia: Psychosocial Issues. Norwich: Singular Publishing.
65. Davies P, Woolf C. Dysphasia Matters: A Training Package for Medical Professionals [VIDEO]. Creative Film Productions; 1997.
66. Avent, J., Glista, S., Wallace, S. et al. (2005). Family information needs about aphasia. Aphasiology 19 (3–5): 365–375.
67. National Institute for Health Research (2018). Enabling People with Aphasia to Participate in Research: Resources for Stroke Researchers. London: National Institute for Health Research.
68. Anderson, R. (1992). The Aftermath of Stroke: The Experience of Patients and their Families. Cambridge: Cambridge University Press.
69. Luker, J. and Grimmer-Somers, K. (2009). The relationship between staff compliance with implementing discharge planning guidelines, and stroke patients' experiences post-discharge. Internet Journal of Allied Health Sciences and Practice 7 (3): 11.
70. Tilling, K., Sterne, J.A., Rudd, A.G. et al. (2001). A new method for predicting recovery after stroke. Stroke 32 (12): 2867–2873.

71. Cruice, M., Worrall, L., Hickson, L., and Murison, R. (2003). Finding a focus for quality of life with aphasia: social and emotional health, and psychological well-being. Aphasiology 17 (4): 333–353.

72. Hilari, K., Wiggins, R., Roy, P. et al. (2003). Predictors of health-related quality of life (HRQL) in people with chronic aphasia. Aphasiology 17 (4): 365–381.

73. Hilari, K. (2011). The impact of stroke: are people with aphasia different to those without? Disability and Rehabilitation 33 (3): 211–218.

74. Cruice, M., Worrall, L., and Hickson, L. (2006). Quantifying aphasic people's social lives in the context of non-aphasic peers. Aphasiology 20 (12): 1210–1225.

75. Hilari, K. and Northcott, S. (2006). Social support in people with chronic aphasia. Aphasiology 20 (1): 17–36.

76. Northcott, S., Marshall, J., and Hilari, K. (2016). What factors predict who will have a strong social network following a stroke? Journal of Speech, Language, and Hearing Research 59 (4): 772–783.

77. Kauhanen, M.-L., Korpelainen, J., Hiltunen, P. et al. (1999). Poststroke depression correlates with cognitive impairment and neurological deficits. Stroke 30 (9): 1875–1880.

78. Tsouna-Hadjis, E., Vemmos, K.N., Zakopoulos, N., and Stamatelopoulos, S. (2000). First-stroke recovery process: the role of family social support. Archives of Physical Medicine and Rehabilitation 81 (7): 881–887.

79. Boden-Albala, B., Litwak, E., Elkind, M. et al. (2005). Social isolation and outcomes post stroke. Neurology 64 (11): 1888–1892.

80. Ayerbe, L., Ayis, S., Crichton, S. et al. (2014). The long-term outcomes of depression up to 10 years after stroke; the South London stroke register. Journal of Neurology, Neurosurgery and Psychiatry 85 (5): 514–521.

81. Thomas, S.A., Walker, M.F., Macniven, J.A. et al. (2013). Communication and Low Mood (CALM): a randomized controlled trial of behavioural therapy for stroke patients with aphasia. Clinical Rehabilitation 27 (5): 398–408.

82. Northcott, S., Burns, K., Simpson, A., and Hilari, K. (2015). 'Living with aphasia the best way I can': a feasibility study exploring solution-focused brief therapy for people with aphasia. Folia Phoniatrica et Logopaedica 67 (3): 156–167.

83. Lam, J.M. and Wodchis, W.P. (2010). The relationship of 60 disease diagnoses and 15 conditions to preference-based health-related quality of life in Ontario hospital-based long-term care residents. Medical Care 48 (4): 380–387.

84. Hickey, E., Bourgeois, M., and Olswang, L. (2004). Effects of training volunteers to converse with nursing home residents with aphasia. Aphasiology 18 (5–7): 625–637.

85. Fotiadou, D., Northcott, S., Chatzidaki, A., and Hilari, K. (2014). Aphasia blog talk: how does stroke and aphasia affect a person's social relationships? Aphasiology 28 (11): 1281–1300.

86. Brown, K., Worrall, L.E., Davidson, B., and Howe, T. (2012). Living successfully with aphasia: a qualitative meta-analysis of the perspectives of individuals with aphasia, family members, and speech-language pathologists. International Journal of Speech-Language Pathology 14 (2): 141–155.

87. Hinckley, J.J. (2006). Finding messages in bottles: living successfully with stroke and aphasia. Topics in Stroke Rehabilitation 13 (1): 25–36.

CHAPTER 8

Management of Physical Impairments Post-Stroke

Cherry Kilbride[1,2], Rosie Kneafsey[3], and Vicky Kean[4]
[1] Brunel University London, London, UK
[2] Royal Free London NHS Foundation Trust, London, UK
[3] School for Nursing, Midwifery and Health, Coventry University, Coventry, UK
[4] George Eliot Hospital NHS Trust, Nuneaton, UK

KEY POINTS

- A stroke nurse within the team is pivotal to early rehabilitation and the management of physical impairments.
- Patients should be encouraged to use their own movement in the achievement of functional activities to promote positive neuroplastic brain changes.
- Prevention remains the best approach to contracture management.
- Inactive/immobile stroke patients are at risk of adaptive muscle shortening; active intervention is required to minimise changes and prevent loss in range-of-movement.
- Opportunities for practice of task-specific activities should be encouraged in formal therapy sessions and throughout the day by all members of the team and family.
- Members of the nursing team must build meaningful connections and personal engagement with patients and families, thus supporting the therapeutic milieu of the rehabilitation environment.

Stroke Nursing, Second Edition. Edited by Jane Williams, Lin Perry, and Caroline Watkins.
© 2020 John Wiley & Sons Ltd. Published 2020 by John Wiley & Sons Ltd.

This chapter maps to criteria within the following sections of the Stroke-Specific Education Framework (SSEF):

I'm back to work now, and I work in London. You can imagine, it's all a fast pace, and I used to get the bus to the station or walk to the station, jump on the train, get off the train, walk, the majority of the time I used to walk, from London Bridge to Tower Bridge which is a good 20 minute walk. Then walk back, it's nice in the summer doing that. No way; no chance of doing that now. I get the train, which is not the easiest thing to get on when they're packed; because I have to have a seat, so I leave really early. I get into work at 8.30 so I can leave at 4.30, to get a chance of getting a seat. I don't walk any more. I did try to get the Tube, which was a nightmare, because there was a lot of stairs, which I never really realised before, so I ended up getting a taxi, which is not cheap. At the moment I'm very dependent where before I was very independent. I had my own flat, my own car; I was doing what I wanted to do when I wanted to do it. Now I have to more depend on other people; I have to go a slower pace, which in some respects is nice, but London is a very fast pace, you cannot afford to be slow. So I think I probably will have to end up changing my job. Something like this, it makes you take stock of your life.

(Jodie, 31-year-old woman, South London, 6 months post-stroke)

8.1 Introduction

The focus of this chapter is the early management of physical impairments post-stroke. Losing the ability to easily and purposefully move, impinges on individuals' capacity to remain physically independent in daily activities and can have negative impact on quality of life. Being in *control* of movement is a source of autonomy, pride, and dignity, and reduced mobility and movement can have profound psychological and emotional effects. Early rehabilitation, through the promotion of physical activity and the reduction of sedentary behaviour, is key to stroke treatment; nurses have a central role.

Initially, we will review how stroke affects movement (including the role of sensation), and then we will explore moving and handling, risk assessment, therapeutic positioning and seating, early rehabilitation, falls prevention, and the re-education of movement. Rehabilitation activities to promote function, reduce sedentary behaviours, and increase levels of participation are also considered. The importance of ongoing involvement and education of the patient, family, and carers is implicit in everything discussed.

8.2 Movement

Coordinated and purposeful movement arises from the interaction of a complex array of information from the brain, spinal cord, and peripheral receptors in the head, body, and limbs [2]. Post-stroke, this interrelationship between the central and peripheral *control systems* is disrupted, which can lead to problems in carrying out everyday functional activity. Depending on the site and size of the lesion, damage can occur to the long descending tracts from the brain that help control movement, and patients can present with symptoms collectively described as the upper motor neuron syndrome (UMNS).

The UMNS is commonly divided into:

- positive features (e.g. spasticity, clonus, increased tendon reflexes extensor/flexor spasms, associated reactions);
- negative features (e.g. muscle weakness, fatigue, loss of dexterity/coordination); and
- adaptive features (e.g. changes in mechanical and functional properties of muscle and connective tissue) [3, 4]

Clinically, the positive, negative, and adaptive features of the UMNS can present in many ways, with varying degrees of influence on functional recovery. It is now commonly acknowledged that the effect of positive signs on decreased function post-stroke may have been previously overestimated. Indeed, spasticity can help function in some people; for example, increased tone in lower limbs can be utilised when weakness would otherwise impede transfers or walking [5–7]. The bigger impact of negative changes, particularly weakness, and adaptive features is now more widely recognised [8, 9]. Hence, the active management of secondary complications arising from adaptive motor behaviour and the resultant effect on the musculoskeletal system is fundamental early post-stroke.

8.2.1 The Role of Sensation in Movement

Sensation acts as a driver for movement; functional mobility involves the integration of sensory feedback from receptors in the periphery with programmes of movement stored in the central nervous system (CNS) [10]. Following a stroke, sensory functions may be impaired, affecting a person's ability to move. The extent of impairment is dependent on the site and size of the lesion. For example, sensory receptors in muscles and tendons provide information about body and limb position, and this information is conveyed via the dorsal column tract to be processed in the somatosensory area located in the post-central gyrus of the parietal lobe of the brain [2]. Thus, following a middle cerebral artery infarct, resultant cell death can alter the brain's ability to accurately process and interpret sensory information sent from the body, leading to a diminished ability to move. Movement without sensation is possible, but it lacks accuracy, exhibiting increasing clumsiness in the absence of sensory feedback which updates instructions coming from the brain [10]. It is therefore important to be aware of the effect of sensory involvement in the rehabilitation of mobility.

A lot of people when they have strokes, can't feel anything in the side that's affected. I could feel everything, I just couldn't move it. But I could feel everything. And when I was laying there the first day, and they was touching me, I could feel everything. It was so frustrating 'cos I couldn't move.

(Jodie, quoted at the start of this chapter)

8.3 Promoting Physical Activity and Movement After Stroke

As described in Chapter 2, the brain's neuroplastic properties are influenced by sensory inputs received and motor outputs requested [11]. Therapeutic interactions with patients post-stroke can drive positive neuroplastic change for recovery of mobility. It follows that *specific nursing attention should be given to maintaining patients' existing movement and mobility levels, and to promoting and supporting improvements.*

It is essential that the moving and handling of people who have experienced stroke is not treated as a routine or ritualistic task. Rather, nursing teams should play an active part in a structured, multiprofessional, goal-focused approach to rehabilitation. This often begins with the nurse's initial assessment of positioning, mobility, and moving and handlings needs [12, 13]. From this point forwards, a plan of nursing interventions to maintain and promote the individual's movement and mobility should be implemented until a team approach has been established.

A focused approach such as this is particularly pertinent as the problem of *hospital-induced deconditioning and mobility loss can seriously complicate an inpatient stay*, leading to poor long-term patient outcomes [14]. There are numerous contributing factors to in-hospital deterioration in mobility function: the initial condition and associated treatments, prior cognitive impairment or functional difficulty, and multiple co-morbidities [15, 16]. However, unnecessary, extended periods of bed/chair rest, inactivity, and general 'low mobility' [17, 18] are modifiable factors leading to loss of muscle mass, strength, and fitness [19, 20]. In addition, protective or custodial nursing practices and restrictive hospital environments may also worsen functional loss [21–23].

On admission to hospital, stroke patients may be highly dependent on healthcare staff for movement, positioning, and mobility, placing them in an extremely vulnerable position. It is therefore *vital that nursing teams are proactive in encouraging early mobilisation and engagement in physical activity*, rather than waiting for other members of the rehabilitation team to lead and direct nursing activities [12, 18]. For example, patient handling carried out by nurses should be viewed as an important therapeutic component of rehabilitation, not simply a means of getting the individual from A to B. Each time nursing assistance is given with positioning, transfers, or walking, it should be viewed as a therapeutic moment, an opportunity to provide coaching and to build therapy into nursing care. In this way, the nurse's 'therapy integration' and 'therapy carry-on' roles [24] can maximise the value of time-limited therapist–client interactions. Activities such as helping someone to the toilet can form a core component of daily therapy. It is essential that continence issues are effectively managed, but this can be part of rehabilitation for movement or mobility. Benefits can work both ways, with regular physical activity promoting normal bowel habits as well as better night-time sleep.

Supporting the mobility needs of people post-stroke has been identified as an area of specialist nursing, requiring additional skills and knowledge [12]. Moreover, this advanced practical skill must be combined with the ability to connect and communicate effectively [25], along with the aptitude to assess progress towards rehabilitation goals [12]. This is crucial where patients are, for example, depressed or fearful of falling [21]. Patients may choose to restrict their activity levels, requiring the nurse to provide additional emotional support and encouragement to bolster their sense of self-efficacy and achievement. As the following example illustrates, older adults may have more rehabilitation potential than is initially realised, and skilled intervention, timely hospital discharge planning, advocacy, and community support are crucial to an individual's longer-term outcomes.

> *We went to see him in hospital and everyone was just walking past and he was just sat there, in his chair, every day, all the time. He was so sad and low. Once we got him home it was different. The community physio got him playing the golf Wii and he got an exercise bike in the house. Not bad for an 80-year-old. He's back in the garden now and walking to the shops. Not even his family thought it was possible, it is amazing what he has achieved when it all seemed so bleak to start with.*
>
> *(Family member of Harry, an 80-year-old man)*

Nurses may encounter barriers to their full engagement in the rehabilitation process and activities to support mobility and movement. Divided teamwork practices between nurses and physiotherapists may hamper the sharing of skills and knowledge, leading to missed opportunities for rehabilitation. Fear of back injury may result in nurses feeling reluctant to engage in mobility activities [12, 26], and it is important to be aware of safe patient handling principles and their application to rehabilitation practice.

8.3.1 Rehabilitation Handling and Manual Handling Regulations

In the United Kingdom, as in many other countries, moving and handling regulations [27] legally require employers to undertake specific assessments of all manual handling operations, such as patient handling, to identify potential risks of injury to patients or staff. *Where risks are identified, actions must be taken to eliminate or reduce them*, as far as is practical [27]. As a result, many hospitals and community services have introduced 'minimal handling' and 'safer patient handling' policies, to which staff must adhere. Such regulations have improved the working conditions for nursing teams, for example by encouraging the use of adaptive equipment such as standing aids, hoists, slide sheets, and transfer boards. It is important that nursing staff are confident in using this equipment within an individuals' rehabilitation programme. There have been concerns expressed that overuse of patient handling equipment may stifle the rehabilitation process;

a balance must be struck to ensure that nurses keep themselves safe in the workplace and avoid physical injury where possible, whilst at the same time enabling patients to safely practice mobility and transfer skills and promoting physical independence [21, 26].

A central component of successful patient handling and injury prevention is the completion of effective risk assessments. The acronym TILEE is often used as a framework to assist in the risk assessment of load handling activities; this refers to an assessment of the *task*, *individual capability*, *load*, *environment*, and *equipment*. It is vital that appropriate action is taken if risks are identified. Initial risk assessment might suggest a more detailed analysis of the task to identify the best course of action.

8.3.2 Therapeutic Positioning and Seating in the Acute Phase

As stroke can affect a person's ability to move and change position, *therapeutic positioning is a cornerstone of early stroke rehabilitation.* The provision of appropriate external support enables a patient to better cope with the effects of gravity and maintain good postural alignment without using undue muscular activity [28].

Therapeutic positioning, whether in bed or sitting out in a chair, is essential to:

- limit sustained postures;
- maximise function;
- maintain skin integrity and prevent pressure sores;
- maintain soft-tissue length and prevent contractures;
- reduce noxious stimuli and decrease discomfort; and
- promote socialisation [4].

Specialist stroke nurses need a good understanding of therapeutic positioning, although the evidence is largely based on clinical experience [29–31]. A postal survey of 674 UK physiotherapists explored patient positioning post-stroke and found three main reasons underpinning choice of position:

- modulation (alteration) of muscle tone;
- prevention of damage to affected limbs; and
- support to body segments [30].

Sitting in an armchair and side lying on the non-hemiplegic and hemiplegic side were cited as the most frequently used positions. Another survey, of 150 nurses and 25 therapists, reported sitting out in a chair as the preferred position for conscious patients post-stroke, and side lying on the non-hemiplegic side for unconscious patients. There was less agreement about the use of supine, high side lying, and lying on the hemiplegic side [31]. *There is no single correct position, and varying the patient's posture during the day and night* (using T-rolls, pillows, and wedges to achieve this in supine, prone, side lying, and sitting out) *is advocated* [4]. Changing and rotating positions rather than sustaining any one posture is key. Standard positioning charts are useful to promote consistency across the stroke unit or ward team; alternatively, photographs can be used (with patient consent) [4].

A well-positioned patient demonstrates good biomechanical alignment of different parts of the body in relation to one another, which ultimately affects the efficiency of movement [32]. For example, a patient sitting in a flexed position and weight bearing through their sacrum, rather than ischium, thighs and feet is not only at increased risk of pressure sores, but must use excessive muscle activity elsewhere (e.g. head, upper limbs, trunk, or hips) to remain upright. In this situation, patients use their arms to help 'fix' themselves in sitting positions. Poorly designed chairs, soft mattresses, and lack of specialist equipment can present challenges to therapeutic positioning and may require creative use of foot blocks, pillows, or folded blankets to provide external support and attain 90° at hips, knees, and ankles. Aspects of positioning identified by physiotherapists as being the most important are:

- head alignment (neutral, midline, and supported on pillow);
- scapular protraction;
- equal weight bearing between right and left buttocks;
- hip and trunk alignment (i.e. hips at 90°); and
- support of distal components (i.e. hands and feet) [30].

Photographs (taken with informed consent) of the patient are increasingly used to individualise information for specific patient needs, and standard positioning charts can also be individualised by drawing on additional pillows to help postural alignment.

Positioning in the early stages of acute stroke is also carried out as *part of respiratory care for optimal oxygen saturation*. In a systematic review of four studies of 183 stroke patients, body position was shown not to affect oxygen saturation in acute stroke patients without relevant (respiratory) co-morbidities; there was limited evidence that sitting in a chair had any beneficial effect or that lying positions had a deleterious effect on oxygen saturation in patients with respiratory co-morbidities [33]. See Chapter 4 for detail on positioning in the hyper-acute stage.

The orientation and position of the patient within their immediate surroundings can also provide valuable stimulation when visual and perceptual problems are evident. However, in the early stages, with a patient who has marked visual and perceptual deficits, it may be necessary to address them in midline (i.e. straight on and within their visual field). As remediation occurs, stimulation can be provided from the affected side [9].

Special consideration is required for the small number of patients who present with the *contraversive pushing syndrome*, where they lean towards the hemiplegic side, strongly resisting any attempts to passively correct posture towards or across the midline, as they already perceive themselves to be upright [34, 35]. Karnath and Broetz [35] describe an intervention plan to address this impairment that includes helping the patient recognise their altered perception of erect body position by using visual aids (e.g. the upright of a door frame) to check their own verticality.

In summary, therapeutic positioning and seating can maximise function, limit secondary complications, and enhance perceptual awareness, communication, swallow function, and social interaction, and is therefore an essential part of rehabilitation [28, 36]. Readers are referred to Pope [28] for a comprehensive review of posture and seating.

8.4   Promoting Early Rehabilitation

Inactivity has a detrimental effect on body function and can lead to complications such as chest infections, pressure damage, deep vein thrombosis, constipation, and urinary tract infections. Even short periods of immobility will lead to muscle atrophy, loss of subcutaneous fat, contractures, decreased range-of-movement, and activity intolerance [37]. Respiratory difficulties are also common when mobility is limited, and the patient may become dyspnoeic with chest crackles and wheezes and an increased respiratory rate [38]. Some patients may also experience cardiovascular disruption associated with immobility, including orthostatic hypotension, increased heart rate, and peripheral oedema [39–41]. Complications that may be a consequence of, or related to, immobility are detailed in Table 8.1.

To prevent such complications from occurring, it is important that, *following careful assessment of their condition occurring within the first 24 hours of onset* by an appropriately trained professional [13], *patients begin to move and start physical rehabilitation.* The promotion of early rehabilitation is a key aspect in acute stroke care; the National Clinical Guidelines for Stroke recommend people who have difficulty in moving early after stroke, and who are medically stable, be offered frequent, short daily mobilisations (defined as unsupported sitting out of bed, standing, or walking), typically beginning between 24 and 48 hours after stroke onset. Mobilisation within 24 hours of stroke onset should only occur for patients requiring little or no assistance to mobilise [13]. Results from a global randomised controlled trial (AVERT, A Very Early Rehabilitation Trial), involving 56 stroke units in five countries and 2104 stroke patients, underpin this clinical guidance [42]. While questions remain about the dosage and frequency of therapy, *there is agreement on the importance of avoiding sedentary behaviour and physical inactivity post-stroke.* However, for some nurses in acute settings, there can be a clash of priorities within their workload between encouraging patients to walk and change position and the patients' other needs [12]. One study showed that only 27% of 118 patients actually 'walked' whilst an inpatient; those that did walk, only did so for an average of 5.5 minutes [43]. A more recent 3-year longitudinal study indicated little had changed, with patients observed sitting/lying, standing, and walking 94, 4, and 2% of the time, respectively [44]. It is of utmost importance that nurses, as the multidisciplinary team (MDT) members most consistently present, promote and engage in early rehabilitation.

Once the patient is ready to start rehabilitation, a number of parameters should be used to monitor how well he or she tolerates therapy. Stiller and Phillips [45] provide a useful overview of the safety aspects of mobilising acute stage patients. For example, contraindications to mobilising patients include acute infections, unstable angina, pulmonary embolus, and infarction. Patients with a diagnosis of deep vein thrombosis will be prescribed anticoagulation, and mobilisation may be delayed.

TABLE 8.1 Complications that may be related to immobility

System	Presenting problem
Metabolic	Slowed wound healing
	Muscle atrophy
	Decreased amount of subcutaneous fat
	Stasis oedema
Respiratory	Decreased chest wall and diaphragmatic movement
	Limited alveolar ventilation, may result in dyspnoea
	Noisy breathing (wheeze, crackles, crepitation), increased respiratory rate
Cardiovascular	Orthostatic hypotension
	Deconditioning, leading to increased heart rate
	Weak peripheral pulses, cold extremities
	Peripheral oedema
Musculoskeletal	Deep vein thrombosis: erythema, increased diameter in calf or thigh; discomfort/pain
	Decreased range-of-movement
	Joint contracture
	Loss of activity tolerance
	Muscle atrophy
Skin	Damage to skin integrity; pressure ulcer development
Elimination	Difficulty with micturition; scanty, cloudy, or concentrated urine
	Decreased frequency of bowel movements; constipation
	Abdominal distension
	Decreased or increased bowel sounds

If a patient's level of oxygenation deteriorates during mobilisation, the intensity of the activity should be reduced or ceased and oxygen saturation levels monitored. Guidance on oxygen saturation levels and supplementary oxygen can be found in the British Thorax Society National Guidelines [46].

Patients with type 1 diabetes may be vulnerable to unstable blood glucose levels post-stroke, and their blood glucose levels should be monitored in relation to mobilisation activities because these have the potential to reduce glycaemic control. Similar precautions should be taken with patients who may have developed hyperglycaemia post-stroke.

All patients should be monitored to ascertain how well they cope and to spot signs of distress during mobilisation activities. These might include signs of pain or discomfort, perceived exertion, shortness of breath, fatigue, anxiety, skin colouration, sweatiness, and clamminess.

Patients require sufficient energy to actively participate in rehabilitation; nutrition and hydration needs must be met (see Chapter 5), and healthy sleep and rest patterns promoted. Stroke patients with pain may be reluctant to move, and pain relief should be arranged, including in advance of therapy sessions.

8.4.1 Sitting Out of Bed

Patients should be sat out of bed, ideally within 24–48 hours of stroke onset [13, 42], *or within 24 hours of stroke onset for those who require little or no assistance to mobilise.* However, it is important initially not to sit the patient out for too long, because it can become very tiring and may lead to unwanted excessive muscle activity (e.g. overuse of the head in trying to remain upright). Depending on individual needs, the patient might be sat out for approximately 15–20 minutes. Ideally, a range of wheelchairs should be available for use (e.g. tilt in space specialist seating), but often ward chairs are adapted (with pillows, rolled-up towels, and folded blankets) to achieve optimum postures for maintaining length, protecting vulnerable joints such as the glenohumeral joint, and aiding in respiration, communication, and social interaction [28, 36]. Support should be provided for the head, trunk, and hemiplegic upper limb as required, and should be sufficient to maintain good posture and help with carry-over of treatment [47]. If patients have difficulties with seating, they should be referred to a specialist seating service.

8.4.2 Standing

Standing is a key component of early rehabilitation and *should be commenced as soon as the patient's cardiovascular system has stabilised, ideally within 24–48 hours of stroke onset*, or within 24 hours for patients requiring little or no help [9, 42]. Encouraging patients to stand and undertake weight bearing maintains muscle length, and promotes extensor muscle activity to counter the predominance of flexion incurred from prolonged periods sitting [9, 48].

With the exception of standing hoists, the increasing use of mechanical lifting aids to transfer people has raised concerns at potentially reduced opportunities for patients to take weight through their lower limbs. Regular standing through the day can help maintain tone levels, decrease frequency of spasms, assist maintenance of joint range [49], and activate extensor muscles, none of which happens when lying [48, 50, 51]. If a patient has no or only minimal movement, a tilt table can be used [52]; if the patient shows more extensor activity in the trunk and lower limb, then other standing devices such as a motorised standing frame can be introduced [4].

Periods as short as 5 minutes may be tolerated initially. Mechanical ventilation does not preclude standing or sitting, but close monitoring of oxygen saturation and vital signs is required, particularly if autonomic disturbances are exhibited [53]. As the patient progresses, the amount of support can be reduced and the patient can practise standing with the help of one or two team members, or within parallel bars if appropriate and available.

8.4.3 Walking

Depending on the degree of hemiparesis, walking may not be possible in the early stages post-stroke, or it may require additional equipment. The MDT should take the lead from the physiotherapist as to how to help the patient mobilise. For example, diminished movement in the upper limb often precludes the use of a walking frame, yet patients may choose to use a walking stick to help their walking practice, rather than wait until they can walk without one [54].

Lack of dorsiflexion in the ankle may require a temporary ankle–foot orthosis [55] or orthotics [56]. Selective functional electrical stimulation (FES) has been used successfully for foot drop and is recommended in national clinical guidelines [57].

In recent years, partial body weight support treadmill training, including partial body weight support systems, has offered the possibility of active and task-specific gait re-education even for stroke patients with low levels of activity; the harness system provides added security. However, these specialist treadmills tend to be confined to larger physiotherapy departments and rehabilitation units, and are no more effective for improving walking ability (in those that can walk) than other physiotherapy interventions, matched for intensity. Patients who are unable to walk independently at the start of treatment do not seem to benefit [58, 59].

8.4.4 Falls Prevention

Falls are common at all stages of recovery post-stroke due to alterations in balance and coordination and changes in gait pattern [60]. The impact of a fall post-stroke may be significant, psychologically and physically. Not only may a fall result in hip fracture, but it may lead to the individual becoming socially isolated or physically inactive due to fear of falling. A number of factors increase the risk of a fall (detailed in Box 8.1). It is impossible to prevent all falls from occurring, even when a patient is in hospital, but the likelihood of a fall can be reduced. Many hospital and community services produce useful information leaflets for patients and relatives about this. Handling falling or fallen people also presents risks of injury to patients, carers, and staff members. It is inadvisable to try to catch someone falling despite the ethical dilemma this poses.

Box 8.1 | Falls Risk Factors

- Reduced strength and balance, poor gait, physical weakness
- Foot problems and footwear
- Sensory deficits, e.g. visual problems, poor hearing
- Cognitive and perceptual problems, e.g. neglect, altered judgement
- Medical conditions, e.g. acute illness, stroke, postural hypotension
- Fear of falling
- History of falls
- Hurrying, altered environment, space and furniture layout, poor lighting

---

I was getting the breakfast stuff tidied up again, and I came in here and I went down. I knew I was going down, and I hit against this thing [coffee table]. I was bleeding and all. I got as far as the door and I fell again and I couldn't get up.

(Betty, 82 years old, living alone 6 months post-stroke)

People with stroke should be offered falls risk assessment and management as part of their stroke rehabilitation, along with training for them and their family/carers on how to get up after a fall. Assessment of fear of falling should form part of their falls risk assessment [13], which should include [61]:

- history of falls;
- assessment of gait, balance, mobility, and muscle weakness;
- osteoporosis risk;
- functional ability;
- fear of falling;
- visual or cognitive impairment;
- urinary incontinence;
- home hazards;
- neurological and cardiovascular examination; and
- medication review.

A falls prevention intervention can be offered if needed. This could involve modification of risk factors, strength and balance training, changes within the home, referral and vision improvement, and modification of medication. On the rehabilitation ward, safety measures might include using a wheelchair to the toilet and walking back, or positioning a walking aid or chair halfway between the bedside and toilet [62]. People at risk of falls post-stroke should participate in physical activity/exercise, including balance and coordination, at least twice a week [13, 63].

8.5 Re-education of Movement

As described earlier, the loss of movement post-stroke results from the combined effect of positive (i.e. spasticity), negative (i.e. weakness), and adaptive (i.e. contractures) features. Alteration of sensory input from the periphery (i.e. moving the hemiplegic limb) can affect the resultant motor output [2, 11, 64, 65]. Interventions described in this section assist with restoration and maintenance of movement post-stroke and should be taken in addition to those covered in previous sections.

8.5.1 Decreased Range-of-Movement and Contractures

Difficulties moving limbs and joints through full range-of-movement post-stroke may be due to a combination of positive and negative UMNS features and can ultimately lead to loss in range-of-movement and development of contractures

[9, 66]. *Without active intervention, the affected parts of the body tend to remain in shortened positions for prolonged periods, leading to soft tissue changes and loss in range-of-movement* [67]. Contracture is a common secondary complication of hemiparesis and weakness following nervous system damage [68]. Changes in muscle activation and inability to move lead to habitual postures, which contribute to soft tissue shortening and biomechanical changes in muscle. These peripheral (non-neural) mechanisms can compound any central motor dysfunction from the stroke and lead to further movement difficulties [66].

Patients thought to be most at risk of developing contractures are those who:

- are unconscious/have a low score on the Glasgow Coma Scale (GCS) (<9);
- are immobile and have altered muscle tone;
- exhibit shortening with current intervention;
- have fractures and/or pressure damage; and
- are medically unstable and unable to be stood [4].

In addition, patients who show no functional recovery in muscle activity 2–4 weeks post-stroke are also at higher risk of contracture [69]. Decreased range-of-movement and adaptive muscle changes, including contracture, are most commonly seen post-stroke in muscles that cross two joints and in the following areas:

- hip and knee flexors;
- hip adductors;
- calf muscles and Achilles tendon, affecting both the ankle and foot;
- shoulder elevators, adductor and medial rotators;
- elbow flexors and forearm muscles; and
- wrist and finger flexors.

Patients with loss of limb movement are likely to have loss of range-of-movement in the trunk, pelvis, and shoulder girdles [53]. Identification of patients at risk of developing contractures is complex [70, 71], but key indicators include stroke severity and weakness [69, 71] and reduced motor function [71, 72]. The long-term negative effect of contractures is loss of potential function and represents an important area of intervention for all team members; methods for intervention are considered next.

8.5.2 Stretching and Assisted and Passive Movements

Contractures are best treated by prevention, but this is not always possible. Loss of movement post-stroke and inactivity lead to decreased joint range motion; interventions are required to maintain movement in all large and small joints of the body [53]. Current evidence is not strong, but National Stroke Clinical Guidelines recommend *any patient whose range-of-movement at a joint is reduced, or at risk of becoming reduced, should have a programme of passive stretching of all affected joints on a daily basis* and that the programme should be taught to the patient and their carers [13]. If nothing else, passive movements can increase patient comfort. Movements to help maintain range can be carried out in a variety of ways:

- *Active.* Movements performed solely by the patient.
- *Active assisted.* Patient helped by someone else, such as one of the nursing team.
- *Passive.* Movements carried out solely by the therapist, nurse, or carer.

Movements carried out independently by the patient result in larger cortical sensorimotor changes [73, 74], but passive movements have been shown to stimulate brain activity and may be involved in the reorganisation of sensory and motor systems [73, 75]. Therefore, in the absence of voluntary muscle action, passive movements should be carried out as part of rehabilitation, but the preference is always to promote active movement by the patient.

Approaches to handling that may be used for patients with differing levels of muscle activation have been described [4]. Movement should be carried out at different speeds and utilising compression, traction, stretch, and rotational movements, but should never be vigorous or forced due to the risk of heterotrophic ossification (the laying down of bone in muscle).

When taking patients out of their preferred postures, particular attention should be paid to muscles that cross two joints and to patterns of movement. The length and frequency with which sustained muscle stretch should be applied continues to be the subject of clinical uncertainty and debate [76]. A recent systematic review of stretching in spasticity recognised the complexity of the concept and recommended further research [77].

8.5.3 Splinting

The mechanism of action behind the benefits of prolonged stretch is the subject of ongoing research but is thought to encompass both neural and musculo-skeletal processes. An overview of the theoretical basis for splinting in contracture management has been provided by the College of Occupational Therapists (COP) and Association of Chartered Physiotherapists in Neurology (ACPIN) [78]. Although *splinting is commonly seen in practice, underpinning evidence remains the subject of debate* [79, 80]. *If positioning and regular movements are ineffective in preventing adaptive feature of contractures, it may be necessary to consider splinting as an adjunct to treatment* [56, 78].

> I've got no control over that hand at all. It's very numb down that side still, and this, the fingers on this hand are constantly moving, I can't stop them getting into peculiar positions, because I don't feel them doing anything. The therapist fixed that up for me [a splint for the hand and arm], I wasn't sleeping because my hand exercises constantly, and it would wake me up in the night. Anyway I wear this and I get a good night's sleep.
>
> *(Ray, 56 years old, 5 months post-stroke)*

Splinting is defined in national splinting guidelines for the prevention and correction of contractures as the application of a prolonged stretch by a range of devices, such as a splint or cast [78]. It is important to recognise that splinting, especially with non-customised devices, carries risks of pressure and skin damage, so great care is required and nursing input is vital to monitor the skin condition.

There are a number of forms of splinting; three approaches commonly used in stroke patients are [4]:

- *Preventative*. Aims to prevent any loss in range-of-movement, e.g. the use of 'plaster cast' boots or pressure splints [81].
- *Corrective*. Used to increase range-of-movement in the presence of contracture, e.g. cylindrical serial casts, drop out splints, and hinged cast braces can be used to gain activity whilst preventing loss of range-of-movement [56].
- *Dynamic*. Aims to facilitate recovery and assist stability for function, e.g. include ankle–foot orthoses, which can be hinged or fixed [82], and orthotic insoles [56]. Strapping provides an alternative short-term approach, which can be applied to most joints – the ankle and shoulder in particular (see also Section 8.5.1) – although the evidence for efficacy is limited [83].

Botulinum toxin, produced by *Clostridium botulinum*, acts on the neuromuscular junction to help reduce muscle activity; it may be used in conjunction with splinting when tone is high [78]. However, this is unlikely to be needed except in extreme cases in the acute stroke patient, although new evidence is emerging for the early use of botulinum toxin in post-stroke spasticity [84].

8.5.4 Targeted Strengthening Exercise and Sedentary Behaviour

Muscle weakness is now recognised as a cardinal feature post-stroke, and more regard is given to *weakness as a primary factor limiting recovery of physical function* [85, 86]. Difficulties are noted in areas such as generating force, timing and sequencing force production, and sustaining force for functional activity. However, muscle weakness is modifiable through strength training of appropriate intensity [87]. Recent systematic reviews of exercise and strength training post-stroke [88, 89] indicate benefits in muscle strength and function.

As muscle weakness post-stroke is a feature of general motor control impairment, it has been recommended that *strength training should be task-specific, or at least orientated towards characteristics of the task to be learned* [9]. For example, repeating the task of sit-to-stand helps to strengthen the muscles involved in the functional activity whilst practising the action, thus addressing skills to be gained and targeting weak muscles. The task can be varied by executing the task through full, mid, or inner range of the movement, changing speed, or adding resistance by changing the height of the starting position. In addition, there may be a role for *specific* strengthening of muscles in preventing contractures and loss of range-of-movement [90].

Along with weakness, individuals can also show signs of cardiovascular deconditioning with low levels of fitness from enforced inactivity post-stroke [88]. As with any individual planning to undertake a new exercise regime, a risk assessment for cardiorespiratory training should be carried out. A comprehensive text on preparing for exercise post-stroke is available from Dennis et al. [91].

The negative effects of sedentary behaviours (e.g. sitting, lying down) post-stroke are increasingly recognised. People with stroke are generally more sedentary and less active than age-matched controls without stroke [92]. A systematic review [93] of 26 studies and 983 participants concluded that little is known about this growing area of health concern. Physical activity programmes to improve fitness and muscle strength have been successfully carried out without adverse effects in people with stroke screened for contraindications [94].

8.6 Management of the Upper Limb

My right arm, I find combing my hair, taking any weight on the arm, rather – well, trying. But I just get on with it.

(Bill, 72 years old, 5 months post-stroke)

The most common cause of stroke is occlusion of the middle cerebral artery, which is associated with weakness and sensory loss that affects the arm and face more than the leg [95]. Recovery of the upper limb post-stroke ranges from 5 to 52% [96, 97]. Compared with the numbers regaining the ability to walk, estimated at between 70 and 80% of patients [98], the challenge of rehabilitation in this area becomes evident.

Whilst it is generally accepted that most recovery happens in the first few months post-stroke, after which it may plateau [99], further recovery can happen after more than 1 year [100]. A study following 54 patients with first-ever stroke for 4 years and assessing upper limb recovery [101] found that although most of the improvement occurred during the first 16 weeks, in 10 patients it continued thereafter; with 13 patients, meanwhile, recovery of arm function only started after 16 weeks. At 4 years, loss of arm function was still perceived as a major problem by 36 participants. Reasons for poor recovery of the upper limb include:

- learnt disuse [100];
- corticospinal tract damage [95, 102];
- reduced coordination of motor control [103]; and
- the complexity of movement required for activities in the arm and hand, compared with the lower limb [9].

It has also been suggested that other functions are treated and practised at the expense of the upper limb [98, 104]. Further detail is available from Buma et al. [105]. Interventions that provide repetitive and progressive task-specific practice at an appropriate intensity of treatment, and other novel approaches, are relevant to restoration of movement in the upper limb [89, 106].

8.6.1 Managing Shoulder Joint Subluxation and Hemiplegic Shoulder Pain

Shoulder pain post-stroke is common and complicates the recovery of purposeful movement in the arm [107]. Changes in muscle tone, weakness, and loss of range-of-movement can affect normal shoulder posture and soft tissue changes

[108, 109]. Subluxation is a common manifestation of loss of tone in muscles supporting the shoulder joint, because stability is reliant on muscle activity and not ligaments; however, it need not be a cause of pain [110].

A study examining interventions for shoulder subluxation found the collar-and-cuff sling the most common approach, but with low-level evidence. It also identified use of a wheelchair or wheelchair attachments as useful [111]. Taping around the shoulder joint is sometimes used to help decrease inappropriate alignment, reduce subluxation, and increase proprioceptive input, but the mechanisms of this adjunct to treatment are still being debated [83].

Education of staff and family is central [13].

Preventing hemiplegic shoulder pain is a prime concern, but pain is estimated to be present initially after stroke in 17% of patients, increasing to 25% at 6 months [13]. Pain persisted in 47% of 297 people, with sleep disturbed in 58%, and 40% requiring rest to relieve the pain.

The risk of trauma can be reduced, limbs supported, and range-of-movement maintained through use of an integrated care pathway [112]. Figure 8.1 provides a simple example. Overhead arm slings that encourage uncontrolled abduction should be avoided [13]. FES to the supraspinatus and deltoid muscles of the shoulder has been identified as a potential intervention for patients with or at risk of shoulder subluxation [113].

8.6.2 Promoting Task-Specific Training and Practice Opportunities

Repetitive practice that is task-orientated is the foundation of rehabilitation, and it is important that patients have the opportunity to practice outside of formal therapy sessions [9]. There is a direct relationship between practice and learning, with more intensive practice being more beneficial [89, 114, 115]. However, traditional neurorehabilitation interventions have limited effectiveness in promoting motor recovery at the doses typically used [116]. Looking at the dose–response relationship, augmentation of routine therapy input produces additional benefits, with a systematic review indicating a minimum of an additional 16 hours in the first 6 months after stroke [114]. *It is therefore important that all members of the MDT are involved in providing opportunities for patients to practice tasks.* Patients can also be set up with self-monitored practice outside of formal treatment sessions. However, it is essential that the patient can do the exercise and that the exercise is challenging but achievable. A timetable with written instructions, diagrams, photographs, or audiotapes can be helpful, depending on the individual needs of the patient. It is also important that the movements which should be avoided are clearly stated.

The key principle underpinning *task-specific training* is that *restoration of movement should be specific to the task to be mastered, or at least orientated to the characteristics of the task to be performed*, because to a large degree how one action is carried out is dependent on the preceding components [9, 32].

Rehabilitation can be carried out as a *whole-task training* (e.g. walking practice) or as *part or modified training* [32, 117]. For example, with walking, it may be necessary to target a specific impairment, such as weakness in the ankle dorsiflexors, and practise this aspect to address overall improvement in mobility.

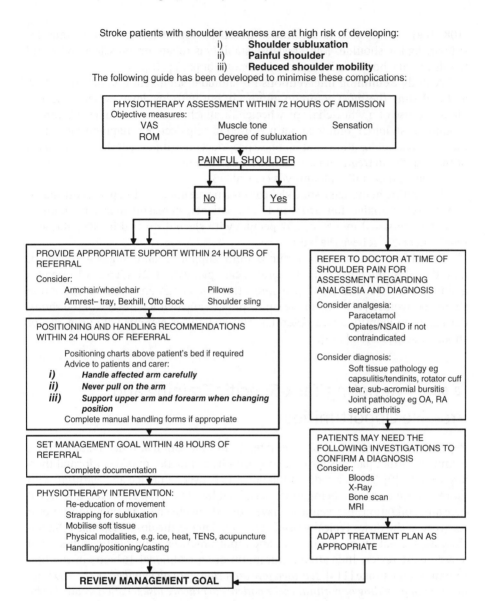

Stroke patients with shoulder weakness are at high risk of developing:

i)   **Shoulder subluxation**
ii)   **Painful shoulder**
iii) **Reduced shoulder mobility**

The following guide has been developed to minimise these complications:

PHYSIOTHERAPY ASSESSMENT WITHIN 72 HOURS OF ADMISSION
Objective measures:

| VAS | Muscle tone | Sensation |
| ROM | Degree of subluxation | |

PAINFUL SHOULDER

No — Yes

No branch:

PROVIDE APPROPRIATE SUPPORT WITHIN 24 HOURS OF REFERRAL

Consider:
Armchair/wheelchair — Pillows
Armrest– tray, Bexhill, Otto Bock — Shoulder sling

POSITIONING AND HANDLING RECOMMENDATIONS WITHIN 24 HOURS OF REFERRAL

Positioning charts above patient's bed if required
Advice to patients and carer:
i)   *Handle affected arm carefully*
ii)   *Never pull on the arm*
iii) *Support upper arm and forearm when changing position*
Complete manual handling forms if appropriate

SET MANAGEMENT GOAL WITHIN 48 HOURS OF REFERRAL

Complete documentation

PHYSIOTHERAPY INTERVENTION:
Re-education of movement
Strapping for subluxation
Mobilise soft tissue
Physical modalities, e.g. ice, heat, TENS, acupuncture
Handling/positioning/casting

Yes branch:

REFER TO DOCTOR AT TIME OF SHOULDER PAIN FOR ASSESSMENT REGARDING ANALGESIA AND DIAGNOSIS

Consider analgesia:
Paracetamol
Opiates/NSAID if not contraindicated

Consider diagnosis:
Soft tissue pathology eg capsulitis/tendinits, rotator cuff tear, sub-acromial bursitis
Joint pathology eg OA, RA
septic arthritis

PATIENTS MAY NEED THE FOLLOWING INVESTIGATIONS TO CONFIRM A DIAGNOSIS
Consider:
Bloods
X-Ray
Bone scan
MRI

ADAPT TREATMENT PLAN AS APPROPRIATE

REVIEW MANAGEMENT GOAL

FIGURE 8.1 Guide for the management of the shoulder in a stroke patient.
Source: Reproduced with thanks to the STEP team, Royal Free NHS Foundation Trust, Hampstead, London.

Equally, with other tasks, such as washing and dressing, it may be necessary to break the task down into component parts in the progression towards functional independence. It is therefore important that opportunities are given to practise tasks. *The effectiveness of motor skill learning is enhanced if the activity is goal-directed and the individual is given active involvement in the learning process* [118].

Self-management is an important aspect of care throughout the rehabilitation process, where the focus is on developing coping skills and working towards personal and meaningful goals. The Bridges stroke self-management programme is an excellent example of co-development with stroke survivors (see [119]).

8.7 Patients' Perspectives on Early Physical Rehabilitation

Patients' experiences of their rehabilitation may not always be positive. Several areas of unmet need have been uncovered, including a lack of information, too little therapy, physical inactivity, boredom, loss of autonomy, and poor pain control [120, 121]. In relation to help with movement, little has been written about patients' views about being 'handled'. Patients may not like being assisted if they do not trust the helper or if assistance involves a mechanical device, or is painful or frightening. For example, older people may view mobility aids as a source of stigma and a threat to dignity and pride [122]. For some patients, suspension in a hoist sling may be extremely uncomfortable; it should always be kept as brief as possible.

Alternatively, some patients may want the nurse to 'do for' or 'care for' them, rather than promote independence [123]. In this situation, sensitive communication will be required to negotiate a balance between listening to patients' wishes and implementing care that is beneficial. It is essential that patients consent to their treatment and are willing participants in their own rehabilitation. Crucially, patients' wishes and opinions should be incorporated into decisions about assistance with mobility and movement. Communication with and active participation of the patient and family members are crucial.

8.8 Conclusion

This chapter has demonstrated the importance of early and proactive management and treatment of physical impairments post-stroke as an integral part of the overall recovery of movement and function. Nurses, in collaboration with the MDT, have a central role to play by combining nursing care with rehabilitation principles and integrating therapeutic activity into everyday activity.

This chapter has reviewed familiar areas of practice, including positioning and seating, falls prevention, and the complexity of assessing risk in moving and handling, as well as providing an exploration of therapeutic interventions that promote physical recovery post-stroke. It is only through continuing professional development of all team members and engagement with service users that rehabilitation can keep pace with new developments and research, enabling change in this challenging but rewarding area of clinical practice.

> I want to be able to walk down the road arm-in-arm with me boyfriend and not have people look at me because I'm limping. And some people say that's bad, you should not worry about what people think. But I think it's good that I worry about what other people think. Because if I didn't, if I didn't give a damn, and thought well it doesn't matter if I limp – come and see me 10 years later, I'd still be limping.
>
> (Jodie, quoted at the start of this chapter)

Acknowledgements

Thank you to the members of the STEP team, and all others who contributed to our learning along the way.

References

1. UK Stroke Forum Education & Training. Stroke-Specific Education Framework, United Kingdom: UK Stroke Forum 2010. Available from: http://www.stroke-education. org.uk/about. [30 November 2018].
2. Marieb, E. and Hoehn, K. (2014). Human Anatomy and Physiology, 9e. San Francisco: Pearson.
3. Sheean, G. (2002). The pathophysiology of spasticity. European Journal of Neurology 9 (Suppl. 1): 3–9; disc. 53–61.
4. Kilbride, C. and Cassidy, C. (2011). Physical management of altered tone and movement. In: Physical Management for Neurological Conditions, 3e (ed. M. Stokes and E. Stack), 289–318. Edinburgh: Elsevier.
5. Barnes, M.P. (2001). Medical management of spasticity in stroke. Age and Ageing 30 (Suppl. 1): 13–16.
6. Thompson, A.J., Jarrett, L., Lockley, L. et al. (2005). Clinical management of spasticity. Journal of Neurology, Neurosurgery and Psychiatry 76 (4): 459–463.
7. Ward, A.B. (2002). A summary of spasticity management-a treatment algorithm. European Journal of Neurology 9 (Suppl. 1): 48–52; disc. 3–61.
8. Ada, L. and Canning, C. (2005). Changing the way we view the contribution of motor impairments to physical disability after stroke. In: Science-Based Rehabilitation: Theories into Practice (ed. K. Refshauge, L. Ada and E. Ellis), 87–108. Edinburgh: Elsevier.
9. Carr, J. and Shepherd, R. (2010). General principles of treatment. In: Neurological Rehabilitation: Optimising Motor Performance, 2e (ed. J.H. Carr, R.B. Shepherd, J. Bernhardt, et al.). Edinburgh: Churchill Livingstone Elsevier.
10. Rothwell, J.C. (2004). Motor control. In: Physical Management in Neurological Rehabilitation, 2e (ed. M. Stokes), 3–20. Edinburgh: Elsevier.
11. Kleim, J.A. and Jones, T.A. (2008). Principles of experience-dependent neural plasticity: implications for rehabilitation after brain damage. Journal of Speech Language and Hearing Research 51 (1): S225.
12. Kneafsey, R., Clifford, C., and Greenfield, S. (2013). What is the nursing team involvement in maintaining and promoting the mobility of older adults in hospital? A grounded theory study. International Journal Nursing Studies 50 (12): 1617–1629.
13. Intercollegiate Stroke Working Party (2016). National Clinical Guidelines for Stroke. London: Royal College of Physicians.
14. Timmer, A.J., Unsworth, C.A., and Taylor, N.F. (2014). Rehabilitation interventions with deconditioned older adults following an acute hospital admission: a systematic review. Clinical Rehabilitation 28 (11): 1078–1086.
15. Buurman, B.M., Hoogerduijn, J.G., van Gemert, E.A. et al. (2012). Clinical characteristics and outcomes of hospitalized older patients with distinct risk profiles for functional decline: a prospective cohort study. PLoS One 7 (1): e1–e8.
16. Folden, S. and Tappen, R. (2007). Factors influencing function and recovery following hip repair surgery. Orthopaedic Nursing 26 (4): 234–241.
17. Brown, C.J., Redden, D.T., Flood, K.L., and Allman, R.M. (2009). The underrecognized epidemic of low mobility during hospitalization of older adults. Journal of the American Geriatrics Society 57 (9): 1660–1665.

18. Doherty-King, B., Yoon, J.Y., Pecanac, K. et al. (2014). Frequency and duration of nursing care related to older patient mobility. Journal of Nursing Scholarship 46 (1): 20–27.
19. Fisher, S.R., Goodwin, J.S., Protas, E.J. et al. (2011). Ambulatory activity of older adults hospitalized with acute medical illness. Journal of the American Geriatrics Society 59 (1): 91–95.
20. Kortebein, P., Symons, T.B., Ferrando, A. et al. (2008). Functional impact of 10 days of bed rest in healthy older adults. Journal of Gerontology, Medical Sciences 63 (10): 1076–1081.
21. Boltz, M., Resnick, B., Capezuti, E., and Shuluk, J. (2014). Activity restriction vs. self-direction: hospitalised older adults' response to fear of falling. International Journal of Older People Nursing 9 (1): 44–53.
22. Resnick, B., Galik, E., Enders, H. et al. (2011). Pilot testing of function-focused care for acute care intervention. Journal of Nursing Care Quality 26 (2): 169–177.
23. Brown, C.J., Williams, B.R., Woodby, L.L. et al. (2007). Barriers to mobility during hospitalization from the perspectives of older patients and their nurses and physicians. Journal of Hospital Medicine 2 (5): 305–313.
24. Long, A.F., Kneafsey, R., Ryan, J., and Berry, J. (2002). The role of the nurse within the multi-professional rehabilitation team. Journal of Advanced Nursing 37 (1): 70–78.
25. Tyrrell, E.F., Levack, W.M., Ritchie, L.H., and Keeling, S.M. (2012). Nursing contribution to the rehabilitation of older patients: patient and family perspectives. Journal of Advanced Nursing 68 (11): 2466–2476.
26. Kneafsey, R., Clifford, C., and Greenfield, S. (2015). Perceptions of hospital manual handling policy and impact on nursing team involvement in promoting patients' mobility. Journal of Clinical Nursing 24 (1–2): 289–299.
27. Health and Safety Executive (1992). Manual Handling: Manual Handling Operations Regulations 1992: Guidance on the Regulations. Sudbury: Health and Safety Executive.
28. Pope, P. (2007). Severe and Complex Neurological Disability: Management of the Physical Condition. Edinburgh: Butterworth-Heinemann.
29. de Jong, L.D., Nieuwboer, A., and Aufdemkampe, G. (2006). Contracture preventive positioning of the hemiplegic arm in subacute stroke patients: a pilot randomized controlled trial. Clinical Rehabilitation 20 (8): 656–667.
30. Chatterton, H.J., Pomeroy, V.M., and Gratton, J. (2001). Positioning for stroke patients: a survey of physiotherapists' aims and practices. Disability and Rehabilitation 23 (10): 413–421.
31. Rowat, A.M. (2001). What do nurses and therapists think about the positioning of stroke patients? Journal of Advanced Nursing 34 (6): 795–803.
32. Shumway-Cook, A. and Woollacott, M. (2012). Motor Control: Translating Research into Clinical Practice, 4e. Philadelphia: Lippincott Williams and Wilkins.
33. Tyson, S.F. and Nightingale, P. (2004). The effects of position on oxygen saturation in acute stroke: a systematic review. Clinical Rehabilitation 18 (8): 863–871.
34. Karnath, H.O., Ferber, S., and Dichgans, J. (2000). The origin of contraversive pushing: evidence for a second graviceptive system in humans. Neurology 55 (9): 1298–1304.
35. Karnath, H.O. and Broetz, D. (2003). Understanding and treating 'pusher syndrome'. Physical Therapy 83 (12): 1119–1125.
36. Clark, J., Morrow, M., and Michael, S. (2004). Wheelchair postural support for young people with progressive neuromuscular disorders. International Journal of Therapy and Rehabilitation 11 (8): 365–373.
37. Allen, C., Glasziou, P., and Del Mar, C. (1999). Bed rest: a potentially harmful treatment needing more careful evaluation. The Lancet 354 (9186): 1229–1233.
38. Rochester, C.L. and Mohsenin, V. (2002). Respiratory complications of stroke. Seminars in Respiratory & Critical Care Medicine 23 (3): 248–260.
39. Bernhardt, J., Dewey, H., Thrift, A.G. et al. (2008). A very early rehabilitation trial for stroke (AVERT): phase II safety and feasibility. Stroke 39 (2): 390–396.

40. Indredavik, B., Bakke, F., Slordahl, S.A. et al. (1999). Treatment in a combined acute and rehabilitation stroke unit: which aspects are most important? Stroke 30 (5): 917–923.

41. Adams, H.P. Jr., Adams, R.J., Brott, T. et al. (2003). Guidelines for the early management of patients with ischemic stroke: a scientific statement from the Stroke Council of the American Stroke Association. Stroke 34 (4): 1056–1083.

42. The AVERT Trial Collaboration Group (2015). Efficacy and safety of very early mobilisation within 24 h of stroke onset (AVERT): a randomised controlled trial. The Lancet 386 (9988): 46–55.

43. Callen, B.L., Mahoney, J.E., Grieves, C.B. et al. (2004). Frequency of hallway ambulation by hospitalized older adults on medical units of an academic hospital. Geriatric Nursing 25 (4): 212–217.

44. Kunkel, D., Fitton, C., Burnett, M., and Ashburn, A. (2015). Physical inactivity poststroke: a 3-year longitudinal study. Disability and Rehabilitation 37 (4): 304–310.

45. Stiller, K. and Phillips, A. (2003). Safety aspects of mobilising acutely ill inpatients. Physiotherapy Theory and Practice 19 (4): 239–257.

46. O'Driscoll, B.R., Howard, L.S., and Davison, A.G. (2008). BTS guideline for emergency oxygen use in adult patients. Thorax 63 (Suppl. 6): vi1–vi68.

47. Chui, M. (1995). Wheelchair seating and positioning. In: Physical Therapy for Traumatic Brain Injury (ed. J. Montgomery). New York: Churchill Livingstone.

48. Massion, J. (1994). Postural control system. Current Opinion in Neurobiology 4 (6): 877–887.

49. Bohannon, R.W. (1993). Tilt table standing for reducing spasticity after spinal cord injury. Archives of Physical Medicine and Rehabilitation 74 (10): 1121–1122.

50. Brown, P. (1994). Pathophysiology of spasticity. Journal of Neurology, Neurosurgery & Psychiatry 57 (7): 773–777.

51. Markham, C.H. (1987). Vestibular control of muscular tone and posture. Journal of Canadian Science and Neurology 14 (Suppl. 3): 493–496.

52. Chang, A.T., Boots, R., Hodges, P.W., and Paratz, J. (2004). Standing with assistance of a tilt table in intensive care: a survey of Australian physiotherapy practice. Australian Journal of Physiotherapy 50 (1): 51–54.

53. Carter, P. and Edwards, S. (2002). General principles of treatment. In: Neurological Physiotherapy: A Problem Solving Approach, 2e (ed. S. Edwards). Edinburgh: Churchill Livingstone.

54. Tyson, S.F. and Rogerson, L. (2009). Assistive walking devices in nonambulant patients undergoing rehabilitation after stroke: the effects on functional mobility, walking impairments, and patients' opinion. Archives of Physical Medicine and Rehabilitation 90 (3): 475–479.

55. Olney, S. (2005). Training gait after stroke: a biomechanical perspective. In: Science-Based Rehabilitation: Theories into Practice (ed. K. Refshauge, L. Ada and E. Ellis), 159–184. Edinburgh: Elsevier.

56. Edwards, S. and Charlton, P. (2002). Splinting and the Use of Orthoses in the Management of Patients with Neurological Disorders, 2e. Edinburgh: Churchill Livingstone.

57. National Institute for Health and Care Excellence (NICE) (2009). Functional Electrical Stimulation for Drop Foot of Central Neurological Origin. London: National Institute for Health and Care Excellence.

58. Nadeau, S.E., Wu, S.S., Dobkin, B.H. et al. (2013). Effects of task-specific and impairment-based training compared with usual care on functional walking ability after inpatient stroke rehabilitation: LEAPS Trial. Neurorehabilitation and Neural Repair 27 (4): 370–380.

59. Mehrholz, J., Pohl, M., and Elsner, B. (2014). Treadmill training and body weight support for walking after stroke. Cochrane Database of Systematic Reviews 1 (Art. No.: CD002840). https://doi.org/10.1002/14651858.CD002840.pub4.

60. Verheyden, G.S., Weerdesteyn, V., Pickering, R.M. et al. (2013). Interventions for preventing falls in people after stroke. Cochrane Database of Systematic Reviews 5 (Art. No.: CD008728). https://doi.org/10.1002/14651858.CD008728.pub2.

61. National Institute for Health and Care Excellence (NICE) (2013). Falls: Assessment and Prevention of Falls in Older People. London: National Institute for Health and Care Excellence.

62. Betts, M. and Mowbray, C. (2005). The Falling and Fallen Person and Emergency Handling, 5e. London: BackCare in collaboration with the Royal College of Nursing and National Back Exchange.

63. Department of Health (2011). UK Physical Activity Guidelines. London: Her Majesty's Stationery Office.

64. Hamdy, S., Rothwell, J.C., Aziz, Q., and Thompson, D.G. (2000). Organization and reorganization of human swallowing motor cortex: implications for recovery after stroke. Clinical Science (London) 99 (2): 151–157.

65. Johansson, B.B. (2000). Brain plasticity and stroke rehabilitation. The Willis lecture. Stroke 31 (1): 223–230.

66. Ada, L., O'Dwyer, N., and O'Neill, E. (2006). Relation between spasticity, weakness and contracture of the elbow flexors and upper limb activity after stroke: an observational study. Disability and Rehabilitation 28 (13–14): 891–897.

67. Goldspink, G. and Williams, P. (1990). Muscle Fibre and Connective Tissue Changes Associated with Use and Disuse. London: Heinemann.

68. Lieber, R. (2010). Skeletal Muscle Structure, Function and Plasticity: The Physiological Basis of Rehabilitation. London: Lippincott Williams & Wilkins.

69. Pandyan, A.D., Cameron, M., Powell, J. et al. (2003). Contractures in the post-stroke wrist: a pilot study of its time course of development and its association with upper limb recovery. Clinical Rehabilitation 17 (1): 88–95.

70. Diong, J., Harvey, L.A., Kwah, L.K. et al. (2012). Incidence and predictors of contracture after spinal cord injury – a prospective cohort study. Spinal Cord 50 (8): 579–584.

71. Kwah, L.K., Harvey, L.A., Diong, J.H.L., and Herbert, R.D. (2012). Half of the adults who present to hospital with stroke develop at least one contracture within six months: an observational study. Journal of Physiotherapy 58 (1): 41–47.

72. Malhotra, S., Pandyan, A.D., Rosewilliam, S. et al. (2011). Spasticity and contractures at the wrist after stroke: time course of development and their association with functional recovery of the upper limb. Clinical Rehabilitation 25 (2): 184–191.

73. Jaeger, L., Marchal-Crespo, L., Wolf, P. et al. (2014). Brain activation associated with active and passive lower limb stepping. Frontiers in Human Neuroscience 8: 828.

74. Lotze, M., Braun, C., Birbaumer, N. et al. (2003). Motor learning elicited by voluntary drive. Brain 126 (Pt 4): 866–872.

75. Nelles, G., Spiekermann, G., Jueptner, M. et al. (1999). Reorganization of sensory and motor systems in hemiplegic stroke patients. A positron emission tomography study. Stroke 30 (8): 1510–1516.

76. Kilbride, C., Hoffman, K., Baird, T. et al. (2013). Contemporary splinting practice in the UK for adults with neurological dysfunction: a cross-sectional survey. International Journal of Therapy and Rehabilitation 20 (11): 559–566.

77. Bovend'Eerdt, T.J., Newman, M., Barker, K. et al. (2008). The effects of stretching in spasticity: a systematic review. Archives of Physical Medicine and Rehabilitation 89 (7): 1395–1406.

78. College of Occupational Therapists (COT) and Association of Chartered Physiotherapists in Neurology (ACPIN) (2015). Splinting for the Prevention and Correction of Contractures in Adults with Neurological Dysfunction. Practice Guideline for Occupational Therapists and Physiotherapists. London: College of Occupational Therapists.

79. Katalinic, O.M., Harvey, L.A., Herbert, R.D. et al. (2010). Stretch for the treatment and prevention of contractures. Cochrane Database of Systematic Reviews 9 (Art. No.: CD007455). https://doi.org/10.1002/14651858.CD007455.pub3.

80. Lannin, N.A. and Ada, L. (2011). Neurorehabilitation splinting: theory and principles of clinical use. Neuro Rehabilitation 28 (1): 21–28.

81. Johnstone, M. (1995). Restoration of Normal Movement After Stroke. Edinburgh: Churchill Livingstone.

82. Tyson, S.F. and Thornton, H.A. (2001). The effect of a hinged ankle foot orthosis on hemiplegic gait: objective measures and users' opinions. Clinical Rehabilitation 15 (1): 53–58.

83. Appel, C., Perry, L., and Jones, F. (2014). Shoulder strapping for stroke-related upper limb dysfunction and shoulder impairments: systematic review. Neuro Rehabilitation 35 (2): 191–204.

84. Lindsay, C., Simpson, J., Ispoglou, S. et al. (2014). The early use of botulinum toxin in post-stroke spasticity: study protocol for a randomised controlled trial. Trials 15: 12.

85. VanWijck, F., Smith, M., Halliday, P., and Mead, G. (2013). Post-stroke problems. In: Exercise and Fitness Training After Stroke (ed. G.E. Mead and F. van Mijck). Edinburgh: Churchill Livingstone Elsevier.

86. Cramp, M.C., Greenwood, R.J., Gill, M. et al. (2006). Low intensity strength training for ambulatory stroke patients. Disability and Rehabilitation 28 (13–14): 883–889.

87. Flansbjer, U.B., Lexell, J., and Brogardh, C. (2012). Long-term benefits of progressive resistance training in chronic stroke: a 4-year follow-up. Journal of Rehabilitation Medicine 44 (3): 218–221.

88. Saunders, D.H., Sanderson, M., Brazzelli, M. et al. (2013). Physical fitness training for stroke patients. Cochrane Database of Systematic Reviews 10 (Art. No.: CD003316). https://doi.org/10.1002/14651858.CD003316.pub4.

89. Veerbeek, J.M., van Wegen, E., van Peppen, R. et al. (2014). What is the evidence for physical therapy poststroke? A systematic review and meta-analysis. PLoS One 9 (2): 1–33.

90. Shortland, A.P., Harris, C.A., Gough, M., and Robinson, R.O. (2001). Architecture of the medial gastrocnemius in children with spastic diplegia. Developmental Medicine and Child Neurology 43 (12): 796–801.

91. Dennis, J., Best, C., Dinan-Young, S., and Mead, G. (2017). Preparing for Exercise After Stroke, 1e. Edinburgh: Churchill Livingstone Elsevier.

92. Rand, D., Eng, J.J., Tang, P.F. et al. (2010). Daily physical activity and its contribution to the health-related quality of life of ambulatory individuals with chronic stroke. Health and Quality of Life Outcomes 8: 8–80.

93. English, C., Manns, P.J., Tucak, C., and Bernhardt, J. (2014). Physical activity and sedentary behaviors in people with stroke living in the community: a systematic review. Phyical Therapy 94 (2): 185–196.

94. Billinger, S.A., Arena, R., Bernhardt, J. et al. (2014). Physical activity and exercise recommendations for stroke survivors: a statement for healthcare professionals from the American Heart Association/American Stroke Association. Stroke 45 (8): 2532–2553.

95. Shelton, F.N. and Reding, M.J. (2001). Effect of lesion location on upper limb motor recovery after stroke. Stroke 32 (1): 107–112.

96. Dean, C. and Mackey, F. (1992). Motor assessment scale scores as a measure of rehabilitation outcome following stroke. Australian Journal of Physiotherapy 38 (1): 31–35.

97. Gowland, C., deBruin, H., Basmajian, J.V. et al. (1992). Agonist and antagonist activity during voluntary upper-limb movement in patients with stroke. Physical Therapy 72 (9): 624–633.

98. Rodgers, H., Mackintosh, J., Price, C. et al. (2003). Does an early increased-intensity interdisciplinary upper limb therapy programme following acute stroke improve outcome? Clinical Rehabilitation 17 (6): 579–589.

99. Kwakkel, G., Kollen, B., and Twisk, J. (2006). Impact of time on improvement of outcome after stroke. Stroke 37 (9): 2348–2353.

100. Taub, E., Miller, N.E., Novack, T.A. et al. (1993). Technique to improve chronic motor deficit after stroke. Archives of Physical Medicine and Rehabilitation 74 (4): 347–354.

101. Broeks, J.G., Lankhorst, G.J., Rumping, K., and Prevo, A.J. (1999). The long-term outcome of arm function after stroke: results of a follow-up study. Disability and Rehabilitation 21 (8): 357–364.

102. Bourbonnais, D. and Noven, S.V. (1989). Weakness in patients with hemiparesis. American Journal of Occupational Therapy 43 (5): 313–319.

103. Diedrichsen, J., Criscimagna-Hemminger, S.E., and Shadmehr, R. (2007). Dissociating timing and coordination as functions of the cerebellum. Journal of Neuroscience Rural Practice 27 (23): 6291–6301.

104. Lang, C.E., MacDonald, J.R., and Gnip, C. (2007). Counting repetitions: an observational study of outpatient therapy for people with hemiparesis post-stroke. Journal of Neurologic Physical Therapy 31 (1): 3–10.

105. Buma, F., Kwakkel, G., and Ramsey, N. (2013). Understanding upper limb recovery after stroke. Restorative Neurology and Neuroscience 31 (6): 707–722.

106. Pollock, A., Farmer, S.E., Brady, M.C. et al. (2014). Interventions for improving upper limb function after stroke. Cochrane Database of Systematic Reviews 11 (Art. No.: CD010820). https://doi.org/10.1002/14651858.CD010820.pub2.

107. Gamble, G.E., Barberan, E., Laasch, H.U. et al. (2002). Poststroke shoulder pain: a prospective study of the association and risk factors in 152 patients from a consecutive cohort of 205 patients presenting with stroke. European Journal of Pain 6 (6): 467–474.

108. Kumar, P. and Swinkels, A. (2009). A critical review of shoulder subluxation and its association with other post-stroke complications. Physical Therapy Reviews 14 (1): 13–25.

109. Turner-Stokes, L. and Jackson, D. (2002). Shoulder pain after stroke: a review of the evidence base to inform the development of an integrated care pathway. Clinical Rehabilitation 16 (3): 276–298.

110. Kumar, P., Saunders, A., Ellis, E., and Whitlam, S. (2013). Association between glenohumeral subluxation and hemiplegic shoulder pain in patients with stroke. Physical Therapy Reviews 18 (2): 90–100.

111. Foongchomcheay, A., Ada, L., and Canning, C.G. (2005). Use of devices to prevent subluxation of the shoulder after stroke. Physiotherapy Research International 10 (3): 134–145.

112. Jackson, D., Turner-Stokes, L., Williams, H., and Das-Gupta, R. (2003). Use of an integrated care pathway: a third round audit of the management of shoulder pain in neurological conditions. Journal of Rehabilitation Medicine 35 (6): 265–270.

113. Manigandan, J.B., Ganesh, G.S., Pattnaik, M., and Mohanty, P. (2014). Effect of electrical stimulation to long head of biceps in reducing gleno humeral subluxation after stroke. NeuroRehabilitation 34 (2): 245–252.

114. Kwakkel, G., van Peppen, R., Wagenaar, R.C. et al. (2004). Effects of augmented exercise therapy time after stroke: a meta-analysis. Stroke 35 (11): 2529–2539.

115. Kwakkel, G. (2006). Impact of intensity of practice after stroke: issues for consideration. Disability and Rehabilitation 28 (13–14): 823–830.

116. Wolf, S.L., Winstein, C.J., Miller, J.P. et al. (2008). Retention of upper limb function in stroke survivors who have received constraint-induced movement therapy: the EXCITE randomised trial. The Lancet Neurology 7 (1): 33–40.

117. Hubbard, I.J., Parsons, M.W., Neilson, C., and Carey, L.M. (2009). Task-specific training: evidence for and translation to clinical practice. Occupational Therapy International 16 (3–4): 175–189.

118. Schmidt, R. and Lee, T. (2011). Motor Control and Learning: A Behavioural Emphasis, 5e. Champaign: Human Kinetics.

119. Bridges Self-Management. Available from: http://www.bridgesselfmanagement.org.uk/ [30 November 2018].

120. Luker, J., Lynch, E., Bernhardsson, S. et al. (2015). Stroke survivors' experiences of physical rehabilitation: a systematic review of qualitative studies. Archives of Physical Medicine and Rehabilitation 96 (9): 1698–1708.e10.
121. Long, A., Kneafsey, R., Ryan, J. et al. (2001). Teamworking in Rehabilitation: Exploring the Role of the Nurse. London: English National Board for Nursing, Midwifery and Health Visiting, London.
122. Rush, K.L. and Ouellet, L.L. (1997). Mobility aids and the elderly client. Journal of Gerontological Nursing 23 (1): 7–15.
123. Kneafsey, R. and Long, A.F. (2002). Multidisciplinary rehabilitation teams: the nurse's role. British Journal of Therapy and Rehabilitation 9 (1): 24–29.

CHAPTER 9

Rehabilitation and Recovery Processes

Jane Williams[1] and Julie Pryor[2,3]

[1] Southern Health NHS Foundation Trust, Southampton, UK
[2] Royal Rehab, Sydney, NSW, Australia
[3] University of Sydney, Sydney, NSW, Australia

KEY POINTS

- Rehabilitation following stroke is a journey that the patient, their family, and their loved ones follow for a variable duration of time.
- Rehabilitation optimises the stroke survivor's participation in their life and surroundings.
- Nursing's contribution to rehabilitation is significant and specific.
- A rehabilitative approach should be commenced as soon as possible after the stroke event.
- Rehabilitation should focus on, and be responsive to, individual patients and their circumstances.

This chapter maps to criteria within the following sections of the Stroke-Specific Education Framework (SSEF):

> *I was frightened as I was no longer in charge of my life. They [the rehabilitation team] helped me not to be frightened.*
> *The stroke team cannot be faulted. They put our lives into a liveable place from the trauma and feeling of being shelved as useless.*
> *(Patients from an NHS hospital stroke service)*

9.1 Introduction

Following stroke, most patients embark on a rehabilitation journey; an 'individual, active and dynamic process' [2] aimed at ameliorating their experience of disability and reducing the burden of care. Awareness of the need to embark on this intensely personal journey can be delayed until realisation occurs that the problems resulting from stroke are not going away [3]. Furthermore, each person's journey is unique, as the significance of the experience of stroke and its meaning for the individual are shaped by individual context and biography [4, 5].

For healthcare professionals, rehabilitation must begin at the patient's first point of contact and inform all decision-making thereafter. This means that rehabilitation is everyone's business [6, 7], requiring all healthcare professionals to possess and act upon an awareness of how what happens today – and what does not happen – affects the patient's desired tomorrow [8]. Rehabilitation is more than a series of intermittent interventions done to patients by health professionals. It is a continuous process underpinned by 'the principle of patient empowerment' [9]. This requires active patient participation [10, 11] in the form of physical, psychological, and biographical work [12] and learning 'how to live a life that is not dominated by their disability' [13]. For many, rehabilitation entails a transition from the old to a new self [13–15] that is enabled by a self-management approach [16, 17] which fosters a 'can do' attitude.

Theories of learning and change are as fundamental to rehabilitation as the understanding of health and illness models. More specifically, rehabilitation focuses on recovery [18] by:

- maintaining and restoring function;
- promoting health; and
- preventing and minimising disability.

9.2 Understanding Rehabilitation

There are two critical ways of understanding rehabilitation: first, as a personal journey, and second, as a type of healthcare. Both were discussed in the previous section, but it is the relationship between the two that is central to the effectiveness of rehabilitation service delivery. Pryor [19] explains:

> *Rehabilitation is a co-production between patients, their family and friends, and the treating clinicians. Rehabilitation is not done by one person to another. All members of the team have strengths. Clinicians use their expertise to guide and support patient work [20]. Patients share the significance they assign to their situation with clinicians. Family and friends are potential sources of a wide range of inputs to the co-production.*

Understanding rehabilitation as a co-production helps us to view it as a complex, multifactorial intervention requiring multiple inputs from skilled, expert individuals and enabling environments. It has proven difficult to explain and explore the process, resulting in the development of many different definitions, service designs, and delivery models. Despite this, the evidence base for various rehabilitation approaches, individual therapies, and service provision methods continues to grow. In the United Kingdom, the National Clinical Guidelines for Stroke [21] provide clinical and commissioning recommendations based on the best available evidence. Examples of international resources include:

- the Canadian Evidence Based Review of Stroke Rehabilitation database [22];
- the Cochrane Stroke Group, including the Database of Research into Stroke (DORIS) [23];
- the American Stroke Association [24];
- the Stroke Foundation in Australia [25];
- the Scottish Intercollegiate Guidelines Network (SIGN) [26]; and
- the UK National Institute for Health and Care Excellence (NICE)'s Stroke Rehabilitation in Adults [27].

The World Stroke Organisation (WSO) provides a comprehensive list of guidelines produced across the globe [28]. The evidence available for clinicians can appear overwhelming; consensus guidelines are an invaluable tool in this regard, and their use may result in improved outcomes [29, 30].

Carlson et al. [31] help us to understand rehabilitation as a philosophy by contrasting 'learn to participate' and 'participate to learn' approaches to rehabilitation. The 'learn to participate' approach is more likely to happen in clinical contexts, whereas the 'participate to learn' approach happens in real-world contexts and increases participation in valued life roles. 'Participate to learn' ensures the transfer of skills learnt in clinical areas to real-life settings. 'Participate to learn' provides a more enriched and enabling rehabilitation environment.

A useful framework for understanding the conceptual underpinnings of rehabilitation is the International Classification of Functioning, Disability and Health (ICF) [32] (see Figure 9.1). It portrays functioning and disability as multifaceted, complex interactive processes, and highlights the role of physical, social, attitudinal, and environmental (along with personal) factors as enablers or barriers to human functioning. The ICF enables us to see that following stroke, a person

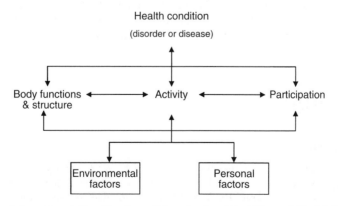

FIGURE 9.1 International Classification of Functioning, Disability and Health (ICF). *Source: Reproduced with permission from the World Health Organization (WHO) [32].*

might have, for example, an impairment of sensation, an activity limitation in eating, and a participation restriction in not being invited to family celebrations. Contextual factors might include personal features such as an outgoing personality and environmental elements such as the attitudes of family members. By asking us to consider enabling environments, ICF is a useful tool for determining the right mix of 'learn to participate' and 'participate to learn' approaches for a particular patient at a particular point in time.

The ICF does not mean that standardised rehabilitation interventions are used for everyone. Rehabilitation uses interventions that may act at a macro or a micro level [33]. This multiplicity of levels of intervention and the many interwoven interactions means that rehabilitation is not an exact science, with a broad range of characteristics capable of influencing outcomes. For example, patient outcomes can be affected at the macro level by characteristics such as team functioning, whereas at the micro level, it might be issues such as the timing of an upper limb training programme [34, 35].

Equally important are patient motivation [36] and the extent of active patient engagement in rehabilitation. Rehabilitation interventions need to integrate and optimise the efforts of the patient and those guiding and supporting them (family, friends, health, and community workers). Importantly, rehabilitation services need to ensure they are patient-centred. From a study of rehabilitation patients, Cott [37] characterises patient-centred rehabilitation as:

- individualization of programmes to the needs of each patient in order to prepare them for life in the real world;
- mutual participation with health professionals in decision-making and goal-setting;
- outcomes that are meaningful to the patient;
- sharing of information and education that is appropriate, timely, and according to the patient's wishes;
- emotional support;
- family and peer involvement throughout the rehabilitation process; and
- coordination and continuity across the multiple service sectors.

The behaviours of healthcare professionals and patients, as well as the interactions between them, contribute to the effectiveness of rehabilitation (Case Study 9.1). 'It is important that professionals communicate effectively so that their interventions are grounded in, and support, the survivor's goals and strategies' [4].

Case Study

Case 9.1 Ian

Ian, a keen golfer, has a stroke resulting in hemianopia. Whilst Ian makes a good recovery in many aspects of physical functioning, the hemianopia continues to affect his golf swing. The early supported discharge (ESD) team finds Ian to be low in mood and his quality of life to be really impacted by the loss of this important activity. The team focuses on tailoring rehabilitation to adjustment to the hemianopia, and brings in the sensory impairment team and orthoptist to help. Ian tries various prisms on his glasses, works with the sight-loss practitioner to improve eye scanning during everyday activities, and uses the practice nets at his local golf centre under the supervision of rehabilitation assistants – a safer environment in which to practise his unpredictable swing! Ian becomes more engaged with rehabilitation, as it is based around his hobby, and gradually adjusts to his impairment.

9.3 Initiation of Rehabilitation

Rehabilitation is not a phase of healthcare or a place. Rehabilitation needs to be a primary focus of care across the emergency department (ED), acute care, rehabilitation wards, and the community. This is a challenge, given the priority demanded for patients' more life-threatening problems. Nonetheless, the evidence in support of what Stucki et al. [38] refer to as 'the new paradigm of "early rehabilitation"' is compelling. In a study of 830 post-stroke (moderate and severe) patients in five US inpatient rehabilitation facilities, Horn et al. [39] found that 'earlier admission to rehabilitation, higher-level activities early in the rehabilitation process, tube feeding and newer medications are associated with better stroke outcomes'. The authors point out that their finding of participation in early gait activities and 'higher-order more challenging therapy activities' even for low-functioning patients challenges conventional thinking in rehabilitation [39]. It seems that improvements in lower-level functions can be achieved by focusing on higher-order activities. Salter et al. [40] found that 'patients admitted to stroke rehabilitation within 30 days of first-ever, unilateral stroke experienced greater functional gain and shorter length of stay than those whose admission to rehabilitation was delayed beyond 30 days'. Most importantly, the commencement of rehabilitation should not be delayed until transfer to a specialised rehabilitation service. 'Fewer days from stroke symptom onset to rehabilitation admission is associated with better functional outcomes at discharge and shorter LOS [length of stay]' [41].

This assumption was more recently tested in the AVERT (A Very Early Rehabilitation Trial) study [42], in which 2104 acute stroke patients were randomly assigned to either very early (within 24 hours) intensive mobilisation or usual care and followed up at 3 months. The median time to mobilisation in the usual care group was also within 24 hours of stroke onset, but the median difference was almost 5 hours later than in the very early mobilisation group. Unexpectedly, 'the very early mobilization protocol was associated with a reduction in the odds of a favourable outcome at 3 months' [42]. This led the researchers to suggest that 'an early lower dose out-of-bed activity regime is preferable to very early, frequent, higher dose intervention' [42].

Another important consideration in relation to rehabilitation initiation is who gets rehabilitation. When rehabilitation is understood as everybody's responsibility, all clinicians intervene to guide and support it. Rehabilitation starts with decisions about which patients are appropriate, which must take into consideration potential and readiness. Rehabilitation potential relates to a prediction of a person's potential to improve in response to rehabilitative care. Exactly what such improvement might entail can be subjective [43], and not all members of a multidisciplinary team (MDT) might agree on the nature of legitimate areas of improvement or the predictions of improvement. In a study of this under-researched aspect of rehabilitation, Burton et al. [43] note that 'rehabilitation potential emerges through the provision (and potential failure) of therapy'. Clinical experience in stroke rehabilitation seems to play a major role in decisions about rehabilitation potential, but it needs to be balanced with what may constitute improvement in the eyes of the individual patient according to the severity of their stroke (e.g. the ability to eat and drink independently for a severe-stroke patient versus the ability to walk without aid for someone who has had a mild event).

Depending on staff in acute care settings to see rehabilitation potential and refer patients for intensive rehabilitation adds another layer of complexity to the initiation of rehabilitation. In a study of eight acute stroke units in Australia [44], factors that influenced referrals to rehabilitation included 'the anticipated discharge destination; severity of stroke; staff expectations of the patient's recovery; and if there was advocacy by families about rehabilitation. Clinicians tended to refer the patients they considered would be accepted by the rehabilitation service'.

9.4 Nursing's Rehabilitation Role

Rehabilitation is the responsibility of every nurse, and as 'rehabilitators par excellence' [45], nurses fulfil the roles of coach [20, 46–49] and travelling companion for patients on their rehabilitation journey, as well as coordinator of input into patient rehabilitation [50]. In the ED, by focusing on the maintenance of function and prevention of complications, nursing contributes to the person's rehabilitation (Box 9.1). In acute care, the main goals of rehabilitation interventions

---

Box 9.1 | Rehabilitative Stroke Nursing Interventions for Emergency and Acute Settings

- Physiological monitoring
- Positioning
- Joint and limb protection
- Recognition, assessment, and management of dysphagia
- Assessment and management of tissue viability
- Prevention of complications (e.g. aspiration pneumonia, venous thromboembolism, constipation, hospital-acquired infections, dehydration, and malnutrition)
- Assessment and management of risk (e.g. falls)
- Promotion of urinary continence without (where possible) catheterisation
- Early education and information sharing (patient and family)
- Consideration of cultural diversity
- Concordance with secondary prevention measures
- Medication management and self-medication programmes
- Commencing collection and collation of background information (housing, leisure, hobbies, etc.)
- Ensuring the patient has adequate rest and sleep
- Psychological support to minimise trauma and support adjustment
- Onward referral to a specialist setting/team

Box 9.2 | Hazards of Hospitalisation

- Hospital-acquired infections
- Weight loss, nutritional and hydration inadequacies
- Loss of physical conditioning (strength and endurance)
- Falls
- Social isolation
- Depression
- Fatigue and sleep disturbance
- Institutionally induced dependence

---

provided by nurses are the conservation and restoration of functioning, prevention of complications, and early mobilisation [38]. AVERT trial results must be considered.

By focusing on conservation of function, nurses can prevent 'imposed dependence' [51]. This is of utmost importance in relation to older people, and whilst not all stroke patients are elderly, it is important to note that hospitalisation is hazardous for older people [52, 53] (Box 9.2). This makes care of the older stroke patient, who is prone to co-morbid health conditions, very complex.

In speciality rehabilitation settings, nursing's contribution is central to optimal patient outcomes. Various studies reveal that nurses in these settings enable patients to reclaim self-care by adopting an informed 'hands-off' approach [20, 48, 54, 55], instead of 'doing for' or 'doing to' patients. Teaching is a significant factor in assisting patients to reclaim self-care [20, 48, 56, 57], as is helping patients and families cope with, and adjust to, what has happened to them [5, 48, 58].

Nursing is well placed to enrich the stroke patient's environment. The enrichment of environments in improving neurobehavioural function shown in animal models has potential in humans. Inactivity is a major concern [59], and environmental enrichment is suggested as a treatment response [60, 61]. The environment can be enriched by initiatives such as eating in a dining room, providing activities and reading materials, and facilitating engagement a range of age-appropriate activities.

Across all settings, nursing is responsible for patient and family education, as well as the coordination of each patient's rehabilitation. This involves:

- explaining the nature and purpose of rehabilitation to patients and families;
- explaining the roles of healthcare professionals, patients, and families in rehabilitation;
- explaining differences between acute care and rehabilitation;
- setting goals relevant to the patient with the patient;
- ensuring timely communication of information between the patient/family and healthcare professionals;
- ensuring timely and appropriate communication of information between healthcare professionals;
- harmonising the efforts of patients and healthcare professionals.

The importance of a coordinated approach to teamwork is highlighted by the Stroke Unit Trialists' Collaboration [62]. Being the only discipline to have a 24-hour presence, and with the responsibility for monitoring patient well-being and the effectiveness of therapeutic interventions provided by the whole team, nursing assumes this responsibility. Sometimes an invisible contribution, coordination is most noticed when it is lacking and therefore reduces the effectiveness of interventions.

9.5 Outcomes of Rehabilitation

The outcomes of rehabilitation interest 'patients [and their families], payers, and society as a whole' [63]. At policy level, reduction in disability and improvement in participation in life by stroke survivors are the ultimate aims of rehabilitation [64]. At the point of rehabilitation service delivery, the desired outcome is achievement of goals mutually agreed by the patient and the healthcare team. These are generally short-term clinical goals that represent the steps required to achieve patients' long-term personal life goals. Clinical goals should be those that rehabilitation services can contribute to within available resources. It is commonly recommended that these goals are specific, measurable, agreed, relevant, and time-limited (SMART). The term 'achievable' has been avoided here, because when being person-centred, we should work with the preference of the patient to determine whether achievable or aspirational goals work best for them.

The patient's ultimate goal is generally to 'return to the existence they had lived before the stroke' [65]. Unfortunately, this is not always possible, regardless of how much rehabilitation intervention is provided. Nonetheless, successful rehabilitation is based on what matters to the person who has had a stroke [4]. An essential starting point is the re-establishment of a person's sense of control over his or her body and life [9].

9.6 Goal–Directed Rehabilitation

The use of goals is a hallmark of rehabilitation. Goal-setting identifies what is important to patients, and a patient's goals provide the rationale for all actions undertaken by healthcare professionals. Engaging patients (or, if unable, their families) in the goal-setting process is an essential first step in the re-establishment of a person's sense of control. Engaging patients should ensure that the patient's priorities become the team's priorities. Through engagement in the process, patients learn about their body structures and functions, as well as the rehabilitation therapies and activities for addressing their impairments, activity limitations, and participation restrictions. Patients may gain a deeper appreciation of what is important to them; this makes the identification of what activities and relationships the patient values an important aspect of the goal-setting process. Additionally, patients learn how to identify functional improvements and goal attainment. Case Study 9.2 illustrates how targeted goal-setting can achieve what is required to enable patients to move from hospital to home.

Case Study

Case 9.2 Molly

Molly has been an inpatient on a stroke rehabilitation ward for 2 weeks. She is experiencing continence problems, and her goal is to achieve night-time control to enable her to go home with the community stroke rehabilitation team.

Various methods are discussed and tried. Molly isn't able to transfer independently, and her husband has health problems which mean he will be unable to assist her. Success is achieved with a female urinal. Molly is able to leave hospital and continue rehabilitation at home.

Although 'evidence regarding the generalisability of goal planning to improve patient outcomes in rehabilitation is inconsistent at best' [66], goal-setting is widely supported as a pragmatic approach that fits with the problem-solving and educational processes of rehabilitation [67]. Effective goal-setting can assist patients to move from pre-contemplation to action [68]. Goals can be a powerful mechanism for enhancing patient ownership of and engagement in their rehabilitation, as well as for evaluating rehabilitation outcomes [69]. Multiple approaches to goal-setting have been used, but the best results are achieved by meeting the patient's individual needs [70]. Most importantly, it is an ethical as well as a practical imperative for rehabilitation to focus on what drives the patient [71].

Given the importance of early rehabilitation, the initial purpose of goal-setting may be to facilitate patient readiness for rehabilitation. By listening, nurses can find out about a patient's life, noting values with a view to understanding the patient's 'idealised self-image', a concept that McGrath and Adams [72] suggest influences a person's actions. Carver and Scheier's control-process model of self-regulation suggests that 'at all times the behaviour [of a patient] is directed toward reducing the discrepancy between the person's goal and existing circumstances' [73]. Siegert et al. [73] make explicit the importance of setting concrete goals enabling patients and healthcare workers to work towards superordinate goals and idealised self-image. Equally important is an appreciation that it is the patient's perception of the rate of progress towards goal achievement in relation to their desired rate that results in a change in emotion or affect [72, 74]. McGrath and Adams [72] report positive changes in the effect of neurological patients following engagement in goal-planning based on Carver and Scheier's model. Negative affect and goal disengagement can arise from slower-than-expected progress towards goal attainment [73].

Mauk's [3, 75] model of post-stroke recovery highlights the importance of setting goals that are appropriate for the patient's stage of recovery. Similar to Prochaska et al.'s [76] transtheoretical model of change, Mauk's model recognises the need for patients to realise that rehabilitation requires them to act. According to Mauk [75], engagement in post-stroke rehabilitation is contingent upon the realisation that 'the effects of his or her stroke may not all go away'. The need for biographical adjustment following stroke may not be apparent to patients during rehabilitation [14]. Tension between lack of patient readiness for rehabilitation and the evidence supporting benefits of early rehabilitation makes a priority of research to determine the most effective ways to use goals to enhance patient rehabilitation. For further detail, see Chapter 10.

Several factors seem to be emerging as central to effective goal-setting with patients:

- Patient engagement in the process is an imperative. Any organisational policy or protocol for goal-setting must be flexible enough to ensure that patients can engage in the manner that best suits them, rather than the manner that best suits the organisation. This includes flexibility about whether the patient meets with one or more healthcare professionals to set goals.
- Discussion should start by establishing the patient's values and long-term goals.
- The process must enable patients to maintain hope that their long-term goals can be achieved. Long-term goals should be revised by patients, not healthcare professionals.
- The link between shorter-term goals and the actions of healthcare professionals must be made explicit to the patient and their family.
- Short-term goals must be measurable.
- Short-term goals should identify who, in addition to the patient and perhaps their family, will be responsible for guiding and supporting the patient to achieve them, and how they will do this.
- For patients who experience variations in their energy, strength, balance, or safety throughout the day or week, short-term goals should be linked to appropriate times of the day or days of the week.
- Progress towards goal achievement must be evaluated regularly so that the next round of goals can be set. One to two weeks seems to be the norm, but this too requires further research.
- Patients and all relevant healthcare professionals must have ready access to their documented goals.
- Goals and evidence of goal attainment can be used as educational tools to make explicit progress towards patients' long-term goals. The use of time-limited and measurable short-term goals enables graphical representations to demonstrate goal achievement across time.

9.7   Recovery Processes

Maximising recovery is the focus of care, and recovery processes are optimised through the adoption of rehabilitation. Planning for rehabilitation should commence as soon as possible, and includes utilising a rehabilitative approach in the acute phase, but proceeding with early and intensive rehabilitation with caution [77]. The exact nature of effective stroke rehabilitation is still not clear, but should address physical, psychological, behavioural, cultural, spiritual, and social issues for the individual and their family. There is evidence that intensity of rehabilitation is vital in the early stages and should be provided by specialist teams [78, 79]. Rehabilitation encompasses natural recovery through central nervous system (CNS) reorganisation (plasticity) and functional recovery, both of which are influenced by rehabilitation (this is further explained in Chapters 2 and 7). Many factors affect progress and recovery, and ensuring that there are opportunities to practise regained skills through consistent management is vital. This is a pivotal role for nurses.

It has been estimated that one-third of stroke patients make significant improvements and a further third survive with continuing severe disability [80]. Despite advances in stroke management, it is estimated that, in the United Kingdom, one in eight will die within the first 30 days after stroke, and one in four within the year [81]. These groups require specific stroke treatment and interventions. Different therapeutic modalities are being researched to demonstrate which are most effective, and for whom. Stroke rehabilitation has been referred to as a 'black box' of interventions [82]. Dobkin and Carmichael [83] conceptualise the interacting principles of 'restitution, substitution, or compensation'. Restitution means that the pre-stroke ability has been restored. Substitution means using another method to achieve the same end, such as learning to write with the previously non-dominant hand. Compensation is a technique used to work around the problem when neither restitution nor substitution is possible or appropriate. An example might be using a hip-hitching movement to facilitate walking.

The World Health Organization (WHO)'s ICF model (see earlier) provides a useful framework to consider a person's adjustment and adaptation to their stroke. The ICF is based on a *biopsychosocial model*, providing a coherent view of different perspectives of health: biological, individual, and social. It can be very helpful in assisting the development of person- and family-centred rehabilitation programmes. Person-centred care is described as a way of thinking and doing things that sees the people using health and social services as equal partners in planning, developing, and monitoring care to make it meet their needs. The central tenet is that by adopting a person-centred care approach, not only will people be helped to receive the care they need, but they and their families will become more active in looking after themselves, resulting in a reduction of some pressures on health and social services [84].

Targeting rehabilitation towards those likely to benefit is challenging. Garraway et al. [85] classified patients into three groups. First, there are those who are likely to make spontaneous recovery without substantial rehabilitation and return home promptly. Second, there are those with poor prognostic indicators (e.g. depressed level of consciousness), who generally do not achieve functional independence and require continuing care. This group may benefit from rehabilitation aimed at reducing their care needs or improving certain aspects of their quality of life (i.e. posture and seating). Third is a middle band of stroke survivors, who are most likely to gain from intensive rehabilitation and make significant functional improvement. A review of the evidence demonstrates significant positive benefit of providing rehabilitation interventions in long-term stroke survivors [86]. However, focusing solely on functional recovery risks overlooking emotional and psychosocial problems [87]. As the ICF model indicates, these factors can play 'a much more important role in stroke outcome than most people realise' [88].

Stroke is considered to be a family illness or 'family dilemma', as both the patient and their family embark on a journey for which they need information and support in physical, emotional, and spiritual terms. How the patient and their family are helped through the acute phases of stroke care will influence their experience in transition to rehabilitation and may affect any future contact with stroke services.

9.8 Transfer to Rehabilitation

Transfer to rehabilitation indicates to patients that healthcare professionals believe further recovery is possible. Nonetheless, transfer from one service or team to another can be very stressful. The move from a familiar to an unfamiliar environment, from known to unknown service providers, requires patients and their families to adjust to new routines and establish relationships with new staff.

To minimise experiences of relocation stress syndrome [89], education about the nature and purpose of rehabilitation and an explanation of the roles of healthcare professionals should be provided to patients and their families. In particular, the differences between acute and rehabilitation settings should be highlighted. Without this knowledge, patients can take several days to understand what to expect from staff and what staff expect of them [48]. It can be helpful to provide this information in written form, with essential contact details included.

Even when this education is provided, some patients are simply not ready to engage in rehabilitation. Some insight into why this may be the case is provided by Mauk's [75] six-phase model of post-stroke recovery (Box 9.3), developed from a study of stroke survivors in the United States [3].

Initially, patients engage in agonising (which is about survival) and fantasising (which is about protection of self from the shock of what has happened) before they realise that the effects of stroke 'may not all just go away' [75]. Mauk reports this as 'the pivotal point in recovery' [75], because positive adaptation cannot occur until the patient has this realisation. Facing this reality enables the patient to own their stroke and to learn what is needed. Nurses can enhance patient readiness to learn by listening to them and their families and helping them make sense of what has happened. Kirkevold [57] refers to this as nursing's interpretive function, whereby nurses help patients and families make sense of what has happened to them, what is currently happening to them, and what may happen to them in the future. Motivational interviewing techniques can also support adjustment through positive reframing [90]. Nurses can be facilitators of personal recovery [14, 56]; additional insights presented in Table 9.1 will assist nurses in this role.

Nurses will be very familiar with the 'roller-coaster ride' articulated by the patient and their close family. Having knowledge of the stroke illness trajectory postulated by Kirkevold [14] enables nurses to anticipate, support, and tailor individual rehabilitation programmes. Focusing on enhanced preparedness and the ability to identify and manage the highs and lows of the post-stroke recovery phases is beneficial for patients and their families.

Box 9.3 | The Six Phases of the Post–Stroke Journey [75]

- Agonising (trying to survive)
- Fantasising (trying to protect self from the reality of the stroke)
- Realising (facing the reality of the aftermath of stroke)
- Blending (beginning to adapt)
- Framing (reflecting on the stroke experience and trying to put it into perspective)
- Owning (beginning to move on with life)

TABLE 9.1 Stroke illness trajectory [13]

Trajectory phase	Approximate time frame	Context	Major adjustment focus	Adjustment/rehabilitation work	Action radius	Trajectory projection
Trajectory onset	1–7 d	Acute medical unit	Body	1. Secure biological integrity 2. Relinquish responsibility to healthcare personnel	Bed, room, hospital unit	Stroke a short-term 'intermission'
Initial rehabilitation	1–8 wk	Hospital rehabilitation unit	Body	1. Hard physical training to conquer body/regain functions (body functions/activities of daily living)	Hospital unit, hospital area	Time-limited 'interlude'
			Biographical	2. Start making sense of stroke and its impact		
			Practical	3. Plan homecoming		
Continued rehabilitation	8 wk–6 mo or more	Outpatient/long-term care/home	Practical	1. Practical adjustment to home (or long-term care), (re)structuring day life	Home, gradual widening of circle of outer world	Long-lasting 'interlude', possibly new episode in life
			Body	2. Trying out body in a 'natural environment' (instrumental activities of daily living and valued activities)		
			Biographic	3. Reinterpreting stroke and its impact (changing time frame of recovery)		
Semistable	6 mo–1 y or more	Home/long-term care	Practical	1. Going on with life for the long-term effects of stroke	(Re)creating boundaries of 'relevant world'	Probably new episode/epoch
			Body	2. Resuming/(re)forming valued activities		
			Biographic	3. Trying to minimise the effects of stroke on life and on self		

Case Study

Case 9.3 John

John is a 63-year-old retired engineer who lives alone. Following transfer to the rehabilitation unit, an introductory meeting is set within the first week. This enables John
and his family to ask more detailed questions about the stroke, likely progress, and the
rehabilitation process. His two grown-up children live away, and a method of communication is agreed to ensure they feel kept up to date. John is happy for his son to be
next-of-kin, and a password system is set up to ensure confidentiality is maintained and
information is provided only to this named relative. This reassures both the family and
John. A further meeting date is set for 2 weeks' time as it is anticipated that John will
require a longer period of rehabilitation. This enables the family to organise the time
to attend.

Much can be done to ensure continuity of care between acute and rehabilitation settings. A visit from rehabilitation staff before transfer out of the acute ward
will ensure that information provided to prepare the patient and their family for
rehabilitation is accurate and that the patient and their family know at least one
familiar face (but preferably more) upon arrival in rehabilitation. Pre-transfer education about rehabilitation allows the patient and their family time to absorb the
information provided, generate questions, and have questions answered before
transfer. A pre-transfer tour of the rehabilitation unit enables the patient and their
family to see rehabilitation in action and may assist them to become ready for the
active role that is expected.

Patients need to understand that, unlike the intermittent nature of acute care
interventions, rehabilitation is a continuous process that requires active participation with all clinical staff [48]. It needs to be made explicit that rehabilitation is
not done *to* patients, but *by* patients. Such explanations can assist patients to take
ownership of their stroke and learn what is needed.

The need to prepare patients for rehabilitation should not be underestimated.
Mismatches between nurses', patients', and families' understandings of rehabilitation have been recognised for many years [49, 91, 92], along with the acknowl-
edgement that patients need to be educated about rehabilitation [20, 48, 93–99].
Case Study 9.3 shows the level of discussion required with families.

9.9 Rehabilitation Provision

9.9.1 Service Models

The WSO's Roadmap to Delivering Quality Stroke Care is an implementation
resource to accompany the WSO Global Stroke Services Guideline and Action
Plan [100]. This roadmap provides the framework for the implementation, monitoring, and evaluation of stroke services globally. It provides standardisation and

consistency for the selection of evidence-based recommendations, approaches to implementation in clinical practice, and the calculation of performance measures to create an environment of continuous quality improvement.

In the United Kingdom, components of an integrated stroke service are described within the National Stroke Strategy [101], as developed from previous documents, notably Standard Five of the National Service Framework for Older People [102], and supported in the National Audit Office report, 'Reducing Brain Damage: Faster Access to Better Stroke Care' [103]. The term 'integrated' refers to a smooth transition between phases of the journey following stroke, encompassing:

- emergency response;
- hyper-acute management;
- acute care;
- rehabilitation;
- transfer to home or residential services;
- longer-term management; and
- stroke prevention.

Debate regarding the organisation of stroke care continues. In 1993, Langhorne et al. [104] produced a meta-analysis which demonstrated that patients managed in a specialised stroke unit were less likely to die. Subsequently, a review by the Stroke Unit Trialists [105] concluded: 'stroke patients who received organised inpatient (stroke unit) care were more likely to be alive, independent and living at home one year after the stroke than those receiving conventional care. The apparent benefits were not restricted to any particular sub group of patients or models of stroke unit care. No systematic increase in length of stay in a hospital or institution was observed.'

Recommendations that care be provided by an organised MDT working within a discrete area continue to be considered best practice [62, 106].

It is thought that the essential characteristics of a stroke unit are [62]:

- coordinated, multidisciplinary rehabilitation;
- staff with a special interest in stroke;
- routine involvement of carers in the rehabilitation process; and
- regular programmes of education and training for the workforce.

We now know that simply having a range of different disciplines involved in service provision is not enough. Integrated teamwork, whereby the whole team is involved in planning, delivering, and evaluating patient care, as well as team performance, produces better outcomes.

The planning of stroke services was previously thought to be 'impossible' [107], due to a lack of information on the exact numbers of stroke patients and the cost of care. The situation improved in the United Kingdom with the advent of the Quality and Outcomes Framework (QuOF) data, collected in primary care from general practitioners (GPs). Planning and organisation of stroke services should be provided across a full range of settings and based on the geography of the area and the demography and epidemiology of the local

---

Box 9.4 | The UK National Picture [109]

- 80% of post-acute stroke services participated in the audit.
- 0% of nurses in participating rehabilitation services have been trained to screen the safety of swallowing.
- Social workers are poorly represented in non-inpatient rehabilitation services.
- Access to psychological support has the longest delays, with a median waiting time of over 10 weeks, and 25% waiting 5 months or more.
- Only 29% of early support discharge teams deliver a 7-day service.
- Many services have time limits in place and should have clear re-referral pathways developed.
- The provision of 6-month reviews is not in place across all areas in the United Kingdom.
- Only 15% of services are commissioned to deliver vocational rehabilitation.

---

population. Comparison of models of stroke care and collaboration in research will enhance the identification of important and effective components of stroke care. High-grade evidence is being facilitated through the UK Clinical Research Network [108].

In the United Kingdom, the 2015 Sentinel Stroke National Audit Programme (SSNAP) indicates progress in relation to rehabilitation service provision for stroke patients. Key findings of this audit are set out in Box 9.4.

In 2016, the Stroke Association document 'A New Era for Stroke' highlighted the considerable progress made in developing stroke services, but also focused attention on continuing wide regional variations. These variations in organisation and access to stroke services have been evident in each round of the UK National Sentinel Stroke Audit, which has also highlighted the importance of rehabilitation:

> *The most expensive medical and rehabilitation care is poor quality care or no care at all. There is good evidence that high quality rehabilitation can reduce the need for longer term formal and informal support and afford people who suffer stroke the best chance of recovery. [110]*

In Australia, inequity of access to rehabilitation following stroke also continues to be a problem. Despite recommendations that all stroke patients, except those receiving palliation, be formally assessed for rehabilitation [25], one study of 2013 and 2014 acute care medical records found no documented rehabilitation assessment for 37% of the 333 stroke patients examined [44]. Only 43% of assessments were conducted by rehabilitation staff. The 2015 national acute stroke audit found that only about two-thirds (68%) of patients were assessed for rehabilitation by a physiotherapist within 24–48 hours of hospital admission [111]. The following year, the national stroke audit of rehabilitation services reported that suitability for rehabilitation was 'commonly assessed by the acute physician (65%) or in conjunction with the whole acute interdisciplinary team (64%)' [112]. This is problematic when it limits patient access to specialist rehabilitation expertise [113].

9.10   Length of Rehabilitation

The length of time for which rehabilitation should be offered is unclear. The Stroke Association [114] calls for all stroke survivors to 'receive an annual review at which remaining disabilities are assessed and appropriate treatment is provided to ensure that recovery is sustained and any potential for further progress is fulfilled'. The long-term problems encountered by stroke survivors and their families will be influenced by the success of early rehabilitation, and cross-organisational working will help to ensure that people receive an appropriate level of support. Desrosiers et al. [115] also note that participation in activities of daily living decline in the years after stroke, and underline the need for provision of ongoing and maintenance rehabilitation programmes.

The effectiveness and ongoing costs of rehabilitation for growing numbers of stroke survivors are unknown. Osberg et al. [107], in their study of characteristics of patients referred to as 'cost outliers' who do not benefit from stroke rehabilitation, conclude that they 'consume a disproportionate share of all inpatient rehabilitation resources'. Gladman and Sackley [80] counter this with references to the costs in terms of quality of life, asking, 'What are small changes in severe disability worth to the patient?'

Living after stroke without creating dependency on services is important. The UK Expert Patient Programme [116] and initiatives in other countries target resources towards self-management and gaining life skills to cope with chronic conditions. True success in rehabilitation surely must be when an individual feels they have the ability to direct and control their lives. The UK National Audit Office [103] states that 'most of the burden of stroke is in the cost of rehabilitation and life after stroke'. It is therefore imperative that hospital-based stroke services provide early rehabilitation by an interprofessional team with the necessary expertise and experience for optimal cost-effectiveness. The National Service Framework for Older People [102] has outlined a stroke pathway which includes early multidisciplinary assessment and a plan for rehabilitation agreed with the patient. The transition from hospital to home forms an important part of post-stroke care, and a Cochrane review of evidence regarding the effectiveness of ESD cites a reduction in long-term dependency, admission to institutional care, and hospital length of stay [23]. However, there is currently no consistency in how rehabilitation services are provided between organisations. Many different types of unit and approach are employed, and SSNAP continues to highlight the greatly differing staffing ratios and disciplines involved. These issues are further highlighted in the National Stroke Strategy [101], and ongoing work is required in consideration of the effectiveness and efficiency of various service models, workforce issues, and training and development requirements.

'A New Era for Stroke' [117] outlines the issues patients continue to experience with access to, and quality of, rehabilitation following a stroke. The personal stories contained within this document are a stark reminder that there is still much to do to ensure patients achieve maximum gain during rehabilitation. The report highlights concerns about support for speech and communication problems; 38% of people with a severe disability reported their physiotherapy to be poor or very poor, nearly 50% of stroke survivors said the support they received for fatigue and memory problems was poor, and 25% waited more than 5 months after discharge from hospital for help with mental health issues.

9.11 Adjustment to Life After Stroke

Whilst formal rehabilitation aims to optimise recovery, for many stroke survivors and their families this is just the start of the long journey of adjustment and coping with residual deficits. The literature about adjustment to life after stroke reflects the many negative or emotive aspects of the experience; for example:

> *The world of a stroke survivor is grounded in experiences of loss and effort which are inextricably connected. [118]*
>   *Stroke constitutes a formidable burden of disability and misery, having severe and long-lasting physical, emotional and social consequences for both patient and family. [119]*

Stroke treatment, and in particular rehabilitation, tends to focus on improving function. In discussions with stroke survivors, they are more likely to define recovery as a return to previously valued activities [120]. These discrepancies may cause tension between the multiprofessional team, the patient, and their family. Bethoux et al. [121] suggest that post-stroke quality of life deteriorates in some aspects over time and warn that some stroke survivors may 'idealise the pre-stroke condition'.

Many personal accounts of the experience of stroke have been published in book, newspaper, magazine, and television documentary format. These insightful stories provide additional information and may increase public awareness about stroke illness. The patient's experience of stroke is likely to be coloured by the amount of recovery they make [122]. The course of an illness has been referred to as a trajectory [123]. In stroke, the trajectory is uncertain, and each patient's experience is unique. Adaptation and acceptance of the stroke is crucial to recovery [124]. The patient's ability to absorb information is very important, and initial conversations with nurses 'constitute a vital contribution to achieving recovery' [125]. Nilsson et al. [126] describe the phenomenon as meeting with stroke and note, 'this experience seems to challenge the whole of the individual's being'. Grasping the situation in which they find themselves takes over the patient's life and continues well after discharge from hospital [14]. Encouraging patients and their families to see 'acquired disability as a time of transition rather than simply of loss' [13] may support them on their post-stroke journey.

These early findings continue to ring true with patients and their families despite development of services. The Stroke Association's report, 'Our Life After Stroke' [127], spotlights the lack of ambition shown by healthcare planners and providers in addressing the needs of people after stroke.

Stroke survivors and their families are often extremely resilient and resourceful. Patient stories are a wonderful way of hearing how individuals have adjusted and learned to get on with life after stroke. Interesting and insightful stories from stroke survivors can be accessed on www.healthtalk.org [128].

> *The bus came along and I went up the steps with my bag and there was an old lady [laughter] just inside. I mean, she must have been about 90 and she said, 'Come on dear, I'll help you'; [laughter] I thought, 'Oh my goodness, you know, there's this dear old lady, years and years older than me, helping me'. And, I did that a few times and I felt very proud of myself. I felt I was independent and then I set myself a goal for walking and we've*

*got a shopping centre which is probably about 10 minutes, 15 minutes'
walk along, you know, when you can walk normally. But on the way,
there's a bus shelter with seats inside and there are some stone walls along
the way as well and then when you get further on into the shopping centre,
there's another bus stop and there's another seat. So I thought, 'One day,
I'll make it to those shops' and I did. One day I made it. I sat at the bus stop
for about a quarter of an hour, to calm myself down and I made it a little
further on and I sat on a wall and I got up and I made it to the next bus
centre, the bus stop and the seat, I sat down. I went in a shop and bought
things and I came back the same way and I did the same thing. I stopped
and I sat, I walked and then when I thought it was really bad, I just stood
where I was and I didn't move and then I continued walking and I, I'd
done it. I'd made it. I'd made it to the shops on my own and I was getting
to feel, and then of course, it was after that I started my driving and I, that
was the real big thing, you know, I was independent.*

(www.healthtalk.org)

9.12 Conclusion

Rehabilitation is a pivotal aspect of a stroke patient's care and has to commence at an appropriate level *immediately* after the stroke occurs to maximise benefit. It is clear that one size does not fit all, and the provision of a person- and family-centred rehabilitation programme will ensure that the stroke survivor is assisted to recover and adjust in the way most meaningful for them. This requires flexibility of service models, periods of timely rehabilitation, an expert workforce, and, most importantly, innovative cross-organisational commissioning to ensure that physical, social, and psychological needs are met.

Resources

Association of Rehabilitation Nurses. Promotes and advances rehabilitation nursing practice through education, advocacy, collaboration, and research to enhance quality of life for those affected by disability and chronic illness: www.rehabnurse.org [129].

Australasian Rehabilitation Nurses' Association. Promotes rehabilitation as an integral part of every nurse's practice. Supports the development and sharing of nursing's body of rehabilitation knowledge, skills, and attitudes for the well-being of individuals and communities: www.arna.com.au [130].

Stroke Foundation. Dedicated to raising awareness, preventing stroke, facilitating research, improving treatment, and making life better for stroke survivors: www.strokefoundation.org.au [131].

World Stroke Organization. The world's leading organisation in the fight against stroke, established in October 2006 through the merger of the International Stroke Society and the World Stroke Federation with the purpose of creating one world voice for stroke: www.world-stroke.org.

References

1. UK Stroke Forum Education & Training. Stroke-Specific Education Framework, United Kingdom: UK Stroke Forum 2010. Available from: http://www.stroke-education.org.uk/about [30 November 2018].
2. Barnes, M.P. and Ward, A.B. (2000). Textbook of Rehabilitation Medicine. Oxford: Oxford University Press.
3. Easton, K.L. (1999). The poststroke journey: from agonizing to owning. Geriatric Nursing 20 (2): 70–75. quiz 6.
4. Alaszewski, A., Alaszewski, H., and Potter, J. (2004). The bereavement model, stroke and rehabilitation: a critical analysis of the use of a psychological model in professional practice. Disability and Rehabilitation 26 (18): 1067–1078.
5. Faircloth, C.A., Boylstein, C., Rittman, M. et al. (2004). Sudden illness and biographical flow in narratives of stroke recovery. Sociology of Health & Illness 26 (2): 242–261.
6. NHS Wessex Strategic Clinical Networks. Rehabilitation is everyone's business: principles and expectations for good adult rehabilitation. Available from: http://www.networks.nhs.uk/nhs-networks/clinical-commissioning-community/improving-adult-rehabilitation-services/principles-expectations [30 November 2018].
7. National Health Service (2016). Commissioning Guidance for Rehabilitation. London: National Health Service.
8. Plaisted, L. (1978). Rehabilitation nurse. In: Disability and Rehabilitation Handbook (ed. R.M. Goldenson). New York: McGraw-Hill.
9. Ozer, M.N. (1999). Patient participation in the management of stroke rehabilitation. Topics in Stroke Rehabilitation 6 (1): 43–59.
10. Demain, S., Wiles, R., Roberts, L., and McPherson, K. (2006). Recovery plateau following stroke: fact or fiction? Disability and Rehabilitation 28 (13–14): 815–821.
11. van Vliet, P.M. and Wulf, G. (2006). Extrinsic feedback for motor learning after stroke: what is the evidence? Disability and Rehabilitation 28 (13–14): 831–840.
12. Pryor, J. and Dean, S. (2012). The Person in Context in Interprofessional Rehabilitation: A Person Centred Approach. Chichester: Wiley-Blackwell.
13. Ellis-Hill, C., Payne, S., and Ward, C. (2008). Using stroke to explore the life thread model: an alternative approach to understanding rehabilitation following an acquired disability. Disability and Rehabilitation 30 (2): 150–159.
14. Kirkevold, M. (2010). The role of nursing in the rehabilitation of stroke survivors: an extended theoretical account. Advances in Nursing Science 33 (1): E27–E40.
15. Kearney MP. Reconfiguring the future: stories of post-stroke transition [Doctorate of Philosophy]. Adelaide: University of South Australia; 2009.
16. Jones, F. (2006). Strategies to enhance chronic disease self-management: how can we apply this to stroke? Disability and Rehabilitation 28 (13–14): 841–847.
17. Hale, L., Jones, F., Mulligan, H. et al. (2014). Developing the Bridges self-management programme for New Zealand stroke survivors: a case study. International Journal of Therapy and Rehabilitation 21 (8): 381–388.
18. Pryor, J. (2014). Rehabilitation, Co-Morbidity and Complex Care in Caring for Older People in Australia: Principles for Nursing Practice. Sydney: Wiley.
19. Pryor, J. (2014). The principles of rehabilitation. Journal of the Australasian Rehabilitation Nurses Association 17 (1): 2–3.
20. Pryor, J. and Smith, C. (2002). A framework for the role of Registered Nurses in the specialty practice of rehabilitation nursing in Australia. Journal of Advanced Nursing 39 (3): 249–257.
21. Intercollegiate Stroke Working Party (2016). National Clinical Guidelines for Stroke. London: Royal College of Physicians.

22. Evidence Based Review of Stroke Rehabilitation. Available from: http://www.ebrsr. com [30 November 2018].
23. Cochrane Stroke Review Group. Available from: www.stroke.cochrane.org [30 November 2018].
24. American Stroke Association. Stroke Resources for Professionals. Available from: http://www.strokeassociation.org/STROKEORG/Professionals/Stroke-Resources-for-Professionals_UCM_308581_SubHomePage.jsp [30 November 2018].
25. Stroke Foundation (2017). Clinical Guidelines for Stroke Management. Melbourne: Melbourne Stroke Foundation.
26. Scottish Intercollegiate Guidelines Network. Management of patients with stroke: identification and management of dysphagia, a national clinical guideline. No. 119. Edinburgh: SIGN; 2010. Available from: https://www.sign.ac.uk/assets/sign119.pdf [30 November 2018].
27. National Institute for Health and Care Excellence (NICE) (2013). Stroke Rehabilitation in Adults: Clinical Guideline (CG162). Manchester: National Institute for Health and Care Excellence.
28. World Stroke Organization. Available from: http://www.world-stroke.org [30 November 2018].
29. Duncan, P.W., Zorowitz, R., Bates, B. et al. (2005). Management of Adult Stroke Rehabilitation Care: a clinical practice guideline. Stroke 36 (9): e100–e143.
30. Reker, D.M., Duncan, P.W., Horner, R.D. et al. (2002). Postacute stroke guideline compliance is associated with greater patient satisfaction. Archives of Physical Medicine and Rehabilitation 83 (6): 750–756.
31. Carlson, P.M., Boudreau, M.L., Davis, J. et al. (2006). 'Participate to learn': a promising practice for community ABI rehabilitation. Brain Injury 20 (11): 1111–1117.
32. World Health Organization (WHO) (2001). International Classification of Functioning, Disability and Health (ICF). Geneva: World Health Organization. Available from: http://www.who.int/classifications/icf/en [30 November 2018].
33. Whyte, J. and Hart, T. (2003). It's more than a black box; it's a Russian doll: defining rehabilitation treatments. American Journal of Physical Medicine and Rehabilitation 20 (369): 374.
34. Kwakkel, G. (2006). Impact of intensity of practice after stroke: issues for consideration. Disability and Rehabilitation 28 (13–14): 823–830.
35. Strasser, D.C., Falconer, J.A., Herrin, J.S. et al. (2005). Team functioning and patient outcomes in stroke rehabilitation. Archives of Physical Medicine and Rehabilitation 86 (3): 403–409.
36. Maclean, N., Pound, P., Wolfe, C., and Rudd, A. (2000). Qualitative analysis of stroke patients' motivation for rehabilitation. British Medical Journal 321 (7268): 1051–1054.
37. Cott, C.A. (2004). Client-centred rehabilitation: client perspectives. Disability and Rehabilitation 26 (24): 1411–1422.
38. Stucki, G., Stier-Jarmer, M., Grill, E., and Melvin, J. (2005). Rationale and principles of early rehabilitation care after an acute injury or illness. Disability and Rehabilitation 27 (7–8): 353–359.
39. Horn, S.D., DeJong, G., Smout, R.J. et al. (2005). Stroke rehabilitation patients, practice, and outcomes: is earlier and more aggressive therapy better? Archives of Physical Medicine and Rehabilitation 86 (12 Suppl. 2): S101–S114.
40. Salter, K., Jutai, J., Hartley, M. et al. (2006). Impact of early vs delayed admission to rehabilitation on functional outcomes in persons with stroke. Journal of Rehabilitation Medicine 38 (2): 113–117.
41. Maulden, S.A., Gassaway, J., Horn, S.D. et al. (2005). Timing of initiation of rehabilitation after stroke. Archives of Physical Medicine and Rehabilitation 86 (12 Suppl. 2): S34–S40.
42. Bernhardt, J., Dewey, H., Collier, J. et al. (2006). A Very Early Rehabilitation Trial (AVERT). International Journal of Stroke 1 (3): 169–171.

43. Burton, C.R., Horne, M., Woodward-Nutt, K. et al. (2015). What is rehabilitation potential? Development of a theoretical model through the accounts of healthcare professionals working in stroke rehabilitation services. Disability and Rehabilitation 37 (21): 1955–1960.

44. Lynch, E.A., Luker, J.A., Cadilhac, D.A., and Hillier, S.L. (2015). Rehabilitation assessments for patients with stroke in Australian hospitals do not always reflect the patients' rehabilitation requirements. Archives of Physical Medicine and Rehabilitation 96 (5): 782–789.

45. Henderson, V.A. (1980). Preserving the essence of nursing in a technological age. Journal of Advanced Nursing 5 (3): 245–260.

46. Staff, A.I., Pryor, J., and Australasian Rehabilitation Nurses Association (2003). Rehabilitation Nursing Competency Standards for Registered Nurses. Melbourne: Australasian Rehabilitation Nurses Association.

47. Price, E. (1997). An Exploration of the Nature of Therapeutic Nursing in a General Rehabilitation Team (Inpatient). Albany: Massey University.

48. Pryor, J. (2005). A Grounded Theory of Nursing's Contribution to Inpatient Rehabilitation. Leigh: Deakin University.

49. Thompson, T. (1990). A Qualitative Investigation of Rehabilitation Nursing Care in an Inpatient Unit Using Leininger's Theory. Michigan: Wayne State University.

50. Burton, C.R. (1999). An exploration of the stroke co-ordinator role. Journal of Clinical Nursing 8 (5): 535–541.

51. Gignac, M.A. and Cott, C. (1998). A conceptual model of independence and dependence for adults with chronic physical illness and disability. Social Science & Medicine 47 (6): 739–753.

52. Mahoney, J.E., Sager, M.A., and Jalaluddin, M. (1998). New walking dependence associated with hospitalization for acute medical illness: incidence and significance. Journals of Gerontology, Series A: Biological Science Medical Science 53 (4): 307–312.

53. Sager, M.A., Franke, T., Inouye, S.K. et al. (1996). Functional outcomes of acute medical illness and hospitalization in older persons. Archives of Internal Medicine 156 (6): 645–652.

54. Hill, M.C. and Johnson, J. (1999). An exploratory study of nurses' perceptions of their role in neurological rehabilitation. Rehabilitation Nursing 24 (4): 152–157.

55. O'Connor, S.E. (2000). Nursing interventions in stroke rehabilitation: a study of nurses' views of their pattern of care in stroke units. Rehabilitation Nursing 25 (6): 224–230.

56. Burton, C.R. (2000). A description of the nursing role in stroke rehabilitation. Journal of Advanced Nursing 32 (1): 174–181.

57. Kirkevold, M. (1997). The role of nursing in the rehabilitation of acute stroke patients: toward a unified theoretical perspective. Advances in Nursing Science 19 (4): 55–64.

58. Long, A.F., Kneafsey, R., Ryan, J., and Berry, J. (2002). The role of the nurse within the multi-professional rehabilitation team. Journal of Advanced Nursing 37 (1): 70–78.

59. Janssen, H., Ada, L., Bernhardt, J. et al. (2014). Physical, cognitive and social activity levels of stroke patients undergoing rehabilitation within a mixed rehabilitation unit. Clinical Rehabilitation 28 (1): 91–101.

60. Janssen, H., Ada, L., Bernhardt, J. et al. (2014). An enriched environment increases activity in stroke patients undergoing rehabilitation in a mixed rehabilitation unit: a pilot non-randomized controlled trial. Disability and Rehabilitation 36 (3): 255–262.

61. White, J.H., Alborough, K., Janssen, H. et al. (2014). Exploring staff experience of an 'enriched environment' within stroke rehabilitation: a qualitative sub-study. Disability and Rehabilitation 36 (21): 1783–1789.

62. Stroke Unit Trialists Collaboration (2013). Organised inpatient (stroke unit) care for stroke. Cochrane Database of Systematic Reviews 9 (Art. No.: CD000197). https://doi.org/10.1002/14651858.CD000197.pub3.

63. Dejong, G., Horn, S.D., Gassaway, J.A. et al. (2004). Toward a taxonomy of rehabilitation interventions: using an inductive approach to examine the 'black box' of rehabilitation. Archives of Physical Medicine and Rehabilitation 85 (4): 678–686.

64. D'Alisa, S., Baudo, S., Mauro, A., and Miscio, G. (2005). How does stroke restrict participation in long-term post-stroke survivors? Acta Neurologica Scandinavica 112 (3): 157–162.

65. Hafsteinsdottir, T.B. and Grypdonck, M. (1997). Being a stroke patient: a review of the literature. Journal of Advanced Nursing 26 (3): 580–588.

66. Levack, W., Taylor, K., Siegert, R.J. et al. (2006). Is goal planning in rehabilitation effective? A systematic review. Clinical Rehabilitation 20 (9): 739–755.

67. Wade, D. (1999). Rehabilitation therapy after stroke. The Lancet 354 (9174): 176–177.

68. van den Broek, M.D. (2005). Why does neurorehabilitation fail? Journal of Head Trauma Rehabilitation 20 (5): 464–473.

69. Levack, W., Dean, S.G., Siegert, R.J., and McPherson, K.M. (2006). Purposes and mechanisms of goal planning in rehabilitation: the need for a critical distinction. Disability and Rehabilitation 28 (12): 741–749.

70. Levack, W. and Dean, S. (2012). Processes in Rehabilitation in Interprofessional Rehabilitation: A Person Centred Approach. Chichester: Wiley Blackwell.

71. McClain, C. (2005). Collaborative rehabilitation goal setting. Topics in Stroke Rehabilitation 12 (4): 56–60.

72. McGrath, J.R. and Adams, L. (1999). Patient-centered goal planning: a systemic psychological therapy? Topics in Stroke Rehabilitation 6 (2): 43–50.

73. Siegert, R.J., McPherson, K.M., and Taylor, W.J. (2004). Toward a cognitive-affective model of goal-setting in rehabilitation: is self-regulation theory a key step? Disability and Rehabilitation 26 (20): 1175–1183.

74. Siegert, R.J. and Taylor, W.J. (2004). Theoretical aspects of goal-setting and motivation in rehabilitation. Disability and Rehabilitation 26 (1): 1–8.

75. Mauk, K.L. (2006). Nursing interventions within the Mauk Model of Poststroke Recovery. Rehabilitation Nursing 31 (6): 257–263, disc. 64.

76. Prochaska, J.O., DiClemente, C.C., and Norcross, J.C. (1992). In search of how people change. Applications to addictive behaviors. The American Psychologist 47 (9): 1102–1114.

77. The AVERT Trial Collaboration Group (2015). Efficacy and safety of very early mobilisation within 24h of stroke onset (AVERT): a randomised controlled trial. The Lancet 386 (9988): 46–55.

78. Diserens, K., Michel, P., and Bogousslavsky, J. (2006). Early mobilisation after stroke: review of the literature. Cerebrovascular Diseases 22 (2–3): 183–190.

79. Indredavik, B., Bakke, F., Slordahl, S.A. et al. (1999). Treatment in a combined acute and rehabilitation stroke unit: which aspects are most important? Stroke 30 (5): 917–923.

80. Gladman, J.R. and Sackley, C.M. (1998). The scope for rehabilitation in severely disabled stroke patients. Disability and Rehabilitation 20 (10): 391–394.

81. Stroke Association (2015). The State of the Nation. London: Stroke Association.

82. Kalra, L. and Eade, J. (1995). Role of stroke rehabilitation units in managing severe disability after stroke. Stroke 26 (11): 2031–2034.

83. Dobkin, B. and Carmichael, T. (2005). Principles of recovery after stroke. In: Recovery After Stroke (ed. M.P. Barnes, B.H. Dobkin and J. Bogousslavsky), 47–66. Cambridge: Cambridge University Press.

84. Health Innovation Network South London. Available from: https://health innovationnetwork.com/ [30 November 2018].

85. Garraway, W.M., Akhtar, A.J., Smith, D.L., and Smith, M.E. (1981). The triage of stroke rehabilitation. Journal of Epidemiology and Community Health 35 (1): 39–44.

86. Teasell, R., Mehta, S., Pereira, S. et al. (2012). Time to rethink long-term rehabilitation management of stroke patients. Topics in Stroke Rehabilitation 19 (6): 457–462.

87. Davidoff, G., Keren, O., Ring, H., and Solzi, P. (1992). Who goes home after a stroke: a case control study. NeuroRehabilitation 2 (2): 53–63.

88. Johnston, M., Kirshblum, S., and Shiflett, S. (1992). Prediction of outcomes following rehabilitation of stroke patients. NeuroRehabilitation 2 (4): 72–97.

89. Gordon, M. (2000). Manual of Nursing Diagnosis. St Louis: Mosby.

90. Watkins, C.L., Auton, M.F., Deans, C.F. et al. (2007). Motivational interviewing early after acute stroke: a randomized, controlled trial. Stroke 38 (3): 1004–1009.

91. Jones, M., O'Neill, P., Waterman, H., and Webb, C. (1997). Building a relationship: communications and relationships between staff and stroke patients on a rehabilitation ward. Journal of Advanced Nursing 26 (1): 101–110.

92. Long, A., Kneafsey, R., Ryan, J. et al. (2001). Team Working in Rehabilitation: Exploring the Role of the Nurse. London: English National Board for Nursing, Midwifery and Health Visiting.

93. Arts, S.E., Francke, A.L., and Hutten, J.B. (2000). Liaison nursing for stroke patients: results of a Dutch evaluation study. Journal of Advanced Nursing 32 (2): 292–300.

94. Berger, M. (1999). Let's visit – on the road to rehabilitation. Journal of Australasian Rehabilitation Nurses Association 2 (2): 7–9.

95. Elesha-Adams, M. and McIntyre, K. (1983). Facilitating the patient's entry into the rehabilitation setting. Rehabilitation Nursing 8 (5): 22–46.

96. Greneger, R. (2003). Relocation stress syndrome in rehabilitation transfers: a review of the literature. Journal of the Australasian Rehabilitation Nurses Association 6: 8–13.

97. Nypaver, J.M., Titus, M., and Brugler, C.J. (1996). Patient transfer to rehabilitation: just another move? Rehabilitation Nursing 21 (2): 94–97.

98. Sheppard, B. (1994). Patients' views of rehabilitation. Nursing Standard 9 (10): 27–30.

99. Sondermeyer, J. and Pryor, J. (2006). 'You're going to rehab': a study into the experiences of patients moving from acute care settings to an inpatient rehabilitation unit. Journal of the Australasian Rehabilitation Nurses Association 9 (2): 23–27.

100. Lindsay, P., Furie, K.L., Davis, S.M. et al. (2014). World Stroke Organization global stroke services guidelines and action plan. International Journal of Stroke 9 (Suppl. A100): 4–13.

101. Department of Health (2007). National Stroke Strategy. London: Department of Health.

102. Department of Health and Social Care (2001). The National Service Framework for Older People. London: Department of Health and Social Care.

103. National Audit Office. Department of Health – reducing brain damage: faster access to better stroke care. Available from: http://www.nao.org.uk/report/department-of-health-reducing-brain-damage-faster-access-to-better-stroke-care [30 November 2018].

104. Langhorne, P., Williams, B.O., Gilchrist, W., and Howie, K. (1993). Do stroke units save lives? The Lancet 342 (8868): 395–398.

105. Stroke Unit Trialists' Collaboration (1997). Collaborative systematic review of the randomised trials of organised inpatient (stroke unit) care after stroke. British Medical Journal 314 (7088): 1151.

106. Cifu, D.X. and Stewart, D.G. (1999). Factors affecting functional outcome after stroke: a critical review of rehabilitation interventions. Archives of Physical Medicine and Rehabilitation 80 (5 Suppl. 1): S35–S39.

107. Osberg, J.S., Haley, S.M., McGinnis, G.E., and DeJong, G. (1990). Characteristics of cost outliers who did not benefit from stroke rehabilitation. American Journal of Physical Medicine and Rehabilitation 69 (3): 117–125.

108. UK Clinical Research Network. Available from: http://www.ukcrc.org/research-infrastructure/clinical-research-networks/uk-clinical-research-network-ukcrn [30 November 2018].

109. Royal College of Physicians (2015). Sentinel Stroke National Audit Programme. London: Royal College of Physicians.

110. Rudd A. Foreword in Royal College of Physicians, Sentinel Stroke National Audit Programme (SSNAP). London: Royal College of Physicians; 2017

111. National Stroke Foundation (2015). National Stroke Audit – Acute Stroke Services Report. Melbourne: National Stroke Foundation.

112. Stroke Foundation (2016). National Stroke Audit – Rehabilitation Services Report 2016. Melbourne: Stroke Foundation.
113. Lynch, E.A., Luker, J.A., Cadilhac, D.A., and Hillier, S.L. (2016). Inequities in access to rehabilitation: exploring how acute stroke unit clinicians decide who to refer to rehabilitation. Disability and Rehabilitation 38 (14): 1415–1424.
114. Stroke Association (1997). Stroke: National Tragedy – National Policy. London: Stroke Association.
115. Desrosiers, J., Rochette, A., Noreau, L. et al. (2006). Long-term changes in participation after stroke. Topics in Stroke Rehabilitation 13 (4): 86–96.
116. Expert Patient Programme. Available from: https://www.sussexcommunity.nhs.uk/services/servicedetails.htm?directoryID=16306 [30 November 2018].
117. Stroke Association (2016). A New Era for Stroke. London: Stroke Association.
118. Secrest, J.A. and Thomas, S.P. (1999). Continuity and discontinuity: the quality of life following stroke. Rehabilitation Nursing 24 (6): 240–246.
119. Mead, J. (1988). King's Fund Forum; Consensus Conference: the treatment of stroke. Physiotherapy 74 (8): 358–359.
120. Doolittle, N.D. (1992). The experience of recovery following lacunar stroke. Rehabilitation Nursing 17 (3): 122–125.
121. Bethoux, F., Calmels, P., and Gautheron, V. (1999). Changes in the quality of life of hemiplegic stroke patients with time: a preliminary report. American Journal of Physical Medicine and Rehabilitation 78 (1): 19–23.
122. Bartlett, D.J., Macnab, J., Macarthur, C. et al. (2006). Advancing rehabilitation research: an interactionist perspective to guide question and design. Disability and Rehabilitation 28 (19): 1169–1176.
123. Wiener, C.L. and Dodd, M.J. (1993). Coping amid uncertainty: an illness trajectory perspective. Scholarly Inquiry for Nursing Practice 7 (1): 17–31, disc. 3–5.
124. Backe, M., Larsson, K., and Fridlund, B. (1996). Patients' conceptions of their life situation within the first week after a stroke event: a qualitative analysis. Intensive and Critical Care Nursing 12 (5): 285–294.
125. Gibbon, B. and Little, V. (1995). Improving stroke care through action research. Journal of Clinical Nursing 4 (2): 93–100.
126. Nilsson, I., Jansson, L., and Norberg, A. (1997). To meet with a stroke: patients' experiences and aspects seen through a screen of crises. Journal of Advanced Nursing 25 (5): 953–963.
127. Stroke Association (2015). Our Lives After Stroke Campaign Report. London: Stroke Association.
128. Health Talk 2016. Available from: http://www.healthtalk.org [30 November 2018].
129. Association of Rehabilitation Nurses. Available from: http://www.rehabnurse.org [30 November 2018].
130. Australasian Rehabilitation Nurses' Association. Available from: http://www.arna.com.au [30 November 2018].
131. Stroke Foundation. StrokeSafe Speakers Australia 2018. Available from: https://strokefoundation.org.au [30 November 2018].

CHAPTER 10

Promoting Continence

Kathryn Getliffe[1] and Lois Thomas[2]

[1] School of Nursing and Midwifery, University of Southampton, Southampton, UK
[2] School of Health Sciences, University of Central Lancashire, Preston, UK

KEY POINTS

- Urinary incontinence is common after a stroke, affecting 32–79% of patients.
- Bowel function is often affected by stroke, with up to 60% of patients in rehabilitation wards experiencing constipation, and more than 30% experiencing incontinence of faeces at 7–10 days.
- Mobility and manual dexterity problems can compound bladder and bowel symptoms by making accessing the toilet difficult. Other problems, such as visual disturbances, aphasia, and the side effects of medication, also contribute to continence difficulties.
- All nurses should be trained in assessment and management of bladder and bowel problems, and should know where to obtain further advice.
- Bladder and bowel care requires active management – this includes a formal assessment and a personalised care plan.

This chapter maps to criteria within the following sections of the Stroke-Specific Education Framework (SSEF):

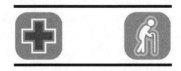

I don't go out, I don't even ask anyone round ... I'm so embarrassed about the smell. I do try and keep myself clean but it gets on to your clothes and furniture. Sometimes I wish that I hadn't survived because it's no life I'm leading now.
(Female stroke survivor)

Stroke Nursing, Second Edition. Edited by Jane Williams, Lin Perry, and Caroline Watkins.
© 2020 John Wiley & Sons Ltd. Published 2020 by John Wiley & Sons Ltd.

10.1 Introduction

Bladder and bowel problems are common following stroke and can have a huge impact on physical, psychological, and social aspects of life for both patients and carers. For many people, involuntary loss of urine or faeces is a sensitive and personal issue, often accompanied by perceptions of loss of dignity and self-respect. The stroke survivor quoted at the start of this chapter shows powerfully the devastating nature of incontinence. Depression is also common in stroke, but is twice as likely in survivors who are incontinent compared with those who are not [2, 3]. Healthcare professionals can do much to help improve and manage bladder and bowel problems, starting with having a good understanding of key issues and completing an early assessment of problems. This chapter examines the causes and contributing factors of bladder and bowel problems in stroke, and discusses assessment and management protocols, together with the underpinning evidence base.

10.2 Prevalence and Causes of Continence Problems Post-Stroke

The prevalence of urinary incontinence (UI) after stroke is high, with studies suggesting around half of people admitted to hospital experience UI, and a third a loss of bowel control [4, 5]. Many (25–50%) are still suffering from UI at discharge and up to 1 year later [6–8]. Longer-term follow-up (on average 9 years post-stroke) suggests up to 17% of survivors remain incontinent [2].

The causes of UI can be varied and complex, including pathophysiological effects of stroke on neural pathways involved in bladder control, and a consequence of functional disability. UI is reported to be more common amongst patients with frontal lobe circulation disorders and subcortical brain lesion [9]. Several studies suggest post-stroke UI may be divided into two clinical categories: 'classical urge UI' and 'UI of persons with perception disorders' [5]. Types of UI are discussed in detail later in this chapter. Perhaps unsurprisingly, the more severe the stroke, the greater the likelihood of UI [10, 11].

UI is widely recognised as an important prognostic indicator of mortality and poor outcome in terms of functional disability, cognition, and discharge destination – home or institutional care [7, 12]. Indeed, UI at 1 week is one of the strongest clinical markers of poor prognosis [13]. UI has been significantly associated with age over 75 years, dysphagia, visual field defect, and motor weakness [7]. Poorer stroke survival is particularly linked with patients with impaired awareness of the need to void [11]. Improvement in UI is common over time [14], suggesting continence problems may be transient in some stroke survivors. Factors predicting early improvements in continence status include less impairment on admission (a Functional Independence Measure [15, 16] score of 60 or more) and the site of the stroke lesion [5, 17].

In the general population, more than one in three people over 40 years of age reported symptoms of bladder problems in a large survey by Perry et al. [18]. This high prevalence suggests many stroke survivors may be vulnerable to exacerbation of pre-existing UI. A recent feasibility trial of a systematic voiding programme delivered in stroke units [19] found 38% (143/413) of patients experienced incontinence prior to their stroke. This should be borne in mind during assessment of continence problems.

Bowel problems post-stroke are more likely to be related to resultant functional disability than direct effects of the stroke. In a study of over 800 stroke patients, constipation affected 60% of those in rehabilitation wards [20], and faecal incontinence (FI) was reported to affect more than 30% of all stroke patients at 7–10 days, 11% at 3 months, 11% at 1 year, and 15% at 3 years [21]. Those with FI at 3 months were at increased risk of long-term placement in a nursing home and death within 1 year. FI may be caused by impaction and overflow, and may be associated more with disability-related factors such as ability to self-toilet than with the brain injury itself [22]. Other common impairments, such as aphasia and cognitive problems, may also indirectly affect bowel function.

10.3 Importance of Continence Care

Good continence care can help mitigate against the effects of stroke, including reducing risk of falls [23]. It also plays a key role in helping restore self-esteem and promoting independence [24], and may be important in reducing barriers to participation in rehabilitation activity. As continence problems are personal, many people are embarrassed and find them difficult to talk about. The attitudes of health professionals can exert a major influence (positive or negative), and it is important to take a proactive, supportive, and well-informed approach. It is particularly important that healthcare professionals do not adhere to a belief that incontinence is an inevitable and non-reversible part of the ageing process.

Failure to adequately assess, treat, and support people with a continence problem negatively impacts on dignity and imposes limitations on lifestyle, employment opportunities, and social functioning. Even if continence cannot be fully restored, there is always the potential for improvement to overall quality of life. Targeting post-stroke continence problems early may reduce the poorer outcomes associated with continuing UI [7, 14].

10.3.1 Clinical Guidelines

UK National Clinical Guidelines for Stroke [25] specify that all wards should have established assessment and management protocols for UI, FI, and constipation in stroke patients (Box 10.1), but many do not. The most recent Sentinel Stroke National Audit Programme (SSNAP) quarterly report, for the period December 2016 to March 2017 [26], found 91.7% of eligible patients had a continence plan drawn up by the time they were discharged from inpatient care. Whilst this percentage has risen in recent successive audits, the authors conclude it is 'unacceptable' that around 6% of patients are not being adequately assessed. Furthermore, the fact that a plan was provided says nothing of whether it was adequate or implemented.

Box 10.1 | National Clinical Guideline for Stroke [25]

A. Stroke unit staff should be trained in the use of standardised assessment and management protocols for UI, FI, and constipation in people with stroke.

B. People with stroke should not have an indwelling (urethral) catheter inserted unless indicated to relieve urinary retention or when fluid balance is critical.

C. People with stroke who have continued loss of bladder or bowel control 2 weeks after onset should be reassessed to identify the cause of incontinence, and be involved in deriving a treatment plan (with their family/carers, if appropriate). The treatment plan should include:

- treatment of any identified cause of incontinence;
- training for the patient and their family/carers in the management of incontinence;
- referral for specialist treatments and behavioural adaptations, if the patient is able to participate; and
- adequate arrangements for the continued supply of continence aids and services.

D. People with stroke with continued loss of urinary continence should be offered behavioural interventions and adaptations such as:

- timed toileting;
- prompted voiding;
- review of caffeine intake;
- bladder retraining;
- pelvic floor exercises; and
- external equipment

prior to considering pharmaceutical and long-term catheter options.

E. People with stroke with constipation should be offered:

- advice on diet, fluid intake, and exercise;
- a regulated routine of toileting;
- a prescribed drug review, to minimise use of constipating drugs;
- oral laxatives;
- a structured bowel management programme which includes nurse-led bowel care interventions;
- education and information for themselves and their family/carers; and
- rectal laxatives, if severe problems persist.

F. People with continued continence problems on transfer of care from hospital should receive follow-up with specialist continence services in the community.

10.4 Bladder Function and Dysfunction

10.4.1 Normal Control of Micturition

Before considering assessment and management of bladder problems and UI in detail, it is important to understand the normal control of micturition. The bladder has two main functions: storage of urine at low pressure and periodic elimination of urine under voluntary control. The major anatomical structures involved in both functions are the:

- bladder (detrusor muscle) and bladder neck;
- urethra and urethral sphincter mechanism (striated muscle); and
- pelvic floor.

During storage of urine, the bladder neck and external sphincter are closed and the detrusor muscle is relaxed (via inhibitory control from higher centres). The bladder stretches to accommodate the increasing volume of urine produced by the kidneys, whilst allowing pressure inside to remain low as the volume increases. During the filling cycle, stretch receptors within the detrusor muscle pass impulses to the spinal micturition centre (via sacral level nerves S2–S4) and then, through the spinal cord (lateral spinothalamic tracts), to the pontine micturition centre and the frontal cortex. At a bladder volume of around 150–250 ml, these impulses are perceived as the desire to void, but they are effectively suppressed by the higher centres until a convenient time. A 'normal' bladder will hold around 400–500 ml of urine before needing to empty. Voluntary voiding requires coordinated relaxation of the external sphincter and bladder neck, followed by detrusor muscle contraction (via parasympathetic stimulation). These two different sets of activities are mediated by three sets of peripheral nerves: pelvic nerves (parasympathetic, cholinergic), hypogastric nerves (sympathetic, adrenergic), and pudendal nerves (somatic). The necessary coordination is achieved via the spinal–pontine spinal reflex, involving the spinal micturition centre (S2–S4) and the pontine micturition centre (the main switching centre between filling and voiding cycles). Voluntary control of voiding appears to be dependent on connections between the frontal cortex and regions within the hypothalamus, as well as the brainstem [27].

10.4.2 Causes of Urinary Incontinence Post-Stroke

There are three mechanisms likely to contribute to symptoms of UI post-stroke [28]:

- disruption of the neuromicturition pathways, resulting in detrusor overactivity and symptoms of urgency and frequency (common terms: 'urge incontinence', 'overactive bladder syndrome', 'bladder hyperreflexia');
- incontinence due to stroke-related cognitive, language, or mobility deficits ('functional incontinence'); and
- concurrent neuropathy or medication use resulting in bladder hyporeflexia (causing urinary retention and incomplete bladder emptying).

10.5 Main Types of UI

The main types of UI are summarised in Box 10.2.

10.5.1 Urge Incontinence

Urge incontinence is the most common type in stroke patients [11, 19], and is characterised by a sudden, compelling urge to void that is difficult or impossible to defer. The problem is caused by overactivity of the detrusor muscle of the bladder, often termed 'overactive bladder syndrome' (OAB), or more specifically, 'bladder hyper-reflexia', where there is a known neurological cause. Neurological damage resulting from stroke may cause loss of inhibitory impulses from the brain, allowing inappropriate activation of the sacral reflex arc and bladder contractions beginning before micturition is voluntarily initiated [29]. Damage above the pons leaves the spinal–bulbar–spinal reflex intact. Coordinated sphincter relaxation and detrusor contraction for voiding is therefore preserved, but the inhibitory input to delay micturition may be lost or impaired. This results in detrusor overactivity, characterised by symptoms of urinary frequency and urgency, with or without urge incontinence. Bladder contractions may occur spontaneously or on provocation (e.g. coughing), or whilst the patient is attempting to inhibit micturition. Contractions may cause major leakage (complete bladder emptying) or partial emptying (frequent small leaks).

Box 10.2 | Main Types of Urinary Incontinence (UI)

Urgency/urge incontinence.[1] The sudden compelling desire to pass urine, which is difficult to defer. Urge incontinence is involuntary leakage accompanied by, or immediately preceded by, urgency. It is often associated with detrusor over-activity, but can be due to other forms of urethra-vesical dysfunction.

Stress incontinence.[1] Involuntary leakage on effort or exertion, sneezing or coughing. Usually caused by pelvic floor weakness or damage, or sphincter incompetence.

Mixed incontinence.[1] Leakage associated with urgency and also with exertion, effort, sneezing, or coughing.

Functional incontinence.[1] Incontinence due to the impairment of physical or cognitive functioning leading to the inability of a usually continent person to reach the toilet in time to avoid unintentional loss of urine.

Neurogenic UI. Loss of urine due to detrusor hyper-reflexia and/or involuntary urethral relaxation in the absence of the desire to void. The bladder empties without warning. The person is unaware of bladder emptying.

Acute urinary retention.[1] A painful, palpable bladder when the patient is unable to pass any urine. Pain may or may not be a presenting feature. Retention may be associated with detrusor overactivity or underactivity.

Chronic urinary retention or voiding symptoms associated with obstruction or underactive detrusor. A non-painful bladder, which remains palpable after the patient has passed urine.

Source: Adapted from Abrams et al. [30].

---

[1] Most common types of UI post-stroke.

If the bladder is not emptied effectively, large residual volumes of urine (100 ml and more) are common. The bladder's overall capacity also decreases, since it no longer has the opportunity to fill completely. Patients with OAB or hyperreflexia usually complain of urgency with little or no warning of the need to void, and may be incontinent of urine before reaching the toilet. In addition, they commonly experience persistent frequency and nocturnal enuresis. Overactivity can be objectively demonstrated by urodynamic studies, which measure pressure changes as they occur within the bladder and urethra during bladder filling. Overactivity is the most frequent urodynamic finding in people who have had a stroke, but the procedure is invasive and is not routinely required for all patients. Recent reviews indicate that bladder training may be a useful intervention [31, 32]; this is discussed further later.

10.5.2 Stress Incontinence

Stress incontinence is characterised by UI upon exertion. It is not a direct consequence of stroke, as its primary cause is weakness of the pelvic floor muscles, or prostatectomy in some men. It may also present as mixed incontinence, with symptoms of both stress and urgency. Stroke may exacerbate existing stress incontinence due to reduced muscle tone and additional mobility problems increasing the amount of exertion required to move.

10.5.3 Mixed Incontinence

Patients with mixed incontinence experience symptoms which include leakage associated with urgency, exertion, and effort such as sneezing or coughing. Mixed incontinence is a common type of UI post-stroke.

10.5.4 Functional Incontinence

Impaired functional status can contribute to UI by inhibiting effective toileting skills even in the absence of physiological bladder dysfunction [19, 33]. Movement, communication, and perception disorders can all impact on continence management. The type and amount of help required to resolve problems requires detailed assessment.

10.5.5 Retention of Urine – Hyporeflexia

Accumulation of urine in the bladder can result from voiding difficulties and incomplete emptying. It is important that urinary retention is identified and treated, as it can lead to urinary tract infection (UTI), hydronephrosis, pyelonephritis, and renal failure. The following symptoms are common indicators of retention:

- constant wetness (dribbling) caused by urinary overflow;
- distended abdomen;
- feeling of incomplete bladder emptying;
- recurrent urine infections; and
- residual volume of more than 100 ml.

Acute retention develops over a short time frame, and can be extremely painful. By contrast, chronic retention due to incomplete emptying can develop over a longer period and may not be associated with pain (Box 10.2).

10.6 Transient Causes of UI

Although UI is common after stroke, it is always important to exclude transient causes early on in the assessment process. UTI is a frequent cause of UI, and urine should be tested for leucocytes and nitrites within 24 hours of admission. Other transient causes may include chest infection and acute or chronic cough; confusion and disorientation; unfamiliar surroundings; and depression and emotional distress (particularly in frail elderly patients). A useful mnemonic for the causes of transient incontinence is DIAPPERS [34] (Box 10.3).

10.7 Assessment of UI and Bladder Dysfunction

10.7.1 Admission Assessment

All patients admitted to hospital with stroke should have a nursing assessment, including urine testing, within 24 hours of admission to identify UI and detect UTI or other abnormality. Aids to communication need to be available, such as the nurse call-bell and picture cards at the bedside. Body-worn pads may be used to provide confidence and comfort, if required. Hand-held urinals are available

---

Box 10.3 | Causes of Transient Incontinence – DIAPPERS [34]

Delirium. Confusion may result from drugs, surgery, or an acute illness.

Infection. Symptomatic urinary tract infections.

Atrophic urethritis/vaginitis. Thinning, friable, irritated tissues that may cause or contribute to incontinence.

Pharmaceuticals. Drugs include sedatives, narcotics, antimuscarinics, calcium-channel blockers (CCBs), loop diuretics, angiotensin-converting enzyme (ACE) inhibitors, non-steroidal anti-inflammatory drugs (NSAIDs), and alpha-receptor agonists/antagonists.

Psychiatric. Severe depression.

Excess urine output. Large fluid intake, caffeinated drinks, and endocrine problems.

Restricted mobility. Arthritis, pain, postprandial hypotension, poor use of assistive devices, fear of falling.

Stool impaction. Can cause both UI and FI.

for male and female use and can be used in bed or in a chair, helping prevent episodes of incontinence due to reduced mobility. Absorbent gel within the urinal can prevent spillage where manual dexterity is a problem.

Patients with bladder problems should have a full continence assessment within 7 days of admission (see national and locally agreed guidelines and standards). This requires time, privacy, and patience. It can be difficult for patients to feel comfortable talking about bladder and bowel activity, and this may be compounded in patients with post-stroke aphasia. The nurse needs to avoid jargon and adopt appropriate body language, eye contact, and a supportive approach to listening to encourage individuals to communicate. Visual formats such as leaflets and diagrams may be helpful. Examples of questions to help characterise the continence problem are given in Box 10.4. Table 10.1 details the nursing assessment of UI.

10.7.2   Frequency and Volume Charting

All patients with UI should have frequency and volume of fluid intake and output recorded for a minimum of 3 days (preferably 5–7 days) following admission or onset of UI, using a validated bladder diary [35]. This will indicate:

- the current pattern of voiding (how often and how much), and determine if particular times are more problematic than others (e.g. dry during the day but wet at night);
- bladder capacity (indicated by the maximum volume voided);
- maximum length of time the patient can hold on between voids during day and night; and
- the number, type, and timing of drinks.

Box 10.4 | Examples of Questions to Help Determine a Pattern of Symptoms and the Type of UI

Questions to determine type of UI:
- Onset: When did UI start?
- Degree: Mild, moderate, severe?
- Frequency: How often in 24 hours?
- Urgency: Able to reach toilet in time?
- Leaking on exertion: On getting up, coughing, sneezing?
- Nocturia: Need to get up for toilet at night?
- Dysuria: Does it hurt to pass urine? (check for UTI)

Voiding difficulties:
- Poor stream: Is the urine flow slow/intermittent?
- Hesitancy: Trouble starting urine flow?
- Straining: Straining to empty the bladder?
- Residual: Is the bladder emptying completely?

TABLE 10.1 Nursing assessment of UI

Intervention	Rationale
Basic nursing assessment within 24 h of admission (all patients)	To identify individuals with UI and instigate early intervention
Urine testing within 24 h of admission (all patients)	To identify presence of leucocytes, nitrites, and protein, which indicate a urinary tract/kidney infection
If results are positive for leucocytes, nitrites, and protein, send an MSU to the laboratory for culture and analysis	To identify appropriate antibiotic treatment if required
If there are other abnormal findings (e.g. glucose), complete assessment as appropriate (e.g. check blood glucose) and refer to medical team	Other disease processes may be present
Frequency/volume and output chart: all patients with UI (including those with a urinary catheter) for a minimum of 5–7 d (following admission or from onset of UI)	To assess: • current pattern of voiding • bladder capacity • maximum length of time the patient can hold on between voids during day/night • number/type of drinks This will show if particular times are problematic (e.g. dry during day but wet at night) and inform schedule for prompted voiding or bladder training
Full assessment of UI should be undertaken within 7 d (from admission or from onset of UI)	To identify problems caused by or contributing to UI
	To determine the type of incontinence and plan appropriate treatment/management
Treatment options will be discussed and agreed with the patient or relevant other person	To promote patient-centred care and reduce anxiety for patient/carer
A plan of care for the treatment and management of UI documented in the patient's notes within 7 d of admission, and treatment initiated and monitored	To improve or manage symptoms of UI and promote ongoing continuity of care
Reassessment/evaluation undertaken and documented at regular intervals according to the plan of care	To identify improvement (and provide positive feedback to patients/carers) or change plan of care

These data can help to confirm the type of UI and, where appropriate, the optimum schedule for bladder training interventions. They also provide a baseline from which to measure improvement once interventions have been initiated. Where possible, patients should be responsible for keeping their own chart.

10.7.3 Full Continence Assessment

There are three issues to consider:

- Is there a failure of bladder storage?
- Is there a failure of bladder emptying?
- Is the problem due to functional disability?

The pattern of symptoms described and the results of the bladder diary will provide a good indication of the type of continence problem. A simple assessment form is shown in Figure 10.1.

10.7.4 Relevant History

People with stroke may have a non-neurological cause for their bladder and bowel symptoms, and if symptoms existed pre-stroke, the underlying cause will need to be investigated. Co-morbid conditions which exacerbate UI include asthma and chronic chest conditions: strain is exerted on the urethral sphincter mechanism by coughing. Other contributing conditions include neurological conditions such as multiple sclerosis and spinal injuries, diabetes (mellitus and insipidus), and dementia.

Previous gynaecological or urological interventions need to be noted and their impact on UI considered; for example, obstetric difficulties can contribute to weak pelvic floor muscles, whilst prostatectomy may leave a post-micturition dribble, possibly due to a weak detrusor contraction or sphincter.

10.7.5 Functional Capacity and Assessment of Toileting Skills

Particular issues to examine include:

- awareness of the need to empty the bladder;
  and the ability to:
- find and get to a toilet or request help;
- manage clothing; and
- maintain appropriate posture for micturition or bowel movement.

The extent and nature of physical and cognitive disabilities are likely to affect the implementation and success of management strategies; therefore, a functional assessment of toileting skills is important. This may include use of a standardised cognitive function test on all patients, such as the Abbreviated Mental Test Score (AMTS) [36]. Where there appears to be a problem, further testing will be required. The Mini-Mental State Examination (MMSE) [37] is the most commonly used instrument for screening cognitive functioning. The test takes only about 10 minutes, but is limited because it will not detect subtle memory losses, particularly in well-educated patients [38]. Chapter 11 addresses cognitive functioning in

Patient name:_____ Hospital no._____

Date of assessment:_____ Name of assessor:_____

Date of onset of urinary incontinence:_____

1. Review the patient's drug chart for drugs that may be implicated in urinary incontinence (diuretics, sedatives etc.)

2. Urine test result (using dipstick)

Leucocytes   positive [ ]   negative [ ]

Nitrites   positive [ ]   negative [ ]

If positive send Mid Stream Urine sample to lab for culture and sensitivity

3. Does the patient have any pain/discomfort related to passing urine?

                         Yes   [ ]   No   [ ]

If yes document in notes, inform medical staff and consider analgesia

4. Does the patient have any of the following indications in the perianal/genital/groin area?

Soreness   Yes   [ ]   No   [ ]

Rash   Yes   [ ]   No   [ ]

Candida   Yes   [ ]   No   [ ]

If yes document in notes and inform medical staff

5. Can the patient hold the urine in the bladder once the desire to pass urine is felt?

                         Yes   [ ]   No   [ ]

If no treat as overactive bladder

6. Is the urinary incontinence initiated or aggravated by coughing, sneezing or standing?

                         Yes   [ ]   No   [ ]

If yes treat as stress incontinence

7. Is the patient independently mobile?

                         Yes   [ ]   No   [ ]

Can the patient use a hand-held urinal unaided?

                         Yes   [ ]   No   [ ]

Can the patient communicate their need to pass urine?

                         Yes   [ ]   No   [ ]

If no to one or more of the last three questions treat as functional incontinence

8. Is the patient able to pass urine spontaneously (bladder scan >500 ml)?

                         Yes   [ ]   No   [ ]

If no treat as acute retention

If yes   **Post-micturition bladder scan result ....ml**

         More than 100 ml [ ]   Less than 100 ml   [ ]

If more than 100 ml treat as incomplete bladder emptying

9. Patient's normal bowel pattern_____

Date of patient's last bowel movement_____

Consider whether the patient may be suffering from constipation.

NB: Patients may be suffering with more than one type of incontinence. A 48-hour frequency/volume chart will help with diagnosis.

FIGURE 10.1 Example of a simple assessment tool to help guide diagnosis.

further detail. Other standardised measures, such as the Barthel Index (BI) [39], are directed towards the ability to perform activities of daily living. The BI can be used to determine a baseline level of functioning and to monitor improvements in activities of daily living over time.

10.7.6   Medications

Many drugs can disturb bladder and bowel function. Polypharmacy can often be a contributing factor, particularly in elderly people with several co-morbid conditions. Some of the most common drug groups that may affect bladder function are diuretics, anticholinergics, sympathomimetics, some antihypertensives, and antiparkinsonism drugs [40].

10.7.7   Social and Environmental Factors

This is an important part of assessment that can be overlooked when patients are in the acute stage. The impact of incontinence on working life, sexual relationships, and family and friends may be dramatic. Many people feel that bowel and bladder functions are personally controllable and that failure to do so is the fault of the person suffering. This is not true, and this must be emphasised to avoid placing feelings of guilt and shame on the family member with the problem. The family must also be encouraged not to feel ashamed or embarrassed to be around the affected member.

It is important that patients, families, and carers are aware of sources of information prior to discharge, such as continence advisory services, the Stroke Association, and the Association for Continence Advice.

10.7.8   Physical Examinations and Tests

Simple palpation of the abdomen is useful to assess for bladder distension or constipation. Observation of skin condition around the symphysis pubis and groin may reveal soreness from UI or wearing pads. A digital rectal examination (DRE) may be used to feel for a faecally loaded rectum, but this is considered an invasive procedure and should not be undertaken without permission and appropriate training [41].

If retention is suspected, the simplest and most accurate non-invasive investigation is an ultrasound scan of the bladder. Training is required before undertaking bladder scanning and interpreting results. Obesity can make scanning difficult or impossible, and constipation or bowel gas can blur the image. If a bladder scan is not possible, the bladder can be drained using an intermittent catheter and the volume measured.

There is no universal agreement on the amount of post-void residual (PVR) that requires intervention. Where a residual is symptomatic (i.e. there is UI, urgency, frequency, or UTI), then action should be taken to address the problem. Tam et al. [42] found an increased risk of UTI when the PVR was more than 100 ml: this appears a reasonable and practical cut-off for instigating further investigation.

10.8 Treatment Strategies and Care Planning for UI

The ultimate aim of treatment is continence; however, this may not always be realistic, and it is important to determine the patient's own goals and motivation when planning a care programme. For some, the goal will be dependent continence: dry with toileting assistance, medication, or pads.

In the early stages post-stroke, it may help patient comfort and confidence to use a body-worn absorbent pad if they are unable to get to the toilet or hold a urinal. However, pad use should be frequently reassessed, because the presence of a pad can contribute to sore skin and slow down access to the toilet, bedpan, or urine bottle.

Although many of the interventions for promoting continence in stroke patients are simple, they can be labour-intensive and their success is dependent on the availability of staff with appropriate skills. Staffing levels within stroke units are associated with patient safety and mortality. In acute stroke units, evidence of a dose–response relationship has been found between nursing ratios at the weekend and patient mortality, with lower nurse/bed ratios associated with higher risk of mortality [43]. The most recent acute organisational audit from the Sentinel Stroke National Audit Programme [44] found only 10% (15/156) of sites met the Royal College of Physicians nurse staffing level standard for Type 1 and 3 (hyper-acute) beds (2.9 nurses/bed and 80:20 ratio of registered to unregistered nurses), and only 15% (14/92) of sites met the criteria for Type 2 (rehabilitation) beds (1.35 nurses/bed and 65:35 ratio of registered to unregistered nurses). The report concludes that 'Current nurse staffing levels are insufficient to provide good care for everyone who needs it, and as we implement guidelines, more skilled nurses will be required rather than less' [44].

10.8.1 Urge Incontinence

Bladder training is used to improve control over frequency, urgency, and urge incontinence [31, 32], although its value in patients with neurogenic detrusor overactivity, rather than idiopathic detrusor instability, is less well established. The first step is to identify the minimum time the patient can hold on between voiding episodes. This can be done by completing an initial baseline frequency/volume chart. The patient then aims to empty their bladder regularly at these intervals (e.g. every hour) throughout the day. If the patient remains dry on this schedule, the interval is increased (usually by 15–30 minutes); progress is monitored and intervals are gradually increased until a 2–3-hour voiding schedule is achieved and incontinence is improved or absent. This technique requires patients to be strongly motivated and able to manage their own toileting. During hospital admission, this technique can be used with patients who may not necessarily be able to manage their own toileting. Nurses can assist patients with bladder training despite dysphasia, functional disability, and even cognitive problems. Ongoing use of frequency and volume charting helps demonstrate progress compared with baseline. Nursing intervention for urge incontinence is outlined in Table 10.2. Bladder training was successfully used to overcome urge incontinence during the day in Case Study 10.1.

TABLE 10.2   Nursing intervention in urge incontinence

Nursing intervention	Rationale
Record frequency volume chart/diary [35] daily	Identify how long the patient is able to wait between episodes of bladder emptying and indicate bladder capacity
Start bladder training at a length of time the patient can manage (based on the frequency/volume chart); encourage the patient to gradually increase the time they are able to 'hold on' by small increments	Encourages the bladder to progressively hold more and more urine until an acceptable time interval (for the individual) is reached; an ongoing frequency/volume chart will provide feedback on progress
Advice on lifestyle measures, e.g. excluding or reducing caffeine (tea, coffee, coca cola, chocolate) and citrus fruits (oranges, lemons, limes); planned weight loss, if appropriate	Substances may exacerbate symptoms [45, 46]; reduction in obesity may improve symptoms [47]
If bladder training programme is unsuccessful or has reached a plateau, medication which reduces bladder contractions may be helpful (e.g. oxybutynin, tolterodine, darifenicin)	May help reduce bladder contractions and aid further progress with bladder training

Case Study

Case 10.1   Mary

Mary is a 79-year-old woman admitted to hospital with right middle cerebral artery infarction. She has left arm and leg weakness, left-sided sensory inattention, and UI. She has been registered blind for the past 4 years, but otherwise was able-bodied, independent, and continent prior to her stroke.

Mary's urinary function is assessed. She reports that she has little or no warning that she needs to pass urine. Monitoring of fluid intake and output shows that she is passing urine every 2 hours on average.

She is commenced on a bladder training programme. She progresses over a period of 2 weeks, managing to reach 3.5 hours between trips to the toilet and remaining dry during the day.

By day, Mary is able to transfer independently on to a commode from her chair, but at night when she wakes needing to use the toilet quickly, she is not safe to transfer on her own – by the time nurses respond, she has often already been incontinent.

Mary is assessed using a female urinal with a drainage bag and is able to use it well despite her poor sight, hemiparesis, and sensory inattention. The care plan specifies that the urinal is to be put within reach on her unaffected side. From this point on, she is dry both day and night and is able to be discharged home with the female urinal.

If bladder training alone is ineffective, a combined approach of bladder training with an anticholinergic medication should be considered. Guidance recommends oxybutynin, tolteradine, or darifenacin as first-line. However, these drugs often take up to 4 weeks to work. Anticholinergics interfere with the parasympathetic innervation of the detrusor muscle by blocking the neurotransmitter acetylcholine, resulting in fewer involuntary contractions. This drug group can cause unpleasant side-effects, including dry mouth, constipation, and blurred vision. To reduce the risk of causing or exacerbating urinary retention, a bladder scan should be carried out prior to prescribing anticholinergic medication to ensure residual urine volume is less than 100 ml.

Patients should not reduce their fluid intake in an effort to reduce UI [47]; this may contribute to constipation, or lead to concentrated urine, which can be a bladder irritant. The recommended daily intake is six to eight glasses of water.

10.8.2 Stress Incontinence

Treatment strategies for stress incontinence are aimed at improving pelvic floor muscle strength and tone [48, 49]. Exercises require concentration, effort, and persistence, and are best initiated after the acute period. Patients should be referred to a continence specialist for assessment of muscle strength, development of an individualised exercise regime, and ongoing support. Nursing intervention for stress incontinence is outlined in Table 10.3.

10.8.3 Mixed Incontinence

In patients with symptoms of both urge and stress incontinence, it is important to deal with the most bothersome symptom first.

TABLE 10.3 Nursing intervention in stress incontinence

Nursing intervention	Rationale
Commence patient diary recording episodes of wetness and associated activity	Highlight particular activities resulting in wetness (e.g. coughing) and monitor progress
Assess patient for ability to undertake pelvic floor education; refer to continence specialist	Pelvic floor exercise effective in reducing amount of leakage [48, 49]
Consider pelvic floor muscle training alongside other behavioural interventions (e.g. bladder training)	Results from a review of combined behavioural interventions [19] found greater perceptions of improvement and the potential for more people to achieve greater levels of improvement
Offer lifestyle advice, e.g. on weight loss and smoking cessation	Smoking is associated with chronic cough

10.8.4   Nocturia

Nocturia is a common problem, particularly in older people, and is characterised by waking one or more times during sleep to void [50]. It is often an accompaniment to an overactive bladder [51]. Nocturia can be defined as the need to wake and pass urine at night (in contrast to nocturnal enuresis, where urine is passed unintentionally during sleep). One episode of nocturia per night is considered within normal limits. Treatment for nocturia and nocturnal enuresis starts with management of fluid intake, particularly avoiding drinking large volumes within 1–2 hours of going to bed. Problems may also be reduced by careful timing of diuretic use to ensure the resultant diuresis is completed during the day.

Nocturia can be helped by medication with desmopressin acetate (DDAVP), a synthetic antidiuretic hormone (ADH). ADH causes less urine to be excreted by the kidneys and reduces the volume of urine in the bladder [52]. Blood pressure and blood electrolytes should be monitored regularly, as desmopressin leads to sodium retention.

10.8.5   Functional Incontinence

Management of functional incontinence should focus on recognition and treatment of transient conditions in the first instance (see Box 10.3). Physical disability may mean that toileting cannot be managed independently, and a range of aids and strategies may be helpful to facilitate mobility, toilet access (including wheelchair access), maintenance of balance, and adjustment of clothing. Advice on easy-to-remove clothing (loose jogging trousers, Velcro fly fastening etc.) may help; patients should be referred to a continence specialist or occupational therapist for more detailed help with aids and appliances. Poor eyesight, confusion, or cognitive impairment may lead to problems identifying toilet facilities or a lack of awareness of the appropriate places where urine (or faeces) should be passed. Good signposting and clearly identified toilets (e.g. large pictures of a toilet on the door) are practical solutions. In Case Study 10.1, training in the use of a female urinal resolved nocturia. Nursing intervention for functional incontinence is outlined in Table 10.4.

Post-stroke patients with UI commonly show low ability to focus in comparison to patients without UI. Attention-focused training may help stimulate renewal of bladder control [53].

10.8.6   Toileting Programmes

Scheduled toileting can be beneficial in reducing episodes of incontinence following stroke (summarised in Box 10.5 and Table 10.5). These programmes have been the subject of a series of Cochrane reviews:

- *Habit training* is a toileting schedule based on the patient's usual pattern of voiding, determined from frequency and volume charting. Intervals shorter than the patient's normal pattern are selected, and toileting is planned prior to the time when incontinence episodes are expected. Habit training has

TABLE 10.4 Nursing intervention in functional incontinence

Nursing intervention	Rationale
Nurse call-bell within easy reach, printed picture/text cards at bedside if required	Help patient express elimination needs
Hand-held urinals (with absorbent gel, if required)	Can be used in a bed or chair; absorbent gels help prevent spills
Frequency/volume chart	Monitor progress and aid planning and adjustment of treatment
Regular toileting regime based on results of intake/output monitoring	Patient given opportunity to use toilet on a regular basis
Body-worn pads and pants of appropriate size, if required	Provide confidence and comfort until continent
Advice on adapted or easy-to-remove clothing	Quick, easy access to toileting

---

Box 10.5 | Key Components of Assessment of UI

- Relevant medical, surgical, and obstetric history.
- Urinary/bowel symptoms and how they differ from usual patterns.
- Onset of symptoms and relation to specific activities.
- Medications.
- Cognitive ability and communication skills.
- Functional capacity (mobility, hearing, vision etc.).
- Aids and appliances used/needed.
- Attitude to problem, how symptoms affect daily living and desire for treatment.
- Social and environmental factors.
- Urinalysis.
- Urinary frequency/volume chart, recorded for 3–5 days.
- Fluid intake.
- Constipation.
- Abdominal palpation (urinary retention; constipation).
- Post-voiding residual urine (bladder scan).
- Skin health/soreness/rash in perianal, genital, groin area.
- Functional assessment of toileting skills.

NB: Patients may be suffering from more than one type of UI.

---

been used primarily in institutional settings with cognitively and physically impaired adults, as well as in home settings [54, 57]. Evidence of effectiveness is inconclusive.

- *Prompted voiding* is a regime that can be used to teach people with or without cognitive impairment to initiate their own toileting through requests for help and positive reinforcement from carers. The individual is prompted to void at regular intervals, commonly every 2 hours [55].
- *Timed voiding* is a fixed voiding schedule (usually every 2–4 hours) that remains unchanged. It is used mainly in neuropathic conditions to prevent

TABLE 10.5   **Toileting programmes**

Regimen	Possible patients	Approach
Bladder training [32]	Overactive bladder syndrome, bladder hyperreflexia Well-motivated, physically and mentally able to manage toileting	Gradual increase in interval between voiding (often only 15–30 min at a time) until satisfactory pattern achieved
Habit training [54]	Some mental awareness, physical disabilities	Assigned toileting schedule (e.g. 2-hourly); schedule adjusted to fit patient's voiding pattern
Prompted voiding [55]	Cognitive and physical disabilities	Prompted to void at regular intervals
Timed voiding [56]	Spinal cord injury, cognitive and physical disabilities	Fixed times, may include techniques to trigger voiding

incontinence by regular bladder emptying before bladder capacity is exceeded [56]. Evidence of effectiveness is inconclusive.

- Toileting assistance programmes are the subject of a further Cochrane review that is nearing completion [58].

10.9   Management and Containment of Incontinence

Despite advances in the treatment of bladder problems, incontinence (or fear of incontinence) commonly persists, and some form of containment using aids or appliances may be necessary. For men, there are two main options: a penile sheath or absorbent pads and pants; for women, pads and pants are the main method available. Absorbent pads can increase patient comfort and confidence during a treatment programme. The variety of pads on the market is wide, although choice may be limited in hospital settings [59]. It is important to use the correct size, shape, and absorbency level, and to ensure pads are fitted according to the manufacturer's instructions. For patients at home or in long-stay institutional settings, there may be additional choices in terms of pad design (e.g. inserts placed inside tight-fitting pants, pull-ups). Continence advisory services and patient support organisations such as PromoCon (UK) will offer advice on containment strategies and supplies.

10.9.1   Treatment and Management of Urinary Retention

A patient with *acute retention* may not be able to pass urine at all, or only small amounts. The bladder needs to be drained by in/out catheterisation as soon as the problem is identified. Frequent monitoring aimed at preventing overdistension of the

TABLE 10.6 Nursing intervention in incomplete bladder emptying

Nursing intervention	Rationale
Exclude faecal impaction	A full bowel may obstruct the urethra
Consider medication	Some drugs may have an effect on bladder tone
Intermittent catheterisation (IC) where post-micturition bladder scan shows residual of >100 ml	Less traumatic to urethra and less risk of infection than indwelling catheter; preserves normal bladder function of filling/emptying
If IC not appropriate, refer to medical staff/appropriate person	Indwelling urethral or suprapubic catheter may need to be inserted

bladder should continue, with regular bladder scans and further catheterisation for volumes over 400 ml. For patients with incomplete emptying, causing *chronic retention*, an intermittent catheterisation (IC) regime will need to be implemented. If IC is impractical or unsuccessful, it may be necessary to insert an indwelling catheter. In all cases of retention, the patient's medication should be reviewed, as some drugs (e.g. sedatives, anticholinergics) may affect bladder tone. It is also wise to consider whether the patient might be constipated: pressure on the bladder neck and urethra from a full bowel can cause retention. A DRE may be necessary to confirm constipation, but should only be performed by someone trained in this skill [41]. Nursing management of incomplete bladder emptying is outlined in Table 10.6.

10.9.2 Intermittent Catheterisation (IC)

In hospital, IC is normally a sterile procedure, but patients with sufficient dexterity can be taught to self-catheterise when they go home using a clean procedure. The frequency of IC varies between individuals, but as a guide it should be carried out sufficiently often to maintain the bladder volume below 500 ml. For many patients with urinary retention, this will mean three to four times a day or more; for those with incomplete emptying, it may be only once daily, alternate days, or less. In hospital, a common regime for patients with incomplete bladder emptying is performing IC twice daily (first thing in the morning and last thing at night). This will help to prevent UTI and promote continence during both day and night. IC should only be initiated after the patient has passed urine, when they have more than 100 ml residual urine, and when they are symptomatic (urgency, frequency, or UTI). Residual volumes should be monitored by regular bladder scans; if the residual falls consistently below 100 ml, IC can be stopped.

All treatments should be discussed and agreed with the patient, if possible. IC may be inappropriate in some cases (e.g. urethral trauma or obstruction, unusual anatomy, or when patients find the procedure unacceptable). In such cases, it may be necessary to insert an indwelling catheter; reasons should be clearly documented in the patient's notes.

10.9.3 Indwelling Catheterisation

The National Clinical Guideline for Stroke [13] states: 'Patients should not have an indwelling (urethral) catheter inserted unless indicated to relieve urinary retention or where fluid balance is critical.' Rates of catheterisation are no longer recorded within the Sentinel Stroke National Audit Programme, but the 2011 National Sentinel Audit [13] found 20% of patients were catheterised in the first week after stroke. A recent feasibility trial of a systematic voiding programme for UI after stroke [19] found nearly half of patients in the two intervention arms were catheterised in the acute stage (139/289, 48.1%). However, this percentage is of those recruited, and it cannot necessarily be extrapolated to all people admitted to the stroke unit.

Problems with UI cannot be assessed and treated whilst a catheter is in place, and many stroke patients are catheterised unnecessarily, usually in emergency departments (EDs) and assessment wards. Often, there is no record of why they were catheterised; this was the case for 1 in 10 patients identified as having a catheter in the 2011 National Sentinel Stroke Audit [13]. Although indwelling catheters can provide an effective way of draining the bladder, they are rarely completely trouble-free, and they should only be used where other options are inappropriate or unsuccessful [59]. Common catheter-associated complications include:

- leakage;
- tissue trauma and inflammatory reactions;
- catheter-associated infection (CAUTI) [60]; and
- recurrent blockage caused by mineral deposits (more common in long-term use).

A variety of catheter materials are available, and selection will depend on whether catheterisation is expected to be long- or short-term (more or less than 14 days). Catheter valves may help maintain bladder tone and capacity, particularly in patients in whom the catheter may be removed in the future [61]. Patients who go home with a catheter will need a long-term product made of silicone, hydrogel-coated latex, or silicone elastomer-coated latex. These materials are designed to reduce friction during insertion and removal, and to be more comfortable in situ. Patients will also need appropriate education and ongoing support, including written guidance on how to manage the catheter and drainage equipment, how to replenish supplies, and when to seek help.

10.10 Bowel Problems and Care

As with bladder problems, bowel problems following stroke can arise from neurological damage or as a consequence of impaired functional capacity. Stroke patients may experience alterations in bowel function related to brain damage and loss of cortical inhibition, resulting in function akin to reflex bowel action (as seen after spinal cord injury). Cortical awareness of the urge to defecate and anal sphincter control may both be impaired, leading to urgency and FI, both of which can have highly detrimental effects on quality of life and social interactions. Patients may also be prone to overflow FI due to constipation and faecal impaction.

Constipation can occur through delayed colonic transit [62], the general effect of reduced mobility and swallowing function on gut function, or medication [63, 64].

10.10.1 Bowel Assessment

All patients with bowel problems should have a thorough assessment to determine the type of problem, probable cause and contributing factors, and treatment plan. A careful history of normal bowel habits is important, because there may have been pre-stroke constipation or other problems. A history of long-term laxative use may suggest unresolved constipation problems. It may also be a contributory factor to current problems, if the bowel is no longer responsive to laxative medication.

A bowel habit diary kept over 5–7 days (Figure 10.2) will provide a good indication of the pattern of activity or presence of constipation. Many people find it difficult to explain the type and consistency of their stools, and scales such as the Bristol Stool Form Scale (Figure 10.3) provide a helpful classification [65, 66]. A record of dietary intake may also be useful, as lack of fibre and/or poor fluid intake can contribute to constipation. Medications also need to be reviewed for potential effect on constipation.

10.10.1.1 Examination
Abdominal palpation may help to identify a full bowel, and for some patients a DRE may be required to assess rectal loading/faecal impaction and the constituency of the faecal material (which may be hard or soft). Any abnormalities of the perineal or perianal area should be observed, such as rectal prolapse and haemorrhoids. The normal state of the rectum is empty; therefore, a lack of faecal matter on DRE does not necessarily signify absence of constipation.

10.10.1.2 Faecal Impaction
Faecal impaction describes the condition where constipation has become so severe that a large mass of faeces cannot be passed. Faeces then accumulate in the rectum and may back up in the sigmoid colon and even as far as the transverse and ascending colon. Occasionally, impaction may be due to soft, poorly formed faeces as a consequence of too much osmotic

BOWEL HABIT DIARY – record accurately for 5–7 days				
Name:				
Date/time	Bristol Stool type	Urge to go felt?		Accident or soiling	Comments e.g. laxatives
		Yes	No		

FIGURE 10.2 Example of a bowel habit diary.

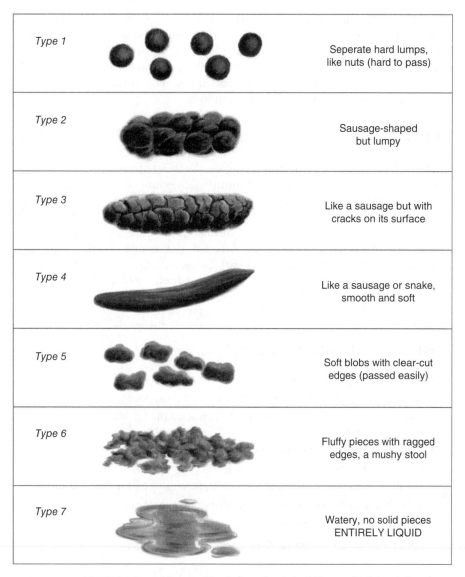

Type 1		Seperate hard lumps, like nuts (hard to pass)
Type 2		Sausage-shaped but lumpy
Type 3		Like a sausage but with cracks on its surface
Type 4		Like a sausage or snake, smooth and soft
Type 5		Soft blobs with clear-cut edges (passed easily)
Type 6		Fluffy pieces with ragged edges, a mushy stool
Type 7		Watery, no solid pieces ENTIRELY LIQUID

FIGURE 10.3   The Bristol stool form scale. *Source: Lewis and Heaton [65]. Reproduced with permission from Taylor & Francis Ltd. www.tandfonline.com.*

laxative. In an attempt to soften hard, impacted faeces, the bowel produces mucus, resulting in faecal impaction with overflow (spurious diarrhoea).

10.10.2   Treatment and Management of Bowel Problems

10.10.2.1   Constipation   Constipation severity varies from slight (causing minimal disruption to life) to severe (impacting upon physical, psychological, and social well-being). Treatment plans will also vary from relatively simple dietary, exercise, and lifestyle advice to planned evacuations. The aim of an individualised planned programme is to reduce constipation without causing FI. The programme is tailored to the individual's needs, taking into consideration ability to toilet and carer requirements. A predictable bowel habit means that constipation and FI can be avoided and daily activities can be organised with greater confidence [67]. Box 10.6 summarises advice on constipation [68].

10.10.2.2 Correct Positioning and Optimum Timing
Patients can be encouraged to take advantage of the morning gastrocolic reflex by having a hot drink soon after waking and sitting on the toilet around 20 minutes later. In people who are resting, colonic intraluminal pressure activity rises markedly during and after food, but this increase is rarely associated with the propulsive activity found in physically active people. It is helpful to ensure patients are sitting correctly on the toilet in order to raise their intra-abdominal pressure during defecation; they should lean forward if possible, ideally with their knees slightly higher than their hips [70]. Some patients may need support to adopt and maintain this position. Patients may benefit from advice on the most effective way to open their bowels:

Box 10.6 | Treating Constipation

- Begin by relieving faecal loading/impaction, if present.
- Set realistic expectations for treatment of chronic constipation.
- Advise people about lifestyle measures – increasing dietary fibre, adequate fluid intake, and exercise.
- Adjust any constipating medication if possible.
- Laxatives are recommended:
  - if lifestyle measures are insufficient, or whilst waiting for them to take effect;
  - for people taking a constipating drug that cannot be stopped;
  - for people with other secondary causes of constipation; and
  - as 'rescue' medicines for episodes of faecal loading.
- If laxative treatment is indicated:
  - start treatment with a bulk-forming laxative whilst maintaining good hydration;
  - if stools remain hard, add or switch to an osmotic laxative;
  - use macrogols as first choice of osmotic laxative;
  - use lactulose if macrogols are not effective or not tolerated;
  - if stools are soft but still difficult to pass or there is inadequate emptying, add a stimulant laxative;
  - adjust the dose, choice, and combination of laxative according to symptoms, the speed with which relief is required, the response to treatment, and individual preference; and
  - gradually titrate the dose of laxative upwards (or downwards) to produce one or two soft formed stools per day.

Source: Adapted from National Institute for Health and Care Excellence (NICE) [69].

- employ abdominal bracing (make the waist wide);
- relax and bulge the tummy muscles;
- let go – without straining, relax and widen the back passage;
- don't hold your breath; and
- finish – draw up the back passage firmly.

10.10.2.3   Lifestyle Advice
The link between dietary fibre and bowel movement is well recognised. Insoluble dietary fibres swell as they absorb water from the gut, resulting in bulky faeces that move more easily through the colon. To be effective, a high-fibre diet needs to be accompanied by adequate fluid intake. Many stroke patients experience eating and drinking difficulties (see Chapter 5); these can also contribute to constipation.

Increased exercise and mobility may help alleviate constipation, but the patient's capacity for exercise will depend on the impact of the stroke. A period of immobility is thought to contribute to weakening of abdominal wall muscles, leading to difficulty in raising intra-abdominal pressure.

10.10.2.4   Laxatives
Laxatives are the most commonly prescribed pharmacological intervention for the management of constipation, and it is important to understand their mode of action. Treatment decisions need to take into consideration whether the constipation is acute or chronic and whether there is impaction of faeces. There are four main types of laxative:

- bulk-forming laxatives;
- osmotic laxatives;
- stimulant laxatives; and
- stool softeners.

Bulk-forming laxatives supplement the fibre content of the diet. They must be taken with fluid, as they work by absorbing liquid and swelling. The resultant increase in bulk increases peristalsis, decreasing the transit time through the colon. The reduction in the amount of time the faeces are in contact with the colon also reduces the amount of fluid absorbed from them, helping keep the stool soft. However, these laxatives are not the best option for stroke patients who are dysphagic or who require altered-consistency fluids. The most commonly used preparations are from ispaghula husk (Fybogel) and sterculia (Normacol).

Osmotic laxatives act like a sponge to draw water into the colon for easier passage of stool. They need to be taken with large quantities of water, and generally produce a semi-fluid stool. Continued use can lead to electrolyte imbalances and dehydration. Products include macrogols (polyethylene glycol preparations, e.g. Movicol), lactulose, magnesium hydroxide, magnesium sulphate (Epsom salts), micro-enemas, and phosphate enemas. Movicol is the treatment of choice in stroke patients: it is effective for both acute and chronic constipation, well tolerated, and does not cause stomach cramps [71]. Enemas may be useful in treating impacted faeces but should not be used as a routine treatment.

Stimulant laxatives work by stimulating the nerve endings in the muscular wall of the colon. They increase peristalsis and secretion of fluid into the colon, helping to soften and lubricate the stool. They usually work within 6–12 hours and should be used short-term only, when bulk-forming laxatives have proven ineffective. These medications can cause severe stomach cramps, which can be distressing. Continued use of stimulant laxatives can reduce muscle tone in the colon and lead to potassium depletion and dehydration. Common preparations include senna, bisacodyl, and glycerol. Biscodyl may be given in suppository form; glycerol suppositories may also act as rectal stimulants. All suppositories should be placed alongside the bowel wall, since they need heat to dissolve; placed within the faecal matter, they will remain intact and ineffective.

Stool softeners provide moisture to the stool and prevent dehydration. They work by lowering surface tension, allowing water and fats to penetrate hardened faeces. The most commonly used softener is docusate sodium.

10.10.2.5 Faecal Incontinence

FI is not only an extremely unpleasant symptom, but can also contribute to decubitus ulcers, UTI, and emotional and psychological disturbances. The most common cause of FI is constipation leading to impaction and spurious diarrhoea. Chronic constipation may cause pelvic floor damage, resulting in incompetent anal sphincters. Other common causes include inflammatory bowel diseases and laxative abuse. In stroke patients, FI may result from neurological damage. In all cases, sensitive assessment should help identify causes and appropriate action [52].

10.11 Conclusion

The consequences of stroke can have a direct effect on bladder and bowel function. Incontinence has a major and enduring impact on all aspects of life. It should not be accepted as an untreatable consequence of ageing or disease. All nurses should be trained in the assessment and management of bladder and bowel problems.

Bladder and bowel care requires active management and regular review. Close involvement and cooperation of families and carers with patients and members of the multidisciplinary team (MDT) are important to ensure the development, implementation, and evaluation of an individually tailored, feasible, and acceptable continence management plan.

Useful Organisations (UK)

Bladder & Bowel Community
    Helpline (general enquiries): 01926 357 220
    Email: help@bladderandbowel.org
    Web site: www.bladderandbowel.org

Bladder & Bowel UK
    Helpline: 0161 607 8219
    Email: bladderandboweluk@disabledliving.co.uk

Web site: www.bbuk.org.uk

Offers information on continence products

Disability Rights UK

Web site: https://www.disabilityrightsuk.org/shop/official-and-only-genuine-radar-key

Co-ordinates the National Key Scheme for wheelchair accessible toilets, supplying keys

References

1. UK Stroke Forum Education & Training. About the SSEF. Available from: http://www.stroke-education.org.uk/about [30 November 2018].
2. Jørgensen, L., Engstad, T., and Jacobsen, B.K. (2005). Self-reported urinary incontinence in noninstitutionalized long-term stroke survivors: a population-based study. Archives of Physical Medicine and Rehabilitation 86 (3): 416–420.
3. Meader, N., Moe-Byrne, T., Llewellyn, A., and Mitchell, A.J. (2014). Screening for poststroke major depression: a meta-analysis of diagnostic validity studies. Journal of Neurology, Neurosurgery, and Psychiatry 85 (2): 198–206.
4. Lawrence, E.S., Coshall, C., Dundas, R. et al. (2001). Estimates of the prevalence of acute stroke impairments and disability in a multiethnic population. Stroke 32 (6): 1279–1284.
5. Pettersen, R. and Wyller, T.B. (2006). Prognostic significance of micturition disturbances after acute stroke. Journal of the American Geriatrics Society 54 (12): 1878–1884.
6. Barrett, J.A. (2002). Bladder and bowel problems after stroke. Reviews in Clinical Gerontology 12 (3): 253–267.
7. Patel, M., Coshall, C., Rudd, A.G., and Wolfe, C.D.A. (2001). Natural history and effects on 2-year outcomes of urinary incontinence after stroke. Stroke 32 (1): 122–127.
8. Williams, M.P., Srikanth, V., Bird, M., and Thrift, A.G. (2012). Urinary symptoms and natural history of urinary continence after first-ever stroke – a longitudinal population-based study. Age and Ageing 41 (3): 371–376.
9. Turhan, N., Atalay, A., and Atabek, H.K. (2006). Impact of stroke etiology, lesion location and aging on post-stroke urinary incontinence as a predictor of functional recovery. International Journal of Rehabilitation Research 29 (4): 335–338.
10. Brittain, K., Peet, S.M., Potter, J., and Castleden, C.M. (1999). Prevalence and management of urinary incontinence in stroke survivors. Age and Ageing 28 (6): 509–511.
11. Pettersen, R., Stien, R., and Wyller, T.B. (2007). Post-stroke urinary incontinence with impaired awareness of the need to void: clinical and urodynamic features. British Journal of Urology International 99 (5): 1073–1077.
12. Thomas, L.H., Cross, S., Barrett, J. et al. (2008). Treatment of urinary incontinence after stroke in adults. Cochrane Database of Systematic Reviews 1 (Art. No.: CD004462). https://doi.org/10.1002/14651858.CD004462.pub3.
13. Royal College of Physicians (2011). National Sentinel Stroke Clinical Audit 2010 Generic Report. London: Royal College of Physicians.
14. Marinkovic, S.P. and Badlani, G. (2001). Voiding and sexual dysfuntion after cerebrovascular accidents. Journal of Urology 165 (2): 359–370.
15. Forer, S. and Granger, C.V. (1987). Functional Independence Measure. Buffalo: The Buffalo General Hospital State University of New York at Buffalo.

16. Linacre, J.M., Heinemann, A.W., Wright, B.D. et al. (1994). The structure and stability of the Functional Independence Measure. Archives of Physical Medicine and Rehabilitation 75 (2): 127–132.

17. Ween, J.E., Alexander, M.P., D'Esposito, M., and Roberts, M. (1996). Factors predictive of stroke outcome in a rehabilitation setting. Neurology 47 (2): 388–392.

18. Perry, S., Shaw, C., Assassa, P. et al. (2000). An epidemiological study to establish the prevalence of urinary symptoms and felt need in the community: the Leicestershire MRC incontinence study. Journal of Public Health 22 (3): 427–434.

19. Thomas LH, French B, Sutton CJ, Forshaw D, Leathley MJ, Burton CR, et al. ICONS: Identifying Continence OptioNs after Stroke: an evidence synthesis, case study and exploratory cluster randomised controlled trial of the introduction of a systematic voiding programme for patients with urinary incontinence after stroke in secondary care. Programme Grants Applies Research No. 3.1; 2015.

20. Robain, G., Chennevelle, J.M., Petit, F., and Piera, J.B. (2002). Incidence of constipation after recent vascular hemiplegia: a prospective cohort of 152 patients. Revue Neurologique 158 (5 Pt 1): 589–592.

21. Harari, D., Coshall, C., Rudd, A.G., and Wolfe, C.D.A. (2003). New-onset fecal incontinence after stroke. Prevalence, Natural history, risk factors, and impact. Stroke 34 (1): 144–150.

22. Harari, D., Norton, C., Lockwood, L., and Swift, C. (2004). Treatment of constipation and fecal incontinence in stroke patients: randomized controlled trial. Stroke 35 (11): 2549–2555.

23. Brown, J.S., Vittinghoff, E., Wyman, J.F. et al. (2000). Urinary incontinence: does it increase risk for falls and fractures? Journal of the American Geriatrics Society 48 (7): 721–725.

24. Department of Health and Social Care (2010). Essence of Care 2010. Leeds: Department of Health and Social Care.

25. Intercollegiate Stroke Working Party (2016). National Clinical Guidelines for Stroke. London: Royal College of Physicians.

26. Royal College of Physicians (2017). Sentinel Stroke National Audit Programme (SSNAP). London: Royal College of Physicians.

27. Fowler, C.J. (2006). Integrated control of lower urinary tract – clinical perspective. British Journal of Pharmacology 147 (Suppl 2): S14–S24.

28. Gelber, D.A., Good, D.C., Laven, L.J., and Verhulst, S.J. (1993). Causes of urinary incontinence after acute hemispheric stroke. Stroke 24 (3): 378–382.

29. National Institute for Health and Care Excellence (NICE). Urinary Incontinence in Neurological Disease: Assessment and Management. Clinical guidelines CG148. National Institute for Health and Clinical Excellence; 2012

30. Abrams, P., Andersson, K.E., Birder, L. et al. (2010). Fourth international consultation on incontinence recommendations of the international scientific committee: evaluation and treatment of urinary incontinence, pelvic organ prolapse, and fecal incontinence. Neurourology and Urodynamics 29 (1): 213–240.

31. Roe, B., Ostaszkiewicz, J., Milne, J., and Wallace, S. (2007). Systematic reviews of bladder training and voiding programmes in adults: a synopsis of findings from data analysis and outcomes using metastudy techniques. Journal of Advanced Nursing 57 (1): 15–31.

32. Wallace, S.A., Roe, B., Williams, K., and Palmer, M. (2004). Bladder training for urinary incontinence in adults. Cochrane Database of Systematic Reviews 1 (Art. No.: CD001308). https://doi.org/10.1002/14651858.CD001308.pub2.

33. Ouslander, J.G. and Schnelle, J.F. (1993). Assessment, treatment, and management of urinary incontinence in the nursing home. In: Improving Care in the Nursing Home: Comprehensive Reviews of Clinical Research (ed. L.Z. Rubenstein and D. Wieland), 131–159. Thousand Oaks: SAGE.

34. Resnick, N.M. (1990). Initial evaluation of the incontinent patient. Journal of the American Geriatrics Society 38 (3): 311–316.
35. Bright, E., Cotterill, N., Drake, M., and Abrams, P. (2014). Developing and validating the international consultation on incontinence questionnaire bladder diary. European Urology 66 (2): 294–300.
36. Hodkinson, H.M. (1972). Evaluation of a mental test score for assessment of mental impairment in the elderly. Age and Ageing 1 (4): 233–238.
37. Folstein, M.F., Folstein, S.E., and McHugh, P.R. (1975). Mini-mental state. A practical method fro grading the cognitive state of patients for the clinician. Journal of Psychiatric Research 12 (3): 189–198.
38. Tombaugh, T.N. and McIntyre, N.J. (1992). The mini-mental state examination: a comprehensive review. Journal of the American Geriatrics Society 40 (9): 922–935.
39. Collin, C., Wade, D., Davies, S., and Horne, V.T. (1988). The Barthel ADL Index: a reliability study. International Disability Studies 10 (2): 61–63.
40. Tsakiris, P., Oelke, M., and Michel, M.C. (2008). Drug-induced urinary incontinence. Drugs & Aging 25 (7): 541–549.
41. Royal College of Nursing (2012). Management of Lower Bowel Dysfunction, Including DRE and DRF. London: Royal College of Nursing.
42. Tam, C., Wong, K., and Yip, W. (2006). Prevalence of incomplete bladder emptying among elderly in convalescence wards: a pilot study. Asian Journal of Gerontology and Geriatrics 1 (2): 66–71.
43. Bray, B.D., Ayis, S., Campbell, J. et al. (2014). Associations between stroke mortality and weekend working by stroke specialist physicians and registered nurses: prospective multicentre cohort study. PLoS Medicine 11 (8): 1–11.
44. Royal College of Physicians (2016). Sentinel Stroke National Audit Programme (SSNAP). London: Royal College of Physicians.
45. Robinson, D., Giarenis, I., and Cardozo, L. (2014). You are what you eat: the impact of diet on overactive bladder and lower urinary tract symptoms. Maturitas 79 (1): 8–13.
46. Wells, M.J., Jamieson, K., Markham, T.C.W. et al. (2014). The effect of caffeinated versus decaffeinated drinks on overactive bladder: a double-blind, randomized, crossover study. Journal of Wound Ostomy & Continence Nursing 41 (4): 371–378.
47. National Institute for Health and Care Excellence (NICE). Urinary Incontinence in Women. Quality Standard (QS77). 2015.
48. Dumoulin, C., Hay-Smith, E.J.C., and Mac Habée-Séguin, G. (2014). Pelvic floor muscle training versus no treatment, or inactive control treatments, for urinary incontinence in women. Cochrane Database of Systematic Reviews 5 (Art. No.: CD005654). https://doi.org/10.1002/14651858.CD005654.pub3.
49. Bø, K., Talseth, T., and Holme, I. (1999). Single blind, randomised controlled trial of pelvic floor exercises, electrical stimulation, vaginal cones, and no treatment in management of genuine stress incontinence in women. British Medical Journal 318 (7182): 487–493.
50. van Kerrebroeck, P., Abrams, P., Chaikin, D. et al. (2002). The standardisation of terminology in nocturia: Report from the standardisation sub-committee of the International Continence Society. Neurourology and Urodynamics 21 (2): 179–183.
51. Marinkovic, S.P., Gillen, L.M., and Stanton, S.L. (2004). Managing nocturia. British Medical Journal 328 (7447): 1063–1066.
52. National Institute for Health and Care Excellence (NICE). Faecal Incontinence in Adults. Quality Standard (QS54). 2014.
53. Pettersen, R., Saxby, B.K., and Wyller, T.B. (2007). Poststroke urinary incontinence: one-year outcome and relationships with measures of attentiveness. Journal of the American Geriatrics Society 55 (10): 1571–1577.
54. Ostaszkiewicz, J., Chestney, T., and Roe, B. (2004). Habit retraining for the management of urinary incontinence in adults. Cochrane Database of Systematic Reviews 2 (Art. No.: CD002801). https://doi.org/10.1002/14651858.CD002801.pub2.

55. Eustice, S., Roe, B., and Paterson, J. (2003). Prompted voiding for the management of urinary incontinence in adults. Cochrane Database of Systematic Reviews 3 (Art. No.: CD002113). https://doi.org/10.1002/14651858.CD002113.

56. Ostaszkiewicz, J., Johnston, L., and Roe, B. (2004). Timed voiding for the management of urinary incontinence in adults. Cochrane Database of Systematic Reviews 1 (Art. No.: CD002802). https://doi.org/10.1002/14651858.CD002802.pub2.

57. Colling, J., Owen, T.R., McCreedy, M., and Newman, D. (2003). The effects of a continence program on frail community-dwelling elderly persons. Urologic Nursing 23 (2): 117–122.

58. Ostaszkiewicz, J., Eustice, S., Roe, B. et al. (2013). Toileting assistance programmes for the management of urinary incontinence in adults (Protocol). Cochrane Database of Systematic Reviews 6 (Art. No.: CD010589). https://doi.org/10.1002/14651858.CD002802.pub2.

59. Getliffe, K.A. and Dolman, M. (2007). Catheters and containment products. In: Promoting Continence: A Clinical and Research Resource, 3e (ed. K.A. Getliffe and M. Fader), 259–308. Edinburgh: Elsevier Science.

60. Harbarth, S., Sax, H., and Gastmeier, P. (2003). The preventable proportion of nosocomial infections: an overview of published reports. Journal of Hospital Infection 54 (4): 258–266.

61. Fader, M., Pettersson, L., Brooks, R. et al. (1997). A multicentre comparative evaluation of catheter valves. British Journal of Nursing 6 (7): 359–367.

62. Ho, Y. and Goh, H. (1995). Anorectal physiological parameters in chronic constipation of unknown aetiology (primary) and of cerebrovascular accidents – a preliminary report. Annals of the Academy of Medicine, Singapore 24 (3): 376–378.

63. Winge, K., Rasmussen, D., and Werdelin, L.M. (2003). Constipation in neurological diseases. Journal of Neurology, Neurosurgery, and Psychiatry 74 (1): 13–19.

64. Craggs M, Vaizey C. Neurophysiology of the bladder and bowel. In: Fowler CJ (ed.). Neurology of Bladder, Bowel, and Sexual Dysfunction. Oxford: Butterworth-Heinemann; 1999.

65. Lewis, S.J. and Heaton, K.W. (1997). Stool form scale as a useful guide to intestinal transit time. Scandinavian Journal of Gastroenterology 32 (9): 920–924.

66. Heaton, K.W., Radvan, J., Cripps, H. et al. (1992). Defecation frequency and timing, and stool form in the general population: a prospective study. Gut 33 (6): 818–824.

67. Wiesel, P. and Bell, S. (2004). Bowel dysfunction: assessment and management in the neurological patient. In: Bowel Continence Nursing (ed. C. Norton and S. Chelvanayagam), 181–203. London: Beaconsfield Publishers.

68. National Institute for Health and Care Excellence (NICE). Lower Urinary Tract Symptoms in Men: Management. 2015.

69. National Institute for Health and Care Excellence (NICE). Constipation Management. Clinical Knowledge Summaries. Available from: https://cks.nice.org.uk/constipation [30 November 2018].

70. Bladder & Bowel Community. Welcome to the Bladder & Bowel Community. Available from: http://www.bladderandbowel.org [30 November 2018].

71. Corazziari, E., Badiali, D., Bazzocchi, G. et al. (2000). Long term efficacy, safety, and tolerability of low daily doses of isosmotic polyethylene glycol electrolyte balanced solution (PMF-100) in the treatment of functional chronic constipation. Gut 46 (4): 522–526.

CHAPTER 11

Emotional and Cognitive Changes Following a Stroke

Peter Knapp[1] and Elizabeth Lightbody[2]
[1]Hull York Medical School, University of York, York, UK
[2]Faculty of Health & Wellbeing, University of Central Lancashire, Preston, UK

KEY POINTS

- Mood and behavioural changes are common following a stroke.
- Changes are distressing for patients, families, and friends.
- If unrecognised and untreated, these changes will have a negative impact on the patient's recovery.
- Early recognition, assessment, and onwards referral to an appropriate clinician are key.

This chapter maps to criteria within the following sections of the Stroke-Specific Education Framework (SSEF):

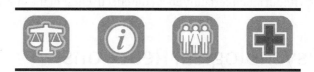

Stroke Nursing, Second Edition. Edited by Jane Williams, Lin Perry, and Caroline Watkins.
© 2020 John Wiley & Sons Ltd. Published 2020 by John Wiley & Sons Ltd.

I just feel I might as well be dead. The only thing is I don't want to die alone, you see, it's different when you've got loved ones, nice to have them there when it does happen, but when you're on your own it easy could happen, couldn't it? Any time. What I find the most terrible, it's a day, a day's long, every day when you're on your own. If I could get out it would be better, what people don't understand, there's no pleasure in giving yourself a lot of pain, just to go out … It all goes back to this, you see. I can't help it, I just think, all day. I can't help it, my children say, come on, Dad, you've got to cheer up, eat your food, that would be similar advice I would give to someone in my position, but it's not so easy carried out. You can sit and say, and really think you're giving good advice but, and you'd like to think you could do what they say, I know they mean it with all their love, all sincerity, eat your food or you'll be bad, but unless you're a marvellous man I don't think you could do it.

(Richard, 72 years old, 6 months post-stroke, South London)

11.1 Introduction

Stroke can have many different effects on patients' mood, cognitions, and behaviour. Many of these changes can be distressing for both the patient and their close relatives. They commonly impact on other outcomes after a stroke, such as physical recovery, the return to normal social activities, and longer-term health. Many changes to mood and behaviour are transient, but some are long-lasting.

The care provided to patients with mood and behavioural changes has altered dramatically over the last 20 years. There has been an increased recognition of the prevalence of mood disorders and a shift away from the view that mood disorder after stroke is inevitable (and therefore not responsive to intervention), towards one where most people have some psychological reaction to the onset of stroke, and that mood disorders are pathological.

The increased recognition of mood disorders, behavioural changes, and cognitive impairment and their effects on patients, has resulted in the development of new interventions, a greater number of professionals skilled to intervene, and increased research evidence on intervention effectiveness. Despite this, the care provided to patients with mood and cognitive impairments after stroke often remains suboptimal. Psychological disorder and distress continue to be under-recognised, some disorders are incorrectly diagnosed and treated, and the relative lack of a research base means that nurses and doctors may be treating disorders in their patients without much certainty about the effectiveness of the interventions [2].

11.2 Psychological Reactions to the Onset of Stroke

Stroke onset, particularly of a first stroke, can be distressing and worrying. For many patients, the stroke comes without warning, resulting in emergency hospital admission and inpatient stay. If the stroke causes a loss of function, the patient is more likely to be unsettled and to react emotionally [3].

It is common for patients to experience worry, confusion, and tearfulness in the first few days after stroke. In this, stroke differs little from many other conditions [3, 4]. Patients may have concerns about practical aspects of their lives, often centred on their roles and responsibilities (e.g. worries about how their spouse will manage at home, who will run the family business, or who will look after their pets). Following a stroke, patients must deal with change and uncertainty. It is common to be unsettled by change, and worries about the future can be distressing. The patient will understandably be concerned about how long-lasting any disability will be, and what effects it will have on their ability to live as they did before. This is sometimes termed 'role crisis' or 'role anxiety': concerns about the ability or future ability to fulfil normal roles (e.g. partner, parent, employee, social club committee member).

Early emotional reactions to stroke can also include frustration, irritability, and anger. Such reactions may distress patients' relatives and can be difficult for staff to deal with, and they are sometimes wrongly explained as being due to a 'personality change' after stroke. A more robust explanation is that irritability, frustration, worry, and anger are understandable responses to the onset of a condition that has the potential to be life-changing and disabling.

11.3 Coping with Stroke

Models of coping theories can help to explain patients' reactions. Coping theory, for example, explains responses to a threatening event – whether anticipated (such as a driving test or dental treatment) or unanticipated (such as bereavement or illness) [5]. People cope (i.e. manage to deal with a changing situation) by drawing on skills and experience they have used before. If they respond successfully to the onset of disabling illness, it may be because they have successfully adapted skills developed years earlier (e.g. when becoming unemployed or dealing with family difficulties). That is, people cope successfully by drawing on personal resources to deal with new demands [6].

However, problems will arise when demands are too great and overwhelm the ability to cope, or when the available personal resources are insufficient or ineffective. It is in this situation that people will benefit from additional external resources, which might be financial (e.g. disability benefits), instrumental (e.g. help with personal or household tasks), or psychological (e.g. emotional support from friends or, more formally, from a counsellor).

Not all coping is effective, however, and people's responses to a threatening situation may be maladaptive. Examples include: increased emotional dependence on others, repeated reassurance seeking, and avoidant behaviours (such as denying the disability or seeking comfort in alcohol or drugs). As with successful coping, maladaptive coping can be patterned, in that people use it as a conventional response to a threat. Such coping responses are unlikely to be successful, particularly in response to a stroke, which may require concentrated effort by the patient to achieve recovery.

11.4 Depression

The emotional outcome most often associated with stroke is depression (or depressed mood), and its frequency after stroke has led some to suggest that post-stroke depression (or PSD) is a distinct type [7]. This view holds that depressed mood is physiological in origin, caused by the neurological damage from the stroke. Some lesions (left hemispheric, particularly frontal lesions) are more likely to lead to depressed mood than those located elsewhere in the brain. However, a systematic review of studies of lesion location and mood after stroke showed that there is no robust evidence that depressed mood after stroke is caused by a lesion in any particular area or side of the brain, suggesting that depression is multifactorial in origin [8].

Clinical depression is a syndrome; that is, a cluster of symptoms or signs. Symptoms include lowered mood (or affect) lasting at least a month, which causes distress. Diagnostic signs also include changed sleep pattern and/or appetite, a lack of pleasure in activities, negative thinking (including about one's self-worth), and lack of energy. That is, clinical depression is a significant pattern of disordered mood and associated symptoms, and is more than a feeling of sadness or consistent tearfulness, distressing though these behaviours can be to the patient and their relatives [9].

Depressed mood is more common in people after a stroke than in people of a similar age without stroke. However, this increase is probably not specific to stroke: higher rates of depression are also seen in people with other disabling conditions. There have been several studies that have looked at the rate of depression after stroke. A systematic review and meta-analysis of observational studies (61 studies) found that 31% of stroke survivors were depressed at any time point up to 5 years after stroke [10]. However, there was considerable variation in frequency (5–84%) between studies. Differences in patient populations, study design, time since stroke, and the way that depression was assessed may account for the large variations in reported rates.

Some people may develop depression early after their stroke; others develop it later [11, 12]. There is a suggestion (based on anecdote) that depression is often provoked by returning home after hospital. This onset might be explained by the patient desiring to go home and holding that as a target during the long weeks of inpatient rehabilitation, and then finding the return anticlimactic. The difficulty of living at home with a disability may also turn out to be a depressing reality. The studies also suggest that depressed mood can be relatively short-lasting in many patients and may remit spontaneously, perhaps once the patient is able to adjust psychologically to their disability.

Given the frequency of depression after stroke, early identification and management of those at high risk is important. A systematic review found that depression is associated with pre-stroke depression, more severe neurological deficit, and significant physical disability both in the acute phase and later after stroke [13]. However, the association between depression and cognitive impairment was less strong. The authors found no consistent association between depression and age, gender, lesion location, or stroke sub-type [13]. As the majority of studies included in the review excluded those with communication deficits, the relationship between depression and communication impairment is less clear. It is reported that patients with communication problems experience a greater risk of depression than those with normal communication, with 73% meeting DSM-III-R criteria for depression at 3 months after stroke, and 68% meeting criteria at 12 months [14]. Aphasia has also been shown to be a significant predictor of distress at 1 and 6 months after stroke [15].

Depression tends to occur more often in patients with low levels of perceived social support [16]. The absence of close, confiding relationships seems to be particularly important. Depression is also more likely in those who find it difficult to adjust to a new situation. Examples include having an expectation of recovery that is unrealistically optimistic and adopting an overly negative and generalised attitude (i.e. thinking that most things will turn out badly).

11.4.1 Diagnosing and Screening for Depression

Depressed mood after stroke should be diagnosed by clinical interview undertaken by a health professional with appropriate mental health training or experience [17]. Ideally, this would be a psychiatrist or clinical psychologist, although in the United Kingdom it is most often undertaken by a stroke physician or general physician. Since depression occurs in the first year in about 30% of stroke patients, all patients admitted to hospital after stroke should be assessed at various stages throughout the stroke pathway, particularly at transition points. Conducting a lengthy clinical interview with all patients is unrealistic and unnecessary, and there are brief screening measures that can be used to identify patients at risk of depression.

Identifying depression can be challenging after a stroke, partly due to the overlap between the symptoms of stroke and those of depression, but also because of neurological impairments such as memory and communication problems. However, there are several validated tools for use with stroke patients, including those with communication problems.

A recent review suggested a number of instruments that may help in assessing PSD. Table 11.1 outlines the proportion of patients correctly identified using these

TABLE 11.1 Accuracy of screening tools in detecting depression following a stroke [18]

Tool	Proportion of those depressed correctly identified (%)	Proportion of those not depressed correctly identified (%)	Probability that those who screen positive are depressed (%)	Probability that those who screen negative are not depressed (%)
CES-D	75	88	75	88
HDRS	84	83	71	91
PHQ-9	86	79	67	92
BDI	86	64	54	90
PHQ-2	79	76	62	88
HADS-D	85	69	57	90
HADS-T	72	86	72	86
GDS-15	74	80	65	86
MADRS	85	79	67	91

CES-D, Center of Epidemiological Studies-Depression Scale; HDRS, Hamilton Depression Rating Scale; PHQ, Patient Health Questionnaire; BDI, Beck Depression Inventory; HADS, Hospital Anxiety and Depression Scale; GDS, Geriatric Depression Scale; MADRS, Montgomery Asberg Depression Rating Scale.

tools, the most promising being the Center of Epidemiological Studies-Depression (CESD) Scale, Hamilton Depression Rating Scale (HDRS), and Patient Health Questionnaire (PHQ-9) [19]. Other tools commonly utilised include the General Health Questionnaire-12 (GHQ-12) [20] and the Geriatric Depression Scale (GDS) [21], which have also been validated in stroke populations [22]. However, none of the tools are satisfactory for case-finding. Therefore, these tools should not be used in isolation; those who screen positive should be followed up with a more detailed clinical assessment in order to make a diagnosis.

Asking a patient about their mood and whether or not they are experiencing emotional difficulties is uncomfortable for some nurses. The situation can be explained to the patient and their relatives by the use of a 'permission-giving' preamble such as:

We know that many people who have had a stroke feel low or emotional. Do you mind if I ask you a few questions about how you feel?

or

Sometimes after stroke, people think that the situation will never improve. Have you had thoughts like that?

For those who are unable to complete standardised screening tools, observational tools, visual analogue scales, or pictorial scales might help. There is also evidence that a simple question (e.g. 'Do you often feel sad or depressed?') can be as effective as a questionnaire with 9 or 12 items [23, 24]. However, in patients with more severe cognitive or communication difficulties, language-based assessments are problematic. This has led to the development of alternative methods of assessment, as presented in Table 11.2.

Whilst these are the most practical methods of assessment in those with cognitive and communication problems, taken alone they are not dependable as a method of assessment. Multiple sources of information should be utilised in those who are unable to complete self-report measures [33], including information from carers, whose observations can accurately detect depressed mood [24], and speech and language therapists (SLTs) [34].

Following assessment, the outcome or score should be recorded in the patient's notes, even if it indicates that they are unlikely to have a mood disorder. A positive screen is not enough to warrant the initiation of treatment, as screening tools tend to produce false-positive scores (as seen in Tables 11.1 and 11.2) with people who don't have depression but who score highly on the measure [35]. This, and the knowledge that some depressed mood remits without treatment, suggests that mood after stroke is best assessed on two separate occasions a few weeks apart [36], to allow the assessment of change over time. If a patient scores highly on both occasions, this information should be recorded in the notes and the details passed on to the doctor or nurse in charge of their care. A referral should be made to the clinician responsible for undertaking a psychiatric clinical interview and assessing the patient for possible treatment. The obvious exception to this 'double screening' rule is the patient whose depression is so severe (perhaps including suicidal thoughts) that treatment

TABLE 11.2 Accuracy of observational screening tools in detecting depression following a stroke

Tool	Proportion of those depressed correctly identified (%)	Proportion of those not depressed correctly identified (%)	Probability that those who screen positive are depressed (%)	Probability that those who screen negative are not depressed (%)	Study
DISCs	60	87	75	77	Turner-Stokes et al. [25]
Smiley faces	76	77	74	79	Lee et al. [26]
SODS	64–86	56–62	36–65	62–95	Lightbody et al. [24], Watkins et al. [27], Bennett et al. [28]
SADQ 10	70–77	77–78	40	95	Leeds et al. [29], Sackley et al. [30]
SADQ-H	68–100	78–79	57–58	85–100	Bennett et al. [28], Hacker Vicki et al. [31]
VAMS	81	51	31	86	Stern [32], Bennett et al. [28]

DISCs, Depression Intensity Scale Circles; SODS, Signs of Depression Scale; SADQ, Stroke Aphasic Depression Questionnaire; VAMS, Visual Analog Mood Scale.

is needed after the first assessment. It is also important that information is fed back to the patient, such as:

> *Thank you for answering those questions. I am a little concerned about*
> *your mood and I want to arrange for a doctor to come to see you to ask you*
> *some more detailed questions about it.*

It is important that depression after stroke is recognised and treated, as it may impact on a patient's engagement in rehabilitation and recovery [37, 38], resulting in longer hospital stays. Depressed patients are also less likely to take medicines as prescribed or to stop smoking, and have decreased involvement in social activity [39], lower quality of life [40], increased suicide rates [41], and decreased chance of survival [42].

11.4.2 Treating Depression

The most common treatment for depression after stroke is antidepressants, as is the case for older patients in general: almost one in seven patients aged 75 and above in general practices in the United Kingdom has received a prescription [43]. The rate may be as high as one in three patients within 1 month of stroke [44]. Antidepressants make a small but significant reduction in scores on depression rating scales, but there is also evidence of increased adverse events [45]. The studies that have reported this have tended to be small and generally not well conducted, so antidepressants should be reserved for patients whose depression is particularly marked or troublesome.

In patients with mild or borderline depression, it may be useful to introduce counselling, hobbies and exercise (if possible), or another social activity (see Case Study 11.1). There is no strong evidence that these therapies are effective [46], but they may help in some patients, and they should be considered as an early alternative to antidepressants. Another alternative to drug treatment is structured psychological treatment (also known as 'talking treatment'). Such treatment can be given by appropriately trained stroke nurses, and brief therapy comprising a few sessions can be effective. A recent meta-analysis of cognitive behavioural therapy (CBT) including 23 studies with 1972 participants found positive effects on depressive symptoms following a stroke [47]. However, the authors stated that the evidence of CBT post-stroke was inconclusive due to the limitations of the studies included [47]. Trials of preventive psychological treatment (problem-solving therapy and motivational interviewing) and case management have shown small but promising effects on reducing the likelihood of being depressed several months later [23, 48]. In those with aphasia, one study showed that behavioural therapy improves mood [49].

Mindfulness is increasingly being offered as a therapeutic intervention. A systematic review of mindfulness-based interventions following transient ischemic attack and stroke showed a positive trend across a range of psychological outcomes, including anxiety, fatigue, and quality of life [50]. However, the studies were small and of poor methodological quality, and further robust trials are required to support the use of mindfulness in clinical practice.

Case Study

Case 11.1 Andrew

Andrew is an 82-year-old male with a large stroke in the left middle cerebral artery territory. He has a marked right-sided weakness and aphasia. Past medical history included previous treatment for depression. The health care assistant notes that Andrew doesn't appear to 'be himself'; over the last week he has been a bit quieter and generally less engaged. They report this to the nurse, who, using a visual communication aide (thumbs up and thumbs down), asks Andrew the single Yale question, 'Do you often feel sad or depressed?' Andrew pointed to the 'thumbs up', indicating that he does feel depressed. The Yale has been shown to identify 85% of cases correctly [23]. However, at the multidisciplinary team (MDT) meeting, the physiotherapists indicate that he is still engaging with therapy, so it is agreed to undertake watchful waiting and rescreen in one week.

A week later, the nurse asks the family to complete the Signs of Depression scale when they come to visit. Andrew scores 4/6 and still answers positively to the Yale question. It is agreed that he should be referred to clinical psychology for further assessment, as he is showing signs of low mood and has several risk factors for depression (previous history of depression, functional impairment, and communication difficulties) [13, 15]. Following assessment, the clinical psychologist agrees that Andrew is showing signs of clinical depression. They suggest that the MDT should promote well-being through supportive conversations using communication aids, talk to Andrew about how he is feeling, and normalise (without minimising) the adjustment process. As Andrew spends a lot of time during the day inactive, they also suggest encouraging engagement in activities. The doctors simultaneously start Andrew on an antidepressant.

Andrew's mood is reviewed weekly at the MDT meetings, with repeat screening ever 2 weeks. Over the next 6 weeks before hospital discharge, Andrew's mood has improved. At the 6-month review, depression is no longer present, and he is able to stop the medication, with regular review by his general practitioner (GP).

Other emerging treatments for PSD include physical exercise [51], music [52, 53], acupuncture, deep breathing, meditation, visualisation, repetitive transcranial magnetic stimulation, and ecosystem-focused therapy [54], but these all require more research.

11.4.3 Emotionalism

Emotionalism or emotional lability refers to uncontrollable crying or laughing. This may be in response to an appropriate stimulus, but out of proportion to the event. It may also occur without any obvious reason. It affects 20–25% of patients in the first 6 months, with 10–15% still affected at 1 year after stroke [55]. It is distinctive and easily recognised, due to the quickly changing nature of emotions (see Case Study 11.2). Its cause is not clear, although it may be neurological in origin, with damage to certain parts of the brain such as the thalamus [56] implicated in its origin. Patients with emotionalism are more likely to have psychological distress [57, 58], and it is also more likely to occur in patients with depressed mood [57, 59].

Case Study

Case 11.2   Sandra

Sandra, an active 55-year-old with three children and eight grand-children, suffers a stroke that leaves her unable to walk and dress independently. Sandra is a determined woman works hard in her rehabilitation sessions. She remains positive in her outlook. However, she becomes emotional when talking about her home and her family. When her children and grandchildren visit, she struggles to talk to them, such is her tearfulness. Some relatives find this embarrassing and distressing, to the point where they prefer not to visit. Sandra's reaction is thought not to be depression – her mood remains positive – but emotional. Staff spend time explaining the condition to Sandra and her relatives, encouraging them not to stay away from visits. Although her mood is not depressed, treatment with an antidepressant medicine is effective. Over the next 3 weeks before hospital discharge, the periods of emotionalism occur less often, and Sandra is able to talk about her family and have visitors with only occasional tears. The emotionalism is no longer present by 2 months post-discharge, and a few weeks later, Sandra is able to stop the medication.

Emotionalism often responds to antidepressant treatment [60, 61], adding further to the view that its cause is neurological. When patients have emotionalism, there is an important nursing role in helping the patient (and their relatives) to deal with it. It can be distressing to experience, and relatives can be upset by it. Patients sometimes avoid emotionally laden situations, such as family visits or trips to places with sentimental significance [62]. Emotionalism can be isolating, particularly if it persists. The social embarrassment caused by public tearfulness can mean that patients avoid socialising, particularly with close family and friends, thus adding to the social isolation [57, 58, 63]. Therefore, patients with emotionalism require close observation.

11.4.4   Anxiety

Anxiety after stroke occurs with similar frequency to depression [64], but is less often recognised and diagnosed. The lack of clinical recognition is also reflected in the research: there are far fewer studies to guide practice than for depression.

Anxiety is a syndrome or clustering of symptoms [9], including an unpleasant, uncontrollable emotional feeling, most commonly fear or apprehension. There are also physical symptoms, such as breathlessness, palpitations, and trembling. Like depression, anxiety varies greatly in its severity. At worst, it is disabling and restricting.

Anxiety can be provoked by a variety of situations, although there are people with 'generalised anxiety' whose symptoms are brought on by no specific provocation. In patients with stroke, anxiety may arise due to a fear of falling (see Case Study 11.3), which can be based on a single real experience that was painful, embarrassing, or distressing. The mood disturbance arises when the patient generalises from that instance to other situations, and so fears falling again. In patients with anxiety, the sensations of fear or apprehension are disproportionate and

Case Study

| Case 11.3 | George |

George, a 70-year-old widower who lives alone, suffers a stroke that leaves him with weakness on his left side, with resultant unsteadiness. Whilst a patient at the stroke unit, he accidentally falls from the toilet whilst trying to take himself back to his bed. The physical injury is minor, but the psychological effect is much greater: he becomes anxious about being left alone in the toilet or elsewhere on the unit. He becomes avoid-ant (e.g. by drinking less water and tea, to reduce the need for trips to the toilet) and less independent, asking staff not to leave him alone when walking in case he falls. This pres-ents a problem, since he is physically ready to return home, but is anxious about being alone in the house. Treatment whilst he is on the unit involves a form of CBT, in which George's cognitions (or thoughts) – that he will come to harm if left alone – are chal-lenged, such as by leaving him alone on the toilet for a short time, then a little longer, and so on. A similar process is undertaken during home visits – leaving George in the house alone for a few minutes at first, then longer. After 3 weeks of this therapy, he is able to return home independently.

unrealistic. Forms of social anxiety may occur after stroke, with patients becoming fearful of social contact with strangers – or any social contact – and avoiding the fear by social withdrawal.

The sudden nature of stroke onset may induce a fear of suffering another stroke, which can cause disabling anxiety symptoms and the avoidance of places and activities linked to stroke onset. Exaggerated fear of recurrence can produce reassurance-seeking behaviour, such as repeatedly asking care staff, 'Am I going to be all right?' Answering 'yes' to such questions when they are asked for the 10th time on a given day may be the easy response, but is unlikely to be helpful. Hearing the answer 'yes' does not help the patient – it does not reduce their fear of 'not being all right' and may even reinforce the reassurance-seeking behaviour (making it more likely that they will ask the question again).

A recent systematic review reported that anxiety occurred in 18% of stroke patients when the condition was assessed by clinical interview, and 25% when as-sessed by rating scale [64]. The rates of occurrence at 1 and >6 months after stroke were similar. Indeed, another study, in which patients were followed up for up to 10 years after stroke, found that even at this stage, anxiety was present in 17–24% of patients, although the cause may not have been attributable to the stroke [65]. Anxiety is more likely in patients with pre-stroke depression, more severe stroke, and dementia or post-stroke cognitive impairment. It is also more likely in youn-ger and female patients, those unable to work after the stroke, and those from lower economic backgrounds [65–67]. Anxiety in the early period after stroke is also a predictor of anxiety later on [67].

There is little strong research evidence to inform treatments for anxiety after stroke [68], so recommendations are based on other settings [17, 69]. In some patients, pharmaceutical treatment can be effective, with antidepressant medicines having a sedating effect that can be beneficial. More likely to have longer-term benefits are structured psychological therapies, such as CBT, although research evaluation is urgently needed [70]. These therapies should be given by appropriately trained practitioners, such as a clinical psychologist or psychiatric nurse.

11.4.5   Post–Traumatic Stress Disorder

Post-traumatic stress disorder (PTSD) is becoming increasingly recognised as a potential response to ill health. Stroke has the potential to be experienced as a traumatic event, and so result in PTSD [71]. However, PTSD's recognition as a sequela of stroke has yet to be fully achieved, despite it occurring in 5–30% of stroke patients [71–76]. The severity of PTSD symptoms is not linked to age, neurological impairment, or disability [72–74], but it is more frequent in women, less educated patients, those who have had peritraumatic responses (feeling nervous or afraid), and those with more negative appraisals of the stroke experience [72, 77]. The extent to which the patient felt frightened at the time of stroke, and how incapacitating they believe it to be, have been found to be significant factors associated with PTSD. However, these studies have generally been cross-sectional, thus limiting our understanding of the cause of the condition.

Clinicians must understand that PTSD can manifest as depression, and that only differential diagnosis and specific treatment are likely to result in improvement. Consequently, when assessing for depression after stroke, clinicians and researchers must be aware that those who screen positive for depression may have PTSD. If not explored further, depression could be inappropriately pursued as the primary treatment goal (see Table 11.3). As advised in National Institute for Health and Care Excellence (NICE) guidance [79], a focus on depression and not PTSD will be unlikely to result in positive change. When PTSD and depression both occur, the PTSD should be addressed primarily, and the depression may dissipate accordingly. There are no specific guidelines relating to the identification and management of PTSD following a stroke. However, NICE guidelines highlight that specific assessment for PTSD should be undertaken in high-risk groups, including those with a history of depression or significant physical illness causing disability. This is highly applicable to the stroke population. In terms of treatment, there is evidence that antidepressants (in particular selective serotonin reuptake inhibitors (SSRIs) [80, 81]), trauma-related behavioural therapy, and eye-movement desensitisation and reprocessing [82, 83] are effective in treating PTSD in the general population.

It is clearly important for people to have a comprehensive psychological assessment after stroke, and for all professionals working with patients after stroke to be aware of the clinical presentation of PTSD. Teasing out the difficulties experienced by individuals following stroke is more complex than is often portrayed in research studies, due to an existing overwhelming focus on depression (see Case Study 11.4). This has implications for the education and training of practitioners.

11.4.6   Cognitive Impairment

The damage caused by stroke to the brain can result in significant impairment associated with sensory or cognitive activity [84]. 'Cognitive' is used by researchers and clinicians to denote thinking, and so cognitive impairment often includes a

TABLE 11.3   **DSM-IV PTSD criteria [78]**

Criterion A

The person has been exposed to a traumatic event in which both of the following were present:

1. person experienced, witnessed, or was confronted with an event or events that involved actual or threatened death or serious injury or threat to the physical integrity of self or others

2. the person's response involved fear, helplessness or horror

Criterion B

The traumatic event is persistently re-experienced in **one** (or more) of the following ways:

1. recurrent/intrusive distressing recollections

2. recurrent distressing dreaming

3. flashbacks

4. psychological distress at exposure to cues

5. physiological reactivity on exposure to cues

Criterion C

Persistent avoidance of stimuli associated with the trauma and numbing of general responsiveness (not present before the trauma) as indicated by **three** (or more) of the following:

1. efforts to avoid thoughts or feelings or talking about the event

2. efforts to avoid activities, places, or people that are reminders

3. inability to recall an important aspect of the trauma

4. diminished interest in activities used to enjoy

5. feeling of detachment or estrangement from others

6. restricted range of affect e.g. unable to feel love or happiness

7. sense of foreshortened future

Criterion D

Persistent symptoms of increased arousal (not present before the trauma) as indicated by **two** (or more) of the following:

1. difficulty falling or staying asleep

2. irritability or outbursts of anger

3. difficulty concentrating

4. hypervigilance

5. exaggerated startle response

Criterion E

Duration of the disturbance is more than 1 month

Criterion F

The disturbance caused clinically significant distress or impairment in social, occupational, or other important aspects of functioning

Full PTSD: Criterion A, Criterion B = 1 or more, Criterion C = 3 or more, Criterion D = 2 or more, Criterion E, and Criterion F

Case Study

Case 11.4   John

John, a 45-year-old who works as a bar manager in a busy bar, has three children and is the main wage earner within his household. He suffers a stroke whilst setting up for work before the bar opens. He is on the floor for about an hour, unable to get up, before he is found. He has marked left-sided weakness. Whilst in hospital, he works hard in rehabilitation and makes a good recovery.

When John returns to the stroke review clinic, the nurse notes that he is anxious, has problems with concentration, and is low in mood. His wife complains that he is always pent-up and irritable, as if he is on guard, and John notes that at night he has difficulty relaxing and falling asleep. He also seems reluctant to return to work, despite having been deemed physically fit to return. Given his symptoms, the nurse feels that John is probably suffering from depression and refers him to his GP, who starts him on antidepressant medication. However, John doesn't respond to treatment.

On his next visit, the nurse completes the Impact of Event Scale, which identifies that John potentially has PTSD, and he is referred on to the clinical psychologist. On assessment, the clinical psychologist diagnoses PTSD. In terms of John's key symptoms, he is re-experiencing the event where he fell to the floor and was unable to get up, and was fearful that he would not be found before he died. He is avoiding returning to work, as being in the work environment immediately rekindles traumatic memories; even just thinking about work increases arousal and makes him feel anxious. With time and treatment from the clinical psychologist, John is able to control his symptoms.

reduction in the efficiency of memory or decision-making. Sensory impairment includes effects on the processing of incoming information, such as visual or auditory information. However, it also includes effects on the way that the brain perceives the world, such as the sophisticated processing work that the brain does in order to perceive, amongst others, three-dimensional vision, the movement of objects, smell, and the taste of food.

After stroke, most patients experience some disturbance of cognitive functioning, although in most, the effects are temporary. A minority of patients have longer-lasting cognitive impairment, producing disabilities of varying severity. This emphasises the importance of being aware of potential problems. It also suggests the need to assess for cognitive impairment soon after stroke, and there are basic measures available that can be used quickly by the non-specialist. A recent review found that only two measures – the Montreal Cognitive Assessment (MoCA) and the Mini-Mental State Examination (MMSE) – were suitable at all levels of cognitive impairment [22], although others are suitable for specific impairments.

11.4.7   Attention Problems

Impairments of attention can have significant effects on a patient's ability to live independently, since attention is needed for almost all cognitive functions. Attention relates to the unconscious focus on particular aspects of the environment.

We are constantly bombarded with different sensory stimuli, and our attentional abilities allow our brain to disregard most of them and focus on what is needed to function effectively.

Attentional deficits have a particular impact on complex and demanding behaviours. For example, a patient with attentional deficits would find it very hard to drive a car. Attentional impairments require the input of neuropsychologists, not just for diagnosis, but also for possible interventions. These may involve some retraining of the brain to identify and focus on certain stimuli whilst rejecting or lowering the volume of others [85].

11.4.8 Memory Impairments

Memory problems after stroke are quite common. Unlike many other cognitive impairments, the patient is often aware of them. Memory problems can respond to treatment, and the patient can be taught relatively straightforward techniques to produce improvements, or at least to compensate for memory loss [86].

Memory can be assessed by standardised assessment measures. If problems are identified, it is important to check that there is no underlying physiological cause (e.g. hypothyroidism), and referral to a specialist is recommended. Therapy sessions and the inpatient ward environment can both be adjusted to better suit the patient's impairment.

11.4.9 Visuospatial Disorders

Disorders of this type include spatial neglect (the disregard of a portion of the vision of the world), perceptual disorders, and motor apraxia and dyspraxia (inability or difficulty in doing activities).

It is hard to give a reliable estimate of the frequency of these disorders, since published rates vary so much. They may occur in around 1 in 10 patients with left-hemisphere stroke and up to half of patients with right hemisphere stroke. Recovery can be quick: the problems often go away after 2–3 weeks, but they may persist. For example, it is suggested that in patients with visuospatial problems after stroke, around 1 in 10 will continue to have these problems 3 months later [87].

Visuospatial disorders can be disturbing and significantly disabling: they interfere with many routine activities and can make it difficult for the patient to live and function independently. The effects of visuospatial problems can cause significant issues during rehabilitation. Not surprisingly, the continuation of these problems tends to increase the chances of longer hospital stay, discharge to residential care, and social isolation [88].

The diagnosis of visuospatial problems may be made by clinical assessment, although there are formal tests that a neuropsychologist may use to clarify the diagnosis. Currently, few interventions are available for visuospatial [89] or perceptual disorders [90], and so the emphasis for the patient will need to be on safety and compensatory techniques. In motor apraxia, interventions have shown benefits on activities of daily living in the short-term, but no evidence is currently available that the benefits persist [91].

11.4.10 Executive Dysfunction

This cognitive impairment has been categorised relatively recently, and it refers to an impact on the ability to organise, plan, and execute (i.e. carry out) tasks and anticipate their consequences. When functioning of this type is impaired, it is termed 'dysexecutive syndrome', and patients may have particular difficulty in planning and organising series of tasks. They may be unable to monitor their behaviour, and, as a result, be unable to adapt well to change. Problems with executive functioning are relatively rare after stroke, but are more commonly seen after subarachnoid haemorrhage. There have been few interventions evaluated thoroughly in research, and none that has shown significant benefit [92].

11.5 Conclusion

It is common for patients to experience mood, cognitive, and behavioural changes after stroke. Many are relatively short-lasting and may remit spontaneously. However, their onset can be distressing for the patient and their relatives, and their presence can provide a challenge during the acute phase of stroke care.

   Mood problems and cognitive impairments are now more frequently recognised and diagnosed, and there is a growing body of evidence to inform treatments. In common with other aspects of stroke care, the emphasis needs to be on early recognition, monitoring, and referral, and on ensuring that the patient understands what is happening and why.

References

1. UK Stroke Forum Education & Training. About the SSEF. Available from: http://www.stroke-education.org.uk/about [30 November 2018].
2. Intercollegiate Stroke Working Party (2016). Stroke Guidelines. London: Royal College of Physicians.
3. Hackett, M.L. and Anderson, C.S. (2005). Predictors of depression after stroke. A Systematic Review of Observational Studies 36 (10): 2296–2301.
4. House, A., Dennis, M., Mogridge, L. et al. (1991). Mood disorders in the year after first stroke. British Journal of Psychiatry 158: 83–92.
5. Pearlin, L.I. and Schooler, C. (1978). The structure of coping. Journal of Health and Social Behavior 19 (1): 2–21.
6. Lazarus, R.S. and Folkman, S. (1984). Stress, Appraisal, and Coping. New York: Springer.
7. Robinson, R.G. (2003). Poststroke depression: prevalence, diagnosis, treatment, and disease progression. Biological Psychiatry 54 (3): 376–387.
8. Carson, A.J., MacHale, S., Allen, K. et al. (2000). Depression after stroke and lesion location: a systematic review. The Lancet 356 (9224): 122–126.
9. World Health Organization (WHO) (2003). The ICD-10 Classification of Mental and Behavioural Disorders: Diagnostic Criteria for Research. Geneva: World Health Organization.
10. Hackett, M.L. and Pickles, K. (2014). Part I: frequency of depression after stroke: an updated systematic review and meta-analysis of observational studies. International Journal of Stroke 9 (8): 1017–1025.

11. Andersen, G., Vestergaard, K., Riis, J.Ø., and Lauritzen, L. (1994). Incidence of post-stroke depression during the first year in a large unselected stroke population determined using a valid standardized rating scale. Acta Psychiatrica Scandinavica 90 (3): 190–195.

12. De Wit, L., Putman, K., Baert, I. et al. (2008). Anxiety and depression in the first six months after stroke. A longitudinal multicentre study. Disability and Rehabilitation 30 (24): 1858–1866.

13. Kutlubaev, M.A. and Hackett, M.L. (2014). Part II: predictors of depression after stroke and impact of depression on stroke outcome: an updated systematic review of observational studies. International Journal of Stroke 9 (8): 1026–1036.

14. Kauhanen, M.L., Korpelainen, J.T., Hiltunen, P. et al. (2000). Aphasia, depression, and non-verbal cognitive impairment in ischaemic stroke. Cerebrovascular Diseases 10 (6): 455–461.

15. Thomas, S.A. and Lincoln, N.B. (2008). Predictors of emotional distress after stroke. Stroke 39 (4): 1240–1245.

16. Morris, P.L.P., Robinson, R.G., Raphael, B., and Bishop, D. (1991). The relationship between the perception of social support and post-stroke depression in hospitalized patients. Psychiatry 54 (3): 306–316.

17. Intercollegiate Stroke Working Party (2016). National Clinical Guideline for Stroke, 5e. London: Royal College of Physicians.

18. Meader, N., Moe-Byrne, T., Llewellyn, A., and Mitchell, A.J. (2014). Screening for poststroke major depression: a meta-analysis of diagnostic validity studies. Journal of Neurology, Neurosurgery and Psychiatry 85 (2): 198–206.

19. Kroenke, K. and Spitzer, R.L. (2002). A new depression diagnostic and severity measure. Psychiatric Annals 32 (9): 509–515.

20. Goldberg, D. and Williams, P. (1988). A User's Guide to the General Health Questionnaire. Windsor: Nfer-Nelson.

21. Yesavage, J.A., Brink, T.L., Rose, T.L. et al. (1983). Development and validation of a geriatric depression screening scale: a preliminary report. Journal of Psychiatric Research 17 (1): 37–49.

22. Burton, L. and Tyson, S.F. (2015). Screening for cognitive impairment after stroke: a systematic review of psychometric properties and clinical utility. Journal of Rehabilitation Medicine 47 (3): 193–203.

23. Watkins, C.L., Auton, M.F., Deans, C.F. et al. (2007). Motivational interviewing early after acute stroke: a randomized, controlled trial. Stroke 38 (3): 1004–1009.

24. Lightbody, C.E., Auton, M., Baldwin, R. et al. (2007). The use of nurses' and carers' observations in the identification of poststroke depression. Journal of Advanced Nursing 60 (6): 595–604.

25. Turner-Stokes, L., Kalmus, M., Hirani, D., and Clegg, F. (2005). The Depression Intensity Scale Circles (DISCs): a first evaluation of a simple assessment tool for depression in the context of brain injury. Journal of Neurosurgery and Psychiatry 76 (9): 1273–1278.

26. Lee, A.C., Tang, S.W., Yu, G.K., and Cheung, R.T. (2008). The smiley as a simple screening tool for depression after stroke: a preliminary study. International Journal of Nursing Studies 45 (7): 1081–1089.

27. Watkins, C., Daniels, L., Jack, C. et al. (2001). Accuracy of a single question in screening for depression in a cohort of patients after stroke: comparative study. British Medical Journal 323 (7322): 1159.

28. Bennett, H.E., Thomas, S.A., Austen, R. et al. (2010). Validation of screening measures for assessing mood in stroke patients. British Journal of Clinical Psychology 45 (3): 367–376.

29. Leeds, L., Meara, R.J., and Hobson, J.P. (2004). The utility of the Stroke Aphasia Depression Questionnaire (SADQ) in a stroke rehabilitation unit. Clinical Rehabilitation 18 (2): 228–231.

30. Sackley, C.M., Hoppitt, T.J., and Cardoso, K. (2006). An investigation into the utility of the Stroke Aphasic Depression Questionnaire (SADQ) in care home settings. Clinical Rehabilitation 20 (7): 598–602.
31. Hacker Vicki, L., Stark, D., and Thomas, S. (2010). Validation of the Stroke Aphasic Depression Questionnaire using the brief assessment schedule depression cards in an acute stroke sample. British Journal of Clinical Psychology 49 (1): 123–127.
32. Stern, R.A. (1997). Visual Analog Mood Scales. Odessa: Psychological Assessment Resources.
33. Gordon, W.A. and Hibbard, M.R. (1997). Poststroke depression: an examination of the literature. Archives of Physical Medicine and Rehabilitation 78 (6): 658–663.
34. Brumfitt, S. and Barton, J. (2006). Evaluating wellbeing in people with aphasia using speech therapy and clinical psychology. International Journal of Therapy and Rehabilitation 13 (7): 305–310.
35. Gilbody, S.M., House, A.O., and Sheldon, T.A. (2001). Routinely administered questionnaires for depression and anxiety: systematic review. British Medcial Journal 322 (7283): 406–409.
36. Hill K. Mood state after stroke and its effect on outcome: a prospective cohort study. UK Stroke Forum. Harrogate: UK Stroke Forum Conference; 2009. pp. 2–4.
37. Chemerinski, E., Robinson, R.G., and Kosier, J.T. (2001). Improved recovery in activities of daily living associated with remission of poststroke depression. Stroke 32 (1): 113–117.
38. Spalletta, G., Guida, G., De Angelis, D., and Caltagirone, C. (2002). Predictors of cognitive level and depression severity are different in patients with left and right hemispheric stroke within the first year of illness. Journal of Neurology 249 (11): 1541–1551.
39. Mayo, N.E., Wood-Dauphinee, S., Cote, R. et al. (2002). Activity, participation, and quality of life 6 months poststroke. Archives of Physical Medicine Rehabilitation 83 (8): 1035–1042.
40. Jaracz, K., Jaracz, J., Kozubski, W., and Rybakowski, J.K. (2002). Post-stroke quality of life and depression. Acta Neuropsychiatrica 14 (5): 219–225.
41. Stenager, E.N., Madsen, C., Stenager, E., and Boldsen, J. (1998). Suicide in patients with stroke: epidemiological study. British Medical Journal 316 (7139): 1206.
42. House, A., Knapp, P., Bamford, J., and Vail, A. (2001). Mortality at 12 and 24 months after stroke may be associated with depressive symptoms at 1 month. Stroke 32 (3): 696–701.
43. Petty, D.R., House, A., Knapp, P. et al. (2006). Prevalence, duration and indications for prescribing of antidepressants in primary care. Age and Ageing 35 (5): 523–526.
44. Ruddell, M., Spencer, A., Hill, K., and House, A. (2007). Fluoxetine vs placebo for depressive symptoms after stroke: failed randomised controlled trial. International Journal of Geriatric Psychiatry 22 (10): 963–965.
45. Hackett, M.L., Anderson, C.S., House, A.O., and Xia, J. (2009). Interventions for treating depression after stroke. Stroke 40 (7): e487–e488.
46. Knapp, P., Young, J., House, A., and Forster, A. (2000). Non-drug strategies to resolve psycho-social difficulties after stroke. Age and Ageing 29 (1): 23–30.
47. Wang, S.-B., Wang, Y.-Y., Zhang, Q.-E. et al. (2018). Cognitive behavioral therapy for post-stroke depression: a meta-analysis. Journal of Affective Disorders 235: 589–596.
48. Williams, L.S., Kroenke, K., Bakas, T. et al. (2007). Care management of poststroke depression: a randomized, controlled trial. Stroke 38 (3): 998–1003.
49. Thomas, S.A., Walker, M.F., Macniven, J.A. et al. (2013). Communication and Low Mood (CALM): a randomized controlled trial of behavioural therapy for stroke patients with aphasia. Clinical Rehabilitation 27 (5): 398–408.
50. Lawrence, M., Booth, J., Mercer, S., and Crawford, E. (2013). A systematic review of the benefits of mindfulness-based interventions following transient ischemic attack and stroke. International Journal of Stroke 8 (6): 465–474.

51. Lai, S.M., Studenski, S., Richards, L. et al. (2006). Therapeutic exercise and depressive symptoms after stroke. Journal of the American Geriatrics Society 54 (2): 240–247.
52. Kim, D.S., Park, Y.G., Choi, J.H. et al. (2011). Effects of music therapy on mood in stroke patients. Yonsei Medical Journal 52 (6): 977–981.
53. Sarkamo, T., Tervaniemi, M., Laitinen, S. et al. (2008). Music listening enhances cognitive recovery and mood after middle cerebral artery stroke. Brain 131 (3): 866–876.
54. Alexopoulos, G.S., Wilkins, V.M., Marino, P. et al. (2012). Ecosystem focused therapy in poststroke depression: a preliminary study. International Journal of Geriatric Psychiatry 27 (10): 1053–1060.
55. Hackett, M.L., Anderson, C.S., House, A., and Halteh, C. (2008). Interventions for preventing depression after stroke. Cochrane Database of Systematic Reviews 3 (Art. No.: CD003689). https://doi.org/10.1002/14651858.CD003689.pub3.
56. Tang, W.K., Chen, Y., Lam, W.W.M. et al. (2009). Emotional incontinence and executive function in ischemic stroke: a case-controlled study. Journal of the International Neuropsychological Society 15 (1): 62–68.
57. Calvert, T., Knapp, P., and House, A. (1999). Psychological associations with emotionalism after stroke. Journal of Neurology, Neurosurgery and Psychiatry 65: 928–929.
58. House, A., Dennis, M., Molyneux, A. et al. (1989). Emotionalism after stroke. British Medical Journal 298 (6679): 991–994.
59. Carota, A., Berney, A., Aybek, S. et al. (2005). A prospective study of predictors of poststroke depression. Neurology 64 (3): 428–433.
60. Hackett, M.L., Yang, M., Anderson, C.S. et al. (2010). Pharmaceutical interventions for emotionalism after stroke. Cochrane Database of Systematic Reviews 2 (Art. No.: CD003690). https://doi.org/10.1002/14651858.CD003690.pub3.
61. Horrocks, J.A., Hackett, M.L., Anderson, C.S., and House, A.O. (2004). Pharmaceutical interventions for emotionalism after stroke. Stroke 35 (11): 2610–2611.
62. Eccles, S., House, A., and Knapp, P. (1999). Psychological adjustment and self reported coping in stroke survivors with and without emotionalism. Journal of Neurology, Neurosurgery and Psychiatry 67 (1): 125–126.
63. Chriki, L.S., Bullain, S.S., and Stern, T.A. (2006). The recognition and management of psychological reactions to stroke: a case discussion. Primary Care Companion to the Journal of Clinical Psychiatry 8 (4): 234–240.
64. Campbell Burton, C.A., Murray, J., Holmes, J. et al. (2012). Frequency of anxiety after stroke: a systematic review and meta-analysis of observational studies. International Journal of Stroke 8 (7): 545–559.
65. Ayerbe, L., Ayis, S.A., Crichton, S. et al. (2014). Natural history, predictors and associated outcomes of anxiety up to 10 years after stroke: the South London Stroke Register. Age and Ageing 43 (4): 542–547.
66. Broomfield, N.M., Scoular, A., Welsh, P. et al. (2013). Poststroke anxiety is prevalent at the population level, especially among socially deprived and younger age community stroke survivors. International Journal of Stroke 10 (6): 897–902.
67. Menlove, L., Crayton, E., Kneebone, I. et al. (2015). Predictors of anxiety after stroke: a systematic review of observational studies. Journal of Stroke and Cerebrovascular Diseases 1 (24): 1107–1117.
68. Campbell Burton, C.A., Knapp, P., Holmes, J. et al. (2010). Interventions for treating anxiety after stroke. Cochrane Database of Systematic Reviews 12 (Art. No.: CD008860). https://doi.org/10.1002/14651858.CD008860.pub2.
69. National Institute for Health and Care Excellence (2014). Anxiety Disorders (NICE Quality Standard QS53). London: National Institute for Health and Care Excellence.
70. Chun, H.Y., Whiteley, W.N., Carson, A. et al. (2015). Anxiety after stroke: time for an intervention. International Journal of Stroke 10 (5): 655–656.
71. Holcroft, L. (2005). Post-Traumatic Stress Disorder after Stroke. Lancaster: University of Lancaster.

72. Bruggimann, L., Annoni, J.M., Staub, F. et al. (2006). Chronic posttraumatic stress symptoms after nonsevere stroke. Neurology 66 (4): 513–516.
73. Merriman, C., Norman, P., and Barton, J. (2007). Psychological correlates of PTSD symptoms following stroke. Psychology, Health & Medicine 12 (5): 592–602.
74. Sembi, S., Tarrier, N., O'Neill, P. et al. (1998). Does post-traumatic stress disorder occur after stroke: a preliminary study. International Journal of Geriatric Psychiatry 13 (5): 315–322.
75. Wealleans G, Watkins CL, Sharma AK, Daniels L (eds). PTSD in survivors of stroke [poster presentation]. Telford: British Association of Stroke Physicians Conference; 2009.
76. Wealleans, G. (1998). Post-Traumatic Stress Disorder in Survivors of Stroke. Liverpool: University of Liverpool.
77. Letamendia, C., Leblanc, N.J., Pariente, J. et al. (2012). Peritraumatic distress predicts acute posttraumatic stress disorder symptoms after a first stroke. General Hospital Psychiatry 34 (5): 439–580.
78. First, M., Frances, A., and Pincus, H.A. (2002). DSM-IV-TR Handbook of Differential Diagnosis. Arlington: American Psychiatric Publishing.
79. National Collaborating Centre for Mental Health (UK) (2005). Post-Traumatic Stress Disorder: The Management of PTSD in Adults and Children in Primary and Secondary Care. Leicester: Gaskell.
80. Stein, D.J., Ipser, J.C., Seedat, S. et al. (2006). Pharmacotherapy for post traumatic stress disorder (PTSD). Cochrane Database of Systematic Reviews 1 (Art. No.: CD002795). https://doi.org/10.1002/14651858.CD002795.pub2.
81. Stein, D.J., Ipser, J., and McAnda, N. (2009). Pharmacotherapy of posttraumatic stress disorder: a review of meta-analyses and treatment guidelines. CNS Spectrum 14 (1 Suppl. 1): 25–31.
82. Bisson, J.I., Roberts, N.P., Andrew, M. et al. (2013). Psychological therapies for chronic post-traumatic stress disorder (PTSD) in adults. Cochrane Database of Systematic Reviews 12 (Art. No.: CD003388). https://doi.org/10.1002/14651858.CD003388.pub4.
83. Bisson, J. and Andrew, M. (2007). Psychological treatment of post-traumatic stress disorder (PTSD). Cochrane Database of Systematic Reviews 3 (Art. No.: CD003388). https://doi.org/10.1002/14651858.CD003388.pub3.
84. Gillespie, D.C., Bowen, A., Chung, C.S. et al. (2014). Rehabilitation for post-stroke cognitive impairment: an overview of recommendations arising from systematic reviews of current evidence. Clinical Rehabilitation 29 (2): 120–128.
85. Loetscher, T. and Lincoln, N.B. (2013). Cognitive rehabilitation for attention deficits following stroke. Cochrane Database of Systematic Reviews 5 (Art. No.: CD002842). https://doi.org/10.1002/14651858.CD002842.pub2.
86. das Nair, R. and Lincoln, N. (2007). Cognitive rehabilitation for memory deficits following stroke. Cochrane Database of Systematic Reviews 3 (Art. No.: CD002293). https://doi.org/10.1002/14651858.CD002293.pub2.
87. Stone, S.P., Patel, P., Greenwood, R.J., and Halligan, P.W. (1992). Measuring visual neglect in acute stroke and predicting its recovery: the visual neglect recovery index. Journal of Neurology, Neurosurgery and Psychiatry 55 (6): 431–436.
88. Jehkonen, M., Laihosalo, M., Kettunen, J.E., and Jehkonen, J.E. (2006). Impact of neglect on functional outcome after stroke – a review of methodological issues and recent research findings. Restorative Neurology and Neuroscience 24 (4–6): 209–215.
89. Bowen, A., Hazelton, C., Pollock, A., and Lincoln, N.B. (2013). Cognitive rehabilitation for spatial neglect following stroke. Cochrane Database of Systematic Reviews 7 (Art. No.: CD003586). https://doi.org/10.1002/14651858.CD003586.pub3.
90. Bowen, A., Knapp, P., Gillespie, D. et al. (2011). Non-pharmacological interventions for perceptual disorders following stroke and other adult-acquired, non-progressive brain

injury. Cochrane Database of Systematic Reviews 4 (Art. No.: CD007039). https://doi.org/10.1002/14651858.CD007039.pub2.

91. West, C., Bowen, A., Hesketh, A., and Vail, A. (2008). Interventions for motor apraxia following stroke. Cochrane Database of Systematic Reviews 1 (Art. No.: CD004132). https://doi.org/10.1002/14651858.CD004132.pub2.

92. Chung, C.A., Pollock, A., Campbell, T. et al. (2013). Cognitive rehabilitation for executive dysfunction in adults with stroke or other adult, non-progressive acquired brain damage: a cochrane systematic review: 123. Cochrane Database of Systematic Reviews 4 (Art. No.: CD008391). https://doi.org/10.1002/14651858.CD008391.pub2.

CHAPTER 12

Stroke and Palliative Care

Taking Ownership

Clare Thetford, Munirah Bangee, Elizabeth Lightbody, and Caroline Watkins
Faculty of Health & Wellbeing, University of Central Lancashire, Preston, UK

KEY POINTS

- Stroke is associated with two distinct trajectories of dying. Whilst some patients die very soon after a stroke, others experience fluctuating decline and recovery before death over an extended period of time.

- Palliative care aims to improve quality of life for patients and their families facing life-limiting illness. It aims to manage pain and other physical symptoms. It also provides support with psychological, social, and spiritual needs.

- The terminology surrounding palliative care is problematic, with distinct terms commonly used interchangeably. This contributes to a lack of understanding, and ultimately can impact care.

- Palliative care within stroke should be provided alongside, rather than instead of, other services which focus upon active treatment and rehabilitation.

- Meeting the palliative care needs of stroke patients requires stroke specialists to develop enhanced knowledge and skills in palliation in order to address the specific challenges that stroke presents. This requires investment from within the stroke field and a commitment to a more holistic approach to care which extends beyond rehabilitation goals.

This chapter maps to criteria within the following sections of the Stroke-Specific Education Framework (SSEF):

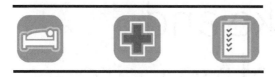

12.1 Introduction

Death rates associated with stroke remain high; 12% of patients die within the first 30 days following a stroke [2], and 25–30% who initially survive die within 12 months [3].

Historically, palliative care has been associated with cancer care [4]. There is, however, increasing recognition of the value of and need for palliative care to support people with a broad range of life-threatening and complex conditions [5, 6], including stroke [7]. Palliative care aims to improve the quality of life of patients and their families facing life-threatening illness [8]. It provides symptom control through identification, assessment, and treatment of pain, alongside physical, psychosocial, and spiritual problems [7].

Patients need not be facing imminent death to benefit from palliative care; indeed, a palliative care approach is potentially beneficial for patients with complex serious conditions, as well as those which are life-limiting, and those patients who are coming to the end of their lives. Palliative care can be provided for months or even years before death [9]. Generally, the patient's usual care team provides palliative care, but specialist palliative care services can offer additional support on decision-making and symptom management [10].

The terminology surrounding palliative care is problematic. The terms 'palliative', 'end of life', and 'last days of life' are intended to describe specific stages of dying and associated time frames, but in practice are used interchangeably, with little recognition or understanding of the differences in what they describe. *Palliative care* describes care for patients with life-limiting conditions, but with no clear or specified time frame. *End of life care* aims to support patients to live as well as possible in their last 12 months of life [11]. Care in the *last days of life* is delivered to people in their final few days of life [12]. Figure 12.1 illustrates how the terms 'end of life care' and 'care in last days of life' sit within the broader concept of palliative care.

These issues surrounding terminology can impact care by creating confusion regarding the type of care that is required to provide appropriate support at specific stages or to meet particular care needs. For example, despite its definition implying a far broader remit, the term 'palliative care' is often used to describe care provided during the last days of life, when a patient is actively dying [13]. The term 'end of life care' is also often used to describe care during the last days of life, rather than its intended meaning of care and support provided when an individual is judged likely to be in their last 12 months of life. The misunderstanding associated with these terms may mean that a patient who would benefit from palliative

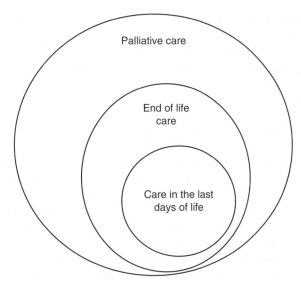

FIGURE 12.1 End of life care and care in the last days of life fit within the broader concept of palliative care. *Source: Adapted from Palliative Care at End of Life. https:// nursekey.com/palliative-care-at-end-of-life.*

care at an earlier stage does not receive that care as their death is not imminent. Uncertainties surrounding the commencement of palliative care approaches in stroke mean that opportunities to improve quality of life are lost [14].

There is also confusion surrounding the descriptions of approaches to care, such as 'pathway', 'operating procedure', and 'guidelines' [15], which are used to support palliative care. This contributes to a lack of clarity regarding requirements, approaches, and processes. In this chapter, we identify a range of challenges in delivering palliative care for stroke patients. We consider generic palliative care pathways and tools, and their suitability in the context of stroke. We conclude with recommendations to guide the development of improved palliative care in stroke.

12.2 Specific Challenges in Stroke

The delivery of timely, effective palliative care is challenging with any patient group. However, stroke poses some significant and unique challenges, associated in particular with uncertainties surrounding prognosis and stroke-specific symptoms [16]. There is increasing recognition of the need to develop condition-specific guidance to support palliative care, including for acute stroke [7]. However, there is a lack of guidance on how to integrate palliative care within stroke, which may account for at least some of the continued neglect of service development this area [4, 17]. This lack of guidance is underpinned by an insufficient evidence base to inform the development of appropriate models of end of life and palliative care in stroke [14].

Stroke can present considerable palliative care needs [16]. Despite patients and families demonstrating a need for the use of palliative care approaches in the earlier stages of dying, there is a lack of processes and guidelines to support healthcare professionals in decisions surrounding commencement of palliative care [18]. These complex decisions require clinicians to consider prognosis, trajectories of dying, and patient and family preferences [19], as well as stroke-specific symptoms and challenges.

12.2.1 Uncertainty in Prognosis

Models of trajectories of dying which are based on cancer and other conditions are reasonably well established [13], and often assume that the trajectory of dying is relatively linear [19]. This implies that prognoses can be made using a range of clinical indicators, enabling a clearer course of progression. Stroke, however, presents clinical trajectories different to those of other disease groups [20], our understanding of which remains limited [19].

Prognostic models within stroke remain underdeveloped [18], and staff recognise the problematic nature of identifying when to commence palliative care approaches in stroke [14]. However, stroke healthcare professionals use a range of signs to identify dying in stroke patients. Common physiological signs include altered blood results, vital signs, and breathing patterns; clinical signs include persistent coma with no significant improvement, no response to sustained treatment, and serious clinical deterioration [13].

There are at least two distinct trajectories of dying associated with stroke [13, 21]. Whilst some patients die suddenly following the onset of stroke, others face 'prolonged dying' associated with a less certain prognosis. These latter patients can experience fluctuating cycles of decline and recovery over an extended period of time before eventually deteriorating and dying. The uncertain prognoses can make recognising a patient who may be dying difficult, which may impact on managing treatment options and the decision whether to sustain or withdraw life-prolonging treatments [22, 23].

The uncertain prognoses associated with stroke mean it is often difficult to predict whether a treatment will be beneficial for patients or will reduce their quality of life. Given the challenges in prognosis, it is especially important that there is effective communication within healthcare teams supporting stroke patients when discussing prognoses, treatment withdrawal, and care decisions [24]. It is also essential for communication with the patient's family to be clear and honest about these uncertainties, in order to support the family in contributing to the decision-making process in a meaningful way [16].

In light of these differing trajectories and associated uncertainties surrounding the identification of dying, palliative care within stroke should be provided alongside, rather than instead of, other services which focus upon active treatment and rehabilitation [25].

12.2.2 Stroke-Specific Symptoms

The sudden onset of stroke often precludes patients having the opportunity to discuss their advanced treatment wishes with their families, especially if they have cognitive or communication problems or altered conscious levels [13, 18].

Treatment decisions concerning patients who are considered to not have capacity must be conducted within the limits and expectations set out in the Mental Capacity Act [26]. Families can find it challenging to make such decisions where they have little knowledge of the patient's wishes. This can be particularly problematic in patients with swallowing problems (dysphagia) [18], which affect about 40% of patients following a stroke. Families often perceive artificial feeding (such as a nasogastric tube or percutaneous endoscopic gastrostomy, PEG) as beneficial. However, in patients with a poor prognosis, artificial feeding may merely prolong an imminent death, and is thus unethical. Careful consideration must be given to the risks and benefits associated with such interventions, which are further complicated by uncertain trajectories of dying. These challenges create the need for staff to provide families with clear communication and support in contributing to treatment decisions [22, 27].

Stroke is associated with a range of symptoms around death which vary from those presenting with other conditions. For example, compared with cancer patients who are dying, stroke patients have a higher prevalence of death rattles, but a significantly lower prevalence of nausea, confusion, dyspnoea, anxiety, and pain [28]. Other symptoms have been identified as being common around the time of dying in stroke; these include dyspnoea, pain, mouth dryness, and respiratory secretions in the last days of life [29, 30]. There is also a growing body of evidence surrounding psychosocial problems after stroke, including anxiety [21], depression, and emotionalism [20]. Family members report less satisfaction with the treatment of psychosocial symptoms of stroke patients who died, compared with other aspects of their care [31], suggesting that further understanding is required concerning how to address these issues and symptoms.

12.2.3 Clinical Guidelines

International clinical guidelines on stroke care acknowledge the need for palliative care. However, these guidelines reflect differing conceptualisations of palliative care and use varying terminology, including 'end of life care' and 'palliative care'. Nevertheless, they appear to indicate a recognition of the wider concept of palliative care, which offers support prior to the last days of life. The UK National Clinical Guidelines for Stroke [32] recommend that high-quality palliative care be provided to stroke patients in acute and long-term care. However, they do not suggest how this should be integrated into stroke care. The American Stroke Association [33] recommends that stroke teams provide palliative care, although specialist palliative care teams should be consulted for complex cases. The Australian Clinical Guidelines for Stroke Management [34] are clear that palliative care is more than end of life care and should be provided to patients who have a poor prognosis or are likely to die. They also suggest that stroke teams should be trained to be able to provide palliative care, with support from specialist palliative care providers in complex cases.

The Australian Guidelines specifically recommend the use of a pathway which manages uncertainties and treatment options to support the delivery of palliative care in stroke. This contrasts somewhat with recent recommendations in the United Kingdom. Care pathways detail the required steps in and elements of the care of patients with specific clinical features, and describe the expected progress of such patients [35]. A UK-based review of the Liverpool Care Pathway (LCP) [15] recommends that the term 'care pathway' be avoided in the context of palliative care. 'Pathway' suggests to families that the patient is on a 'road to death' and that clinicians have in effect made the decision to kill them. There is also confusion within practice regarding how the 'pathway approach' should be used, leading to an interpretation of the LCP as a single document which is to be used rigidly as a 'protocol' to provide care of the dying, rather than as part of an approach; this leads to care that is not appropriate for all individuals or all contexts. A recent Cochrane review of the impact of end of life care pathways on care indicated there was insufficient evidence surrounding their use [36].

12.3   Tools to Support Palliative Care

Several tools, approaches, and pathways have been developed within palliative care, some of which have been implemented in a stroke care setting. In this section, we discuss three palliative care approaches that have been commonly used in the United Kingdom in the last 2 decades: (i) the LCP [37]; (ii) the Gold Standards Framework (GSF) [38]; and (iii) the Assessment, Management, Best practice, Engagement, and Recovery (AMBER) care bundle [39].

12.3.1   Liverpool Care Pathway (LCP)

The LCP was once widely used in the United Kingdom and worldwide [40]. It was developed to provide quality care for patients in the last days of life, with the aim of delivering a hospice model of care in other settings [37]. It comprised three sections, aimed at supporting staff with (i) initial assessment, (ii) ongoing care, and (iii) care after death. Each of these sections considered physical, psychosocial, and spiritual care.

Some limited research has explored the use of the LCP in a range of contexts, including stroke [41]. The LCP has been reported to improve record keeping and to change the way nurses prescribed medications for stroke patients in the last days of life [42]. More recently, families of stroke patients who were dying were reported to have few concerns about the use of the LCP; these focused upon the use of painkillers and sedatives, withdrawal of hydration/nutrition, and consenting family members. They did, however, report difficulties surrounding communication and the management of deaths which took place over an extended period of time. A review of the LCP [15] in response to public concerns acknowledged that it supported the delivery of quality care when it was implemented well, but also reported instances of poor care that were associated with lack of clinical understanding and insufficient communication with families. It found that there was a risk of poor end of life care in acute settings. The review recommended the phasing out of the LCP and replacing it with individualised care plans. The LCP was withdrawn from the United Kingdom in 2014, but continues to be used internationally [13, 36, 40].

12.3.2 Gold Standards Framework (GSF)

The GSF supports care in the final 12 months of life in any care setting, using a range of documents and guidance. It includes Proactive Indicator Guidance (PIG) [43], which provides a flowchart to support identification of the risk of dying, palliative care needs, and decision-making. It appears to accommodate the different trajectories of dying associated with stroke, as it aims to enable the earlier identification of people nearing the end of life who may need palliative care. The PIG follows three main trajectories of illness for expected deaths:

- rapid, predictable decline (associated with cancer);
- erratic, unpredictable decline; and
- gradual decline.

This guidance includes the 'surprise question': Would you be surprised if this patient were to die in the next year, months, weeks, or days? It also prompts consideration of indicators of decline, such as decreased physical activity and specific clinical indicators. The GSF PIG suggests a number of indicators that should be considered in stroke specifically, although it presents these within a trajectory of 'gradual decline' leading to death. It is not clear if these same indicators could be useful in identifying a more rapid or uncertain death with fluctuating cycles of decline and recovery:

- validated scales, such as the National Institute of Health Stroke Scale (NIHSS);
- persistent vegetative, minimal conscious state or dense paralysis;
- medical complications, or lack of improvement within 3 months of onset;
- cognitive impairment/post-stroke dementia; and
- other factors, e.g. old age, male sex, heart disease, stroke sub-type hyperglycaemia, dementia, and renal failure [43]

In UK hospitals, the GSF process has improved the rate of identifying patients in the last year of life [44]. In a London stroke unit, it has been reported to support early identification of patients in the last year of life and to improve coordination of their care [45]. This suggests that the GSF is suitable to use in stroke care, as it supports identification of patients who are likely to die imminently or within a year of the stroke.

12.3.3 AMBER Care Bundle

The AMBER care bundle [39, 46] encourages communication between staff, patients, and families, and supports clinical decision-making when the prognosis is uncertain and patients are identified as being at risk of dying within 1–2 months. It acknowledges the risk of poor outcomes and death, whilst pursuing active treatment. It aims to enable conversations around support, to put supports in place, to meet palliative care needs, and to achieve recovery through treatment and interventions, with regular review.

In UK hospitals, the AMBER care bundle has been reported to increase the number of discussions between clinicians and patients at the time of prognosis, when compared to standard care [47]. Whilst the use of the AMBER care bundle has not been fully explored or evaluated in the context of stroke, in principle it would appear to support the care of stroke patients, in particular through its ability to accommodate uncertainty.

12.3.4 Additional Tools to Support Palliative Care

Following the withdrawal of the LCP, the Leadership Alliance for the Care of Dying People published the 'five priorities of care' which they recommended to support a more individualised approach to care of the dying within the last days of life [48]. This detailed five broad areas of consideration in meeting care needs; it did not include supporting documentation to guide professionals through the processes involved. This lack of documentation and clarity of process has led to practitioners developing local policies and documentation, resulting in large variations in practice [6].

A number of additional tools have been developed in palliative care that focus on a specific stage in the care of the dying:

- *Advance Care Plan (ACP)* [49]. A written document which sets out a patient's wishes, beliefs, values, and preferences about their future care. It provides a guide to help healthcare professionals and anyone else who may be involved in decisions about the patient's care if they become unable to communicate their own preferences. In the United Kingdom, the documentation surrounding Preferred Priorities of Care (PPC) [50] is often used to support ACP, although there are no specific required documents.

- *The Electronic Palliative Care Co-ordination System (EPaCCS)* [51]. An electronic document that records care preferences once an individual is identified as requiring palliative care. The system allows healthcare professionals to share information across care settings and support conversations surrounding end of life care. It is currently being rolled out within the United Kingdom.

- *The Recommended Summary Plan for Emergency Care and Treatment (ReSPECT)* [52]. A personalised care plan that records preferences for care and clinical judgements. It is used in emergencies in which patients do not have capacity to make choices about their treatment.

- *Do Not Attempt Cardiopulmonary Resuscitation (DNACPR)* [52]. The advanced decision not to attempt cardiopulmonary resuscitation on a patient who has stopped breathing, or whose heart has stopped. However, this is surrounded by ethical and legal complexity, with varying legalities and requirements in different countries.

- *A Rapid Discharge Pathway* [53]. Helps to overcome the barriers service providers face in enabling the rapid discharge of a dying patient to allow them to die in their preferred place of care. These barriers include: lack of identification of end of life and resulting lack of discussion with patients and their relatives; difficulty in accessing equipment and care provision; communication challenges with primary care; delays in obtaining medication and transport; and delays in obtaining continuing care funding.

TABLE 12.1 Palliative care pathways and tools in stroke

Care pathway/tool	Purpose	Supporting documentation	Suitability within stroke care
Advance Care Plan	Documents patient wishes about future care, which should be used to inform decisions if they become too unwell to make or communicate decisions	No specific document or content Guidance on what might be included is available from a range of organisations	May support palliative care in stroke, as it accommodates uncertainty Lack of structure means it relies on the patient and those around them to identify possible future scenarios to consider and write in to the plan Stroke can be sudden and often carries many uncertainties
GSF (Gold Standards Framework) and PIG (Proactive Indicator Guidance)	Early identification of patients with palliative care needs Supports advance care planning	Flowchart document to guide earlier identification of patients with palliative care needs	Guidance includes a list of specific stroke clinical indicators of decline Indicators guidance does not address how to deal with uncertainties of stroke or sudden death following stroke
AMBER care bundle	Supports communication and clinical decision making for patients who have an uncertain recovery	Proforma document to guide interventions Document kept in patient notes	Specifically designed to support palliative care needs and decision making in the context of uncertain prognosis Does not address care in the last days of life
EPaCCS (Electronic Palliative Care Co-ordination system)	Records preferences of care, transferrable across different care settings	Digital document shared across healthcare professionals	Could support care over an extended period of time and with uncertain prognosis Potentially particularly useful where there is movement across different care settings, e.g. repeated hospital admissions following discharge to care home Supports advance care planning for patients, which may be helpful in the context of risk of further stroke and general decline

(continued)

TABLE 12.1 Palliative care pathways and tools in stroke *(continued)*

Care pathway/tool	Purpose	Supporting documentation	Suitability within stroke care
ReSPECT (Recommended Summary Plan for Emergency Care and Treatment)	Supports creation of personalised care in advance of medical emergencies Provides information to healthcare professionals in emergency clinical decision making	Summary plan records treatment preferences	Stroke is associated with declining cognition and communication problems ReSPECT aims to support treatment choices when patients do not have capacity through advanced decision making
DNACPR (Do Not Attempt Cardiopulmonary Resuscitation)	Advance decision not to attempt cardiopulmonary resuscitation (CPR) in the event of cardiac arrest or sudden death	Flowchart document and form to record preferred decisions, with supporting guidance	May support clinical decisions of stroke patients facing an uncertain prognosis and prolonged decline, in line with the wishes of the patient
Rapid discharge home	Supports the discharge of patients who wish to die at home where it would not be possible to complete the usual required processes within the timeframe Aims to prevent readmission by ensuring needs are met at home	Document to guide or record areas of care to consider and plans put in place to enable rapid discharge	May enable stroke patients to die at home if they and their family wish, where this would otherwise have not been possible Requires engagement from and coordination of a range of services Management of stroke-related symptoms preceding death and perceived risk of death during transportation may create specific challenges to enabling discharge
SPARC (Sheffield Profile for Assessment and Referral to Care)	Screening tool for referral to specialist palliative care Aims to identify holistic palliative needs of patients	Questionnaire for needs assessment to be completed by the patient or their family	Suitable in identifying palliative care needs in stroke patients [21] Does not provide guidance on how to manage the needs identified

- *Sheffield Profile for Assessment and Referral to Care (SPARC)* [21]. A holistic needs assessment that refers patients who may benefit from additional palliative care. SPARC integrates dimensions of physical symptoms, psychological issues, religious and spiritual issues, independence and activity issues, and family and social issues. This tool has been shown to identify a range of palliative care needs amongst stroke patients.
- *The Best Practice Statement: End-of-Life Care Following Acute Stroke* [54]. The only end of life care guide that specifically addresses stroke. It includes guidance on four areas of palliative care: delivery of stroke services, delivery of care, ethical aspects of care, and family/carer support. It has only been implemented in Scotland, and has not been evaluated. It is also now dated, particularly with regards to recommendations of the use of the LCP.

The use of these tools and approaches within stroke care has not been fully explored. Table 12.1 provides a comparison of palliative care pathways and tools, and a brief consideration of how these may be useful within stroke care.

12.4 Case Studies

Case Studies 12.1–12.3 illustrate how some of these care pathways and tools could be used with stroke patients. We consider how palliative care needs are identified, and the value and limitations of the various tools.

Case Study

Case 12.1 Stella

Stella is admitted to hospital after having a fall and is unable to move her arm. She is 84 years old and lives alone. After initial assessment, doctors are made aware that she has a history of heart disease and is on anticoagulant medication. The doctors suspect a stroke, and a CT scan is ordered. At this stage, Stella is conscious but is unable to communicate verbally. The CT scan confirms that she has suffered an ischaemic stroke. She is transferred to the specialist stroke ward, where she is assessed to have an unsafe swallow.

Stella's daughter arrives later the same day. The doctors take her to a side room and explain that her mother is unable to eat and drink. By this point, Stella is unable to respond to any form of communication and is deemed unable to make treatment decisions. The doctors also advise that she is unlikely to make a full recovery, although they are uncertain of her short-term outcome. Following the Mental Capacity Act [26], Stella's daughter makes decisions on behalf of her mother. After discussions with the doctors, she consents to a PEG tube, which aids Stella in feeding and drinking.

Clinicians consult with the daughter several times regarding the completion of a DNACPR, although she is anxious about the responsibilities she associated with this decision as she has not had any discussions with her mother about her wishes. It is eventually decided that it would be in Stella's best interests to implement the DNACPR. Her daughter states that she does not wish for Stella to stay in hospital; her preferred place of care would be in the community. Acknowledging her high level of care needs, it is decided that a nursing home would be best. A PEG tube is inserted prior to discharge, as this is felt to be a safer, more appropriate longer-term solution to managing her nutritional requirements.

Stella is discharged to a nursing home after several weeks, once a suitable home with a vacancy is identified and the required processes are completed. A few months later, Stella has several further admissions to the hospital with pneumonia and other infections over a period of 3 months. Each time, her prognosis is unclear but she recovers. At the last of these admissions, Stella's condition is judged to have deteriorated considerably, and it is felt that she is likely in her last days of life. She dies in hospital within a week of admission.

Discussion Points

ACP might have helped to guide care decisions; as Stella has an existing serious condition and is of an advanced age there were likely missed opportunities to initiate this. Although a DNACPR is put in place, this is following discussions with her daughter, who assumes this would be her mother's wish. If a RESPECT plan had been completed prior to the stroke, Mrs S's wishes would have been clearer, and her daughter would have been relieved of any uncertainties and anxieties regarding treatment and care preferences. Whilst it is possible to discharge Mrs S to a nursing home in line with the wishes of her daughter, the uncertainty surrounding her prognosis and fluctuating condition, as well as a lack of guidance on care decisions in advance, results in repeated admissions to hospital. ACP, perhaps alongside the use of the GSF, would have facilitated more detailed considerations of palliative care needs and could have been used even after Mrs S was no longer able to communicate. This might have prevented some readmissions and her resultant death in hospital. Whilst the uncertain nature of her prognosis creates challenges in supporting her preferred place of care, if a Rapid Discharge process had been initiated at the point at which it was identified she was in the last days of life, it might have been achievable for her to return to the nursing home and be cared for there.

Case Study

| Case 12.2 | **William** |

William is admitted to hospital after collapsing at home. He is 92 years old and lives with his son. On admission, William has seizures, reduced conscious level, and respiratory secretions. The doctors suspect a stroke and order a CT scan to confirm. The scan shows that he has suffered an intracerebral haemorrhage. At this point, William is unconscious and is transferred to the specialist stroke ward. The doctors discuss with William's son that there are no effective treatment options available. In consultation with his family, a DNACPR order is put in place.

In a further conversation, William's son expresses that his father would not want any life-prolonging treatments. It is agreed that artificial hydration will not commence. William is identified to be in the last days of life based on his unconscious level, the severity of the stroke, and his age. The doctors plan to discuss a preferred place of care with his son the following day. The stroke ward staff manage William's symptoms with intravenous medications and order anticipatory medications. William dies a few hours after being transferred to the stroke ward, with his son by his side.

Discussion Points

The sudden nature of stroke and the associated risk of dying rapidly in this case limited the palliative care tools that could be usefully employed in the short space of time between on-set of stroke and death. Mr W's clinical care is guided by clinical indicators and by his son. However, his preferred place of care is not discussed in sufficient time to explore the possibility of Rapid Discharge home. There doesnot appear to have been an ACP in place; completion of an ACP might have prompted this discussion sooner. Mr W is identified as being in his last days of life; an end of life care pathway might have provided further guidance and supported a more holistic care approach by prompting consideration of a wide range of care and well-being. Although steps are taken to agree on not instigating treatment with the aim of preserving life, these issues do not appear to have been considered in a holistic way, and seem to have had a very clinical focus. The lack of an end of life care pathway or similar tool may suggest that these issues were not considered, or may simply reflect that many areas of practice are undertaken but not documented. The DNACPR provides reassurance to his son that Mr W will not be resuscitated and can die peacefully.

Case Study

Case 12.3   Tony

Tony is 59 years old and lives with his wife. He is admitted to hospital following a sudden weakness and difficulty in walking at home. He has no prior medical conditions and lives a healthy lifestyle. At initial assessment, Tony is unable to speak or swallow and has reduced conscious levels. A CT scan confirms that he has suffered an intracerebral haemorrhage. Clinicians are unsure about his prognosis, and this is communicated to his wife. Tony's condition is monitored closely and a DNACPR order is completed after discussions with his wife.

After 2 days, Tony becomes more alert. He makes attempts at communication by asking for a drink. This indicates to nursing staff that he is improving. The following day, Tony appears to deteriorate again, and following assessment, is treated for pneumonia with antibiotics. Following the course of treatment, Tony is alert and makes attempts at communicating with his family. He is monitored daily and shows signs of improvement. The clinicians update his wife about her husband's condition regularly, although they are unable to provide any certainty regarding his prognosis, in terms of potential quality of life-related outcomes or the risk of dying.

Tony is discharged from hospital, but goes on to have several readmissions due to chest infections. His condition continues to fluctuate over a period of more than 9 months before deteriorating suddenly after a severe heart attack. Taking into account the DNACPR, a decision is made not to attempt to resuscitate, and Tony dies the next day.

Discussion Points

This case demonstrates that cases of sudden, unexpected stroke preclude the prior completion of many palliative care tools and advanced care planning tools. This is especially so in this case, as Tony is relatively young and in good health, with no obvious risk of death to prompt the use of any tools or plans. For Tony, the DNACPR which follows his stroke provides a useful guide to subsequent clinical decision making in a medical emergency, although the RESPECT plan would offer a more thorough consideration. The AMBER care bundle would appear to offer guidance and support care decisions in cases such as Tony's because of its ability to accommodate uncertainty. This would have been helpful here, as it focuses upon treatment with hope of recovery, whilst meeting palliative care needs. A particular strength of the AMBER care bundle is that it requires frequent review of the patient's condition and prognosis in order to inform care decisions, within an overall flexible approach. It would likely be of benefit to employ some other tools alongside the AMBER care bundle; for example, the SPARC tool could have been useful in identifying holistic palliative care needs, although it does not detail how these should be met.

12.5 Discussion: The Value of Existing Palliative Care Approaches and Tools in Meeting the Needs of Stroke Patients and Their Families

The use of care pathways is recommended in stroke care [13, 34]. Tools which guide and support palliative care such as the GSF and AMBER care bundle may be suitable to use with stroke patients who are dying. However, there remains insufficient evaluation of their use in stroke populations in order to fully consider their utility in this context. It is essential that the guidance and tools to support palliative care of stroke patients are sufficiently flexible to accommodate the different trajectories of dying and uncertainties associated with stroke, in addition to enabling the identification and addressing of stroke-specific symptoms.

There is increasing recognition that palliative care is the responsibility of all caregivers [55] and that there cannot be a reliance on specialist palliative care teams to provide or even advise on the care of all end of life patients. We have shown here that stroke presents a range of condition-specific challenges which would be best identified and managed by those who understand stroke best, rather than referring care of those deteriorating or dying on to other care providers once the chances of recovery have diminished.

Whilst it is clear from mortality statistics that palliative care should form core business within stroke care, it remains an underdeveloped area. The underpinning philosophy which guides much stroke research and practice focuses upon recovery and rehabilitation [56]. This appears to be at the cost of enabling holistic consideration of and meeting the needs surrounding palliative care. Evidence presented within this chapter suggests that this is especially the case for those stroke patients who face an uncertain and prolonged dying process, which is often accompanied by distressing symptoms.

Whilst there has been recognition within stroke teams for some time of the need for palliative care to be a key component of stroke care [33], this is yet to be achieved. For palliative care in stroke to be further developed, stroke specialists must embrace their role in this regard and invest in the development of their staff and in further research to inform related strategies and interventions. Previous authors have described the need for greater integration of stroke and palliative care amongst professionals [4, 14], we suggest here that there is a need for stroke care providers to be upskilled to be able to deliver this key element of care as part of their everyday role, supported through specialised palliative care teams in cases which present particular complexity. However, it is unclear how many people who die from stroke are not cared for by a specialised stroke team, and thus further consideration must be given to how the needs of these people can also be met if they are not to be disadvantaged in the care they receive.

In terms of workforce skill development, stroke specialists will require training and development on all aspects of palliative care to manage care for these patients. However, there is no specific or mandatory training for stroke specialists on palliative care. There are elements and modules in two widely available online training resources which relate specifically to palliative care. The Stroke-Specific Education Framework (SSEF, www.stroke-education.org.uk) relates to quality markers outlined in the UK National Stroke Strategy [57]. It includes elements (detailed throughout this chapter) that reflect the knowledge, understanding, skills, and abilities in palliative care that are required by staff to care for people with stroke who require palliative care. This resource is available free to anyone working in stroke. There is also a module on palliative care available for staff to complete on the Stroke Training and Awareness Resources (STARS) Web site (www.strokeadvancingmodules.org). This provides knowledge and skills on care in the last days of life, with guidance on ethical and legal aspects, symptom management, communication, and decision-making processes.

Despite the availability of such resources, we have shown within this chapter an obvious need for further training on palliative care within stroke. Several barriers exist within healthcare, in terms of awareness and knowledge, motivation, practicalities, acceptance and belief, and skills [58]. Each of these barriers must be addressed to bring about real change in the delivery of palliative care in stroke.

12.5.1 Development of Palliative Care in Stroke

Work must be done in the following areas in order to inform the development and implementation of stroke-specific approaches to the delivery of palliative care:

- map current use of existing palliative care approaches and tools (such as the GSF and AMBER care bundle) in stroke;
- explore and assess the utility and limitations of existing palliative care approaches;
- identify and refine the further research that will be required to inform the development of stroke-specific palliative care approaches and implementation; and
- engage in workforce development to enable healthcare staff to provide appropriate palliative care which meets the needs of stroke patients and their families.

12.6 Conclusion

Stroke presents unique challenges in the context of palliative care, and specific guidance is required in order to identify and meet the needs of this population. Given the lack of existing evidence on which to base such guidance, or any interventions, a considerable amount of work is still to be done. This will require commitment and investment from stroke care specialists, as well as the research community, wider healthcare systems, and policy-makers. The successful integration of palliative care approaches within stroke care depends on developing the skills and expertise of stroke specialists and altering mind-sets and conceptualisations regarding what stroke care involves.

Meeting the palliative care needs of stroke patients and their families will require a more holistic approach to the needs of the patient. This will include patient assessment, psychological support, care planning, and symptom control [4]. Although previous considerations of how best to integrate palliative care within stroke presented a great deal of uncertainty [27], we have identified within this chapter a consideration of the utility and possibilities offered by existing approaches, and offered a range of suggestions to drive forward the much-needed developments to firmly embed palliative care within the role and psyche of stroke care professionals. This is set within and contributes towards the wider policy and strategy context of the development of a range of disease-specific palliative care guidelines [7].

References

1. UK Stroke Forum Education & Training. About the SSEF. Available from: http://www.stroke-education.org.uk/about [30 November 2018].
2. Stroke Association (2017). State of the Nation. London: Stroke Association.
3. Katzan, I.L., Spertus, J., Bettger, J.P. et al. (2014). Risk adjustment of ischemic stroke outcomes for comparing hospital performance: a statement for healthcare professionals from the American Heart Association/American Stroke Association. Stroke 45 (3): 918–944.
4. Burton, C.R. and Payne, S. (2012). Integrating palliative care within acute stroke services: developing a programme theory of patient and family needs, preferences and staff perspectives. British Medical Journal Palliative Care 11 (1): 22.
5. Traue, D. and Ross, J. (2005). Palliative care in non-malignant diseases. Journal of the Royal Society of Medicine 98 (11): 503–506.
6. House of Commons Health Committee (2015). End of Life Care. London: The Stationery Office.
7. Marie Curie (2015). Triggers for Palliative Care. London: Marie Curie.
8. World Health Organization. WHO definition of paliative care. Available from: http://www.who.int/cancer/palliative/definition/en [30 November 2018].
9. Sepulveda, C., Marlin, A., Yoshida, T., and Ullrich, A. (2002). Palliative care: the World Health Organization's global perspective. Journal of Pain and Symptom Management 24 (2): 91–96.
10. National Council for Hospice and Specialist Palliative Care Services (2002). Definitions of Supportive and Palliative Care. London: National Council for Hospice and Specialist Care Services.

11. The National Council for Palliative Care (2006). End of Life Care Strategy. London: The National Council for Palliative Care.

12. National Institute for Health and Care Excellence (2017). Care of Dying Adults in the Last Days of Life Quality Standard [QS144]. London: National Institute for Health and Care Excellence.

13. Cowey, E., Smith, L.N., Stott, D.J. et al. (2015). Impact of a clinical pathway on end-of-life care following stroke. Palliative Medicine 29 (3): 249–259.

14. Gardiner, C., Harrison, M., Ryan, T., and Jones, A. (2013). Provision of palliative and end-of-life care in stroke units: a qualitative study. Palliative Medicine 27 (9): 855–860.

15. Neuberger, J., Guthrie, C., Aarononvitch, D. et al. (2013). More Care, Less Pathway: A Review of the Liverpool Care Pathway. Liverpool: Independent Review of the Liverpool Pathway.

16. Payne, S., Burton, C.R., Addington-Hall, J., and Jones, A. (2010). End-of-life issues in acute stroke care: a qualitative study of the experiences and preferences of patients and families. Palliative Medicine 24 (2): 146–153.

17. Creutzfeldt, C.J., Holloway, R.G., and Curtis, J.R. (2015). Palliative care: a core competency for stroke neurologists. Stroke 46 (9): 2714–2719.

18. Alonso, A., Ebert, A.D., Dörr, D. et al. (2016). End-of-life decisions in acute stroke patients: an observational cohort study. British Medcial Council Palliative Care 15 (1): 38.

19. Burton, C.R., Payne, S., Turner, M. et al. (2014). The study protocol of 'initiating end of life care in stroke: clinical decision-making around prognosis'. British Medical Council Palliative Care 13 (1): 55.

20. Creutzfeldt, C.J., Holloway, R.G., and Walker, M. (2012). Symptomatic and palliative care for stroke survivors. Journal of General Internal Medicine 27 (7): 853–860.

21. Burton, C.R., Payne, S., Addington-Hall, J., and Jones, A. (2010). The palliative care needs of acute stroke patients: a prospective study of hospital admissions. Age and Ageing 39 (5): 554–559.

22. de Boer, M.E., Depla, M., Wojtkowiak, J. et al. (2015). Life-and-death decision-making in the acute phase after a severe stroke: interviews with relatives. Palliative Medicine 29 (5): 451–457.

23. Simon, J. (2018). Who needs palliative care? Canadian Medical Association Journal 190 (9): E234–E235.

24. Eriksson, H., Andersson, G., Olsson, L. et al. (2014). Ethical dilemmas around the dying patient with stroke: a qualitative interview study with team members on stroke units in Sweden. Journal of Neuroscience Nursing 46 (3): 162–170.

25. Holloway, R.G., Ladwig, S., Robb, J. et al. (2010). Palliative care consultations in hospitalized stroke patients. Journal of Palliative Medicine 13 (4): 407–412.

26. Mental Capacity Act. Chapter 9: Persons Who Lack Capacity. London: The Stationery Office; 2005.

27. Wee, B., Adams, A., and Eva, G. (2010). Palliative and end-of-life care for people with stroke. Current Opinion in Supportive and Palliative Care 4 (4): 229–232.

28. Eriksson, H., Milberg, A., Hjelm, K., and Friedrichsen, M. (2016). End of life care for patients dying of stroke: a comparative registry study of stroke and cancer. PLoS One 11 (2): 1–10.

29. Mazzocato, C., Michel-Nemitz, J., Anwar, D., and Michel, P. (2010). The last days of dying stroke patients referred to a palliative care consult team in an acute hospital. European Journal of Neurology 17 (1): 73–77.

30. Ntlholang, O., Walsh, S., Bradley, D., and Harbison, J. (2016). Identifying palliative care issues in inpatients dying following stroke. Irish Journal of Medical Science 185 (3): 741–744.

31. Blacquiere, D., Bhimji, K., Meggison, H. et al. (2013). Satisfaction with palliative care after stroke: a prospective cohort study. Stroke 44 (9): 2617–2619.

32. Intercollegiate Stroke Working Party (2016). National Clinical Guideline for Stroke, 5e. London: Royal College of Physicians.

33. Holloway, R.G., Arnold, R.M., Creutzfeldt, C.J. et al. (2014). Palliative and end-of-life care in stroke: a statement for healthcare professionals from the American Heart Association/American Stroke Association. Stroke 45 (6): 1887–1916.

34. Stroke Foundation (2017). Clinical Guidelines for Stroke Management. Melbourne: Melbourne Stroke Foundation.

35. Campbell, H., Hotchkiss, R., Bradshaw, N., and Porteous, M. (1998). Integrated care pathways. British Medical Journal 316 (7125): 133–137.

36. Chan, R.J., Webster, J., and Bowers, A. (2016). End-of-life care pathways for improving outcomes in caring for the dying. Cochrane Database of Systematic Reviews 2 (Art. No.: CD008006). https://doi.org/10.1002/14651858.CD008006.pub2.

37. Ellershaw, J., Smith, C., Overill, S. et al. (2001). Care of the dying: setting standards for symptom control in the last 48 hours of life. Journal of Pain Symptom Manage 21 (1): 12–17.

38. The Gold Standards Framework Centre in End of Life Care. Available from: http://www.goldstandardsframework.org.uk [30 November 2018].

39. Carey, I., Shouls, S., Bristowe, K. et al. (2015). Improving care for patients whose recovery is uncertain. The AMBER care bundle: design and implementation. British Medical Journal Supportive & Palliative Care 5 (4): 405–411.

40. Cauldwell, K. and Stone, P. (2015). The changing nature of end of life care. Indian Journal of Medical and Paediatric Oncology 36 (2): 94.

41. Veerbeek, L., van Zuylen, L., Swart, S.J. et al. (2008). The effect of the Liverpool Care Pathway for the dying: a multi-centre study. Palliative Medicine 22 (2): 145–151.

42. Jack, C., Jones, L., Jack, B.A. et al. (2004). Towards a good death: the impact of the care of the dying pathway in an acute stroke unit. Age and Ageing 33 (6): 625–626.

43. The Gold Standards Framework Centre in End of Life Care. The GSF Proactive Identification Guidance. Shrewsbury: The Gold Standards Framework Centre in End of Life Care; 2016.

44. Thomas K, Armstrong Wilson JA, Tanner T, National Gold Standards Framework Centre. Evidence that Use of Gold Standards Framework Improves Early Identification of Patients in Different Settings. London: National Gold Standards Framework Centre; 2016.

45. Quinn, B. and Thomas, K. (2017). Using the Gold Standards Framework to deliver good end of life care. Nursing Management 23 (10): 20–25.

46. Guy's and St Thomas' NHS Foundation Trust. The AMBER Care Bundle – A Guide for Patients, their Relatives and Carers. London: Guy's and St Thomas' NHS Foundation Trust; 2015.

47. Bristowe, K., Carey, I., Hopper, A. et al. (2015). Patient and carer experiences of clinical uncertainty and deterioration, in the face of limited reversibility: a comparative observational study of the AMBER care bundle. Palliative Medicine 29 (9): 797–807.

48. Leadership Alliance for the Care of Dying People (2014). Once Chance to Get it Right: Improving People's Experience of Care in the Last Few Days and Hours of Life. London: Royal College of Physicians.

49. Department of Health NHS End of Life Care Programme (2008). Advance Care Planning: A Guide for Health and Social Care Staff. Leicester: Department of Health.

50. National End of Life Care Programme. Preferred Priorities of Care. London: National End of Life Care Programme; 2011.

51. NHS Improving Quality (2013). Economic Evaluation of Electronic Palliative Care Co-ordination Systems (EPaCCS) Early Implementer Sites. London: NHS Improving Quality.

52. Fritz, Z., Slowther, A.-M., and Perkins, G.D. (2017). Resuscitation policy should focus on the patient, not the decision. British Medical Journal 356 (j813): 1–16.

53. Montgomery, E. and Whitfield, A. (2012). Rapid discharge at end of life-shared experience from an acute trust [poster presenation]. British Medical Journal Supportive & Palliative Care 2 (Suppl. 1): Poster no. 123.
54. NHS Quality Improvement Scotland, University of Glasgow (2010). Best Practice Statement: End of Life Care Following Acute Stroke. Edinburgh: NHS Quality Improvement Scotland.
55. NHS England. Ambitions for palliative and end of life care. Available from: http://endoflifecareambitions.org.uk/ [30 November 2018].
56. Williams, J., Perry, L., and Watkins, C. (2010). Acute Stroke Nursing. Chichester: Wiley-Blackwell.
57. Department of Health (2007). National Stroke Strategy. London: Department of Health.
58. National Institute for Health and Clinical Excellence (2007). How to Change Practice: Understand, Identify and Overcome Barriers to Change. London: National Institute for Health and Clinical Excellence.

CHAPTER 13

Minimally Responsive Stroke Patients

Elaine Pierce
Independent Lecturer and Researcher

KEY POINTS

- This small group of stroke survivors presents numerous and varied challenges for nurses and the multidisciplinary team (MDT).
- Their high level of dependence and 24/7 needs mean nursing makes a unique contribution to their management and care.
- Irrespective of patients' level of response, their needs should be identified and appropriate rehabilitation provided.
- Privacy, dignity, confidentiality, and fundamental rights should be observed.
- Values, beliefs, and previous wishes should be respected, and relatives and carers should be kept informed, involved in decisions, and supported emotionally.

This chapter maps to criteria within the following sections of the Stroke-Specific Education Framework (SSEF):

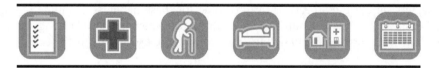

You can bury a son and then move on. You never forget it, but at least he's at peace. But to actually see him go through what he's still going through ... It's so cruel [2]

Stroke Nursing, Second Edition. Edited by Jane Williams, Lin Perry, and Caroline Watkins.
© 2020 John Wiley & Sons Ltd. Published 2020 by John Wiley & Sons Ltd.

13.1 Introduction

Advances in medicine mean that increasing numbers of people survive stroke. However, stroke remains a disease with high levels of enduring disability amongst survivors. This chapter groups together the very small number who survive with prolonged disorder of consciousness (PDoC) such as coma, the vegetative state (VS), and the minimally conscious state (MCS) under the umbrella of the minimally responsive stroke patient. Patients can move from one state to another, or may remain in one state for a considerable period of time. A further minority will survive in a locked-in state, with cognition retained but lacking the physical functional abilities allowing movement and communication. For the locked-in syndrome at least, there is some insight into the patient's experience. This is depicted as traumatic, distressing, depressing, and deeply frustrating by Jean-Dominique Bauby (1997), the editor of the French journal *ELLE*, who experienced it in 1995 [3]. Locked-in syndrome is not a disorder of consciousness, but will also be discussed under the minimally responsive stroke umbrella, because of these individuals' physical limitations.

The language of this field can be emotive and challenging [4]. The term PDoC is used until the patient is formally diagnosed as in a VS, MCS, or locked-in state. The term VS is controversial, with some carers finding it unacceptable, but others finding it helpful in understanding that their loved one is unaware and not suffering. These terms will continue to be used until such time as others are agreed upon and adopted internationally [5].

Patients with PDoC and locked-in syndrome are totally dependent for all their daily needs. It is therefore essential that the multidisciplinary team (MDT), families, partners, friends, and informal carers (hereafter referred to as 'carers') involved all have a good understanding of these conditions and what care is required. These patients and their carers are highly vulnerable and face numerous challenges, given that these conditions are not easy to correctly identify or make prognostic judgements about [6], and are allied with high levels of dependence upon all healthcare services.

This chapter details the pathophysiology, aetiology, presentation, and management of VS and MCS associated with stroke. Two case examples illustrate the treatment and care required for key elements of long-term rehabilitation; other chapters set out the aspects of care required for these patients in common with other stroke patients (e.g. nutrition and hydration, bladder and bowel management, mobility, and moving and handling). Pseudonyms are used for the patients.

13.2 Definitions

Definitions of these states have been established (see Box 13.1). Correctly identifying whether a patient is in coma, VS, MCS, or a locked-in state may not be easy. Misdiagnosis of disorders of consciousness is problematic; up to 43% of VS diagnosed patients are later reclassified with MCS [7]. Misdiagnosis can be a result either of diagnostic error or of a change in the patient's state over time [5, 8].

Consciousness means being in a state of awareness of one's self and the environment, and being responsive to it. Other people can only recognise

---

Box 13.1 | **Definition of Terms**

Coma. A state of presumed profound unconsciousness from which the person: cannot be roused; does not respond to stimuli, including pain; and does not have a normal sleep–wake cycle. It is not usually of a prolonged duration. Coma is not brain death: some brain function remains, and some or all may be recoverable [5]. Coma is not covered in this chapter.

Vegetative state (VS). Can be described as wakefulness without awareness, as there is no environmental awareness or purposeful movement. Patients have a sleep–wake cycle and may respond to stimulation with reflex and spontaneous behaviours such as grasping and grimacing [5].

Minimally conscious state (MCS). Can be described as wakefulness with minimal awareness. There is a wide range of responses, with discernible but inconsistent evidence of consciousness. Cognitively mediated behaviour occurs often enough or for long enough to distinguish it from reflex behaviour; the more complex the response, the easier it is to make this distinction. Responses may vary in patients, and range from a few non-reflex movements to smiling, crying, laughing in response to emotional stimuli, verbalising, and using objects (e.g. a comb) in a meaningful manner. In MCS, the responses do not indicate a capacity for decision making [9].

Locked-in syndrome. Quite distinct from VS and MCS. The patient is aware and awake, but cannot move or communicate due to complete paralysis of nearly all voluntary muscles in the body. It is the result of a brainstem lesion such as a stroke at the level of the basilar artery causing damage to the pons. The term was coined in 1966 [10], and the condition is also referred to as cerebromedullospinal disconnection, de-efferent state, pseudo-coma, and ventral pontine syndrome.

---

consciousness through a person's behaviour. There is no definitive diagnostic test for lack of consciousness; it can only be identified through lack of behaviour that positively indicates consciousness. Patients can remain in VS or MCS for many years or decades. VS becomes described as permanent when it has persisted for more than 1 year post traumatic brain injury or more than 6 months after other brain injury, such as stroke. MCS lasting for more than 4 weeks is classified as continuing MCS [5].

13.3 Assessment and Diagnosis

Initial steps in diagnosis entail establishing causation of the disorder of consciousness and excluding any persisting effect of anaesthesia, drugs, or metabolic disturbance. The possibility of treatable structural causes should be excluded by brain imaging. The criteria for the substantially reduced or lack of consciousness include:

- no evidence of awareness of self or environment;
- no response to visual, auditory, tactile, or other stimuli suggesting conscious purpose;
- no use of language comprehension or meaningful expression;
- an apparent sleep–wake cycle; and
- continuing hypothalamic and brainstem function, ensuring respiration and circulation [5, 11].

Any purposeful movement or evidence of communication or awareness indicates that the patient does not have a disorder of consciousness. Differentiation of VS, MCS, and locked-in syndrome can take time. Repeated observations and evaluation by specialist doctors and the MDT determine whether a simple movement (e.g. finger movement, eye blink, eye movement) seen occasionally is reflexive, simply coincidental, or actually a response to a stimulus such as a command to move the fingers. By contrast, a complex response such as an intelligible word, heard only a few times, may make it clear that the person is conscious. There may be a lag time between the stimulus and the response, further confusing the picture. All assessments must allow sufficient time to be sure whether or not a response was initiated. In locked-in syndrome, the ability to respond is minimal, due to extensive motor paralysis. Detailed assessment is required to identify residual motor function and how best to use this to achieve communication. Accuracy of assessment, management, and, consequently, appropriateness of care depends on understanding and using the correct terminology and applying appropriate training and skills. This will facilitate the tailoring of care to the individual's needs via the combined efforts of the MDT. The MDT should focus on the benefits and effects of assessment, management, and care for the individual and their carers, both in the present and in the longer term [12].

The role of nurses in the assessment process for PDoC in stroke is described briefly. Nurses are involved in, and contribute to, many aspects of assessment, management, and healthcare scenarios (Figure 13.1), including medical support and therapies, as well as nursing activities.

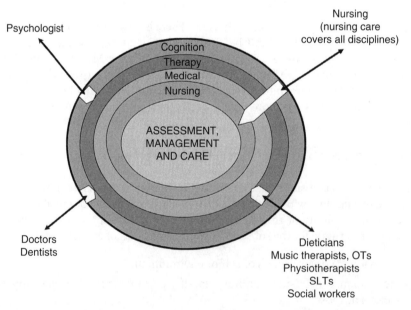

FIGURE 13.1 Staff involved in the assessment and care of minimally conscious state (MCS) individuals: nurses, doctors, dentists, dieticians, music therapists, occupational therapists (OTs), physiotherapists, psychologists, social workers, and speech and language therapists (SLTs).

13.3.1 Prerequisites to Assessment

For individuals who have severe and complex neurodisability, the main reasons for assessment are to identify problems, collect information about what they can or cannot do, and identify how well they can perform a task. Additionally, assessment will show how much of a task they can successfully achieve and the level of support (physical or verbal) they need. With a person who has MCS, the consideration is how and what information can be obtained (e.g. from observations, history, other healthcare professionals, and relatives) in order to prioritise, plan, implement, and evaluate care. In sharing and gathering information, carers should also be assessed, for example in relation to their psychological state. The medical and emotional state of carers is as important as that of the patient. Carers experience a wide variety of psychological reactions and states in response to their family members' circumstances, even without breeching what might be considered 'normal' for the situation [2]. The stress experienced by carers needs to be assessed, because they may require support and professional intervention.

Some important aspects to consider prior to assessment are:

- *Medical stability*. Fitness to be assessed, due to, for example, abnormal nutritional status such as dehydration or malnourishment.
- *Suitability of the environment*. Noise or other distractions could impact the patient's attention.
- *Temperature*. Too hot or too cold could affect how the patient responds.
- *Timing of the assessment*. Preferably, undertaken after the patient has rested (e.g. the patient may be too exhausted to respond after a therapy session).
- *Attributes of the assessor*. This will facilitate correct completion of the assessment and help ascertain the best responses from the patient. See Box 13.2.

Activities should consider cultural and language factors for patients and relatives, especially those of black and minority, culturally and linguistically distinctive ethnic groups.

For people with PDoC referred from acute to specialist stroke rehabilitation units or continuing care institutions, a nursing pre-assessment before arrival may be necessary. Such an assessment typically covers breathing, nutrition, personal care, continence, mobility, communication, orientation, skin integrity, sleeping, medication, motivation, wounds, and behaviours (day and night). A pre-admission meeting with carers for the purpose of introduction and orientation to the services and staff may be beneficial.

13.3.2 Assessment

The preceding considerations are important if the assessment is to be accurate and successful. Many assessments are also utilised in goal setting and for the delivery of care of patients. Assessments should be given priority by all members of the MDT, because findings are crucial for accurate diagnosis and for individual management of disability after the event [13]. Assessment of quality of life should be included amongst standard assessments leading to clinical decisions [14].

Box 13.2 | Attributes of the Assessor

Knowledge and Skills
Have knowledge and skills in dealing with people in MCS and their carers.

Training and Experience
Have training and the experience required to conduct the assessment.

Approach
Be very clear in your approach. The language used should be simple, the stimuli appropriate.

Positioning the patient
Ascertain the best position for the patient in order to obtain the relevant responses. For example, it may be better for the patient to be upright in bed or in a chair rather than lying flat. The patient should be comfortable.

Observation
Be alert to the fact that the patient may be more aware than was first thought. Observe the patient for tiredness, which will affect their responses.

Correct tool
Use the tool or instrument agreed upon by the MDT.

Consistency and limitations
Be consistent and realise the limitations of the patient and of yourself.

Initial assessments should be comprehensive and include a full neurological assessment [15]. UK national stroke guidelines [16] stipulate early (within the first 4 hours) assessment using physical and diagnostic tests for brain injury; swallow function; immediate needs in relation to positioning, mobilisation, moving, and handling; bladder and bowel control; risk of developing skin pressure ulcers; capacity to understand and follow instructions; capacity to communicate needs and wishes; sensory factors (sight and hearing); and nutritional status.

Subsequent assessments should also address motor control and tone, sensation, pain, depression, anxiety and emotionalism, and spatial and perceptual awareness. Oral health, abnormal oral reflexes, and lip biting should be assessed [17]. The purpose of these assessments is to:

- ascertain the arousal levels of the person with PDoC;
- describe their and their carers' actual and potential problems;
- set achievable goals, including the timeframe (it is recommended that goals are agreed and documented by the MDT within 5 days [16]); and
- provide a baseline by which to monitor the person with MCS for changes in condition or management, care, and interventions.

The frequency of assessment depends on the result of the evaluation of each goal set (see Chapter 14). Assessments may need to be repeated: assessors should use their professional judgement as to whether an assessment is necessary and whether the person with PDoC/MCS is medically stable and fit. Assessors should exercise caution to ensure that assessments do not become onerous or burdensome. Clinical assessment is a continuous process, and nurses are crucial to it, since they are in a position to observe patients continuously (e.g. for restlessness and arousal levels) and to monitor changes in behaviour and response. Nurse reporting and communication processes should be standardised, and findings should be shared between and across all members of the MDT [18, 19].

13.3.3 Tools and Measures Used in Assessment, Management, and Care

Tools used should have been tried and tested, and their results must be capable of being used to improve care and patient outcomes [14]. Ideally, tools should be used in specialist centres where staff have been trained in, and are familiar with, their use.

Multidisciplinary rehabilitation programmes utilise a wide range of measures, some of which are discussed in other chapters of this book. Although assessment tools differ, they also have commonalities, for example:

- most require assessment by the MDT;
- several include interviewing the carers, whose input can be invaluable;
- they need to be completed and re-evaluated on a regular basis; and
- the assessment involves stimulating some or all of the senses.

Many commonly used tools, such as the Functional Independence Measure, the Disability Rating Scale, the Rancho Los Amigos Levels of Cognitive Function Scale, the Barthel Index, the Lowenstein Communication Scale, and the Wessex Head Injury Matrix, include aspects of arousal and functional motor, auditory, visual, and communication skills, and are useful in assessing change in responses over time [20–22]. A number of tools have been developed specifically for those with very severe disability or PDoC, such as the:

- **P**utney **A**uditory **C**omprehension **S**creening **T**est (PACST) [23];
- **Mu**sic therapy **A**ssessment **T**ool for Patients in **L**ow-**A**wareness **S**tates (MATLAS) [24];
- **S**ensory **M**odality **A**ssessment **R**ehabilitation **T**echnique (SMART) [25];
- **P**utney **A**uditory **S**ingle **Word** Yes/No Assessment (PASWORD) [26]; and
- **M**ultidisciplinary **E**valuation of **N**euro-**D**ependency (MEND) [27].

The choice of tool depends on its purpose: for example, an assessment tool such as the SMART might be used to assess sense of hearing (and the other senses) alongside the MATLAS, where there is a subtle use of hearing components to assess response and changes in arousal levels to music or music therapy [21].

13.3.4 What Makes a Good Assessment?

Tools used must be based on sound methods, use valid (measure what they purport) and reliable (stable, replicable) approaches, and provide relevant results for the specific patient population [14]. For this patient group, it is particularly important that assessment tools are sensitive enough to detect small increments of change. Simultaneously, tools must not impose unnecessary burden on patients, who are often susceptible to fatigue: they must include only essential items. The balance between the sensitivity and specificity (ability to achieve its purpose with minimal false-positive and false-negative findings) of each tool is complicated by the threshold of tolerance of assessment amongst these patients, which affects the feasibility of the tool's assessment, and its acceptability for all involved. Tools and measures must be user-friendly, easy to complete and interpret, and capable of being completed within a specified (short) time period.

Some assessment tools have ceiling or floor effects, which means that they are not sensitive enough to detect all ranges of change and response, and fail at the extremes of high (ceiling) and, particularly for this group, low (floor) responses. The choice of tools should be agreed within the MDT. The purpose of assessment should dictate which tool is used; the results should inform management and care, which can then be evaluated against assessment outcomes. Tools should be used as an adjunct to rather than a replacement for thorough assessment and clinical judgement.

The responses of someone with MCS may fluctuate and be inconsistent, and it is necessary to be cautious with initial findings and repeat assessments.

13.4 Management and Care

13.4.1 Decision Making

Every individual has the right to make decisions about his or her own treatment and care, but people with MCS are not able to do so. This requires determination of:

- Who holds responsibility for decisions, how that person is appointed, and the nature and limits of their responsibility.
- The role of any previously expressed wishes of the person with MCS. These may have been documented in a non-specific way that guides rather than directs; have been documented formally and specifically; have been expressed informally by others to whom the person had previously made known his or her wishes; or constructed hypothetically based on what others believe the person would have wished.
- The exercise of the professional duty of care of the relevant healthcare professionals [28].

For certain decisions, for a person who lacks capacity and has no one to make decisions on his or her behalf, UK legislation facilitates appointment of an Independent Mental Capacity Advocate [5]. Other countries have similar provisions; for example, Australia has state-based legislation related to guardianship and power of attorney.

With regard to withholding and withdrawal of treatment, formal and informal carers may experience ethical challenges and dilemmas [29]. Few people make their wishes known in an advance statement or advance care plan. The UK

Parliamentary Office of Science and Technology [9] cites judgements and rulings by the courts, including the House of Lords, on the lawfulness of such plans, since the Mental Capacity Act (2005) directs doctors to act in the best interests (medical, welfare, and other) of their patients. Nurses should ensure that they are acquainted with the law of the country in which they practice.

MDT members should take account of one another's findings and adopt a unified, team approach to management and care. Barriers between professional groups, and between staff and patients, can be avoided through awareness of approach, body language, attitude, verbal language, tone, and pace, whether communicating or delivering care. Something as simple as the unnecessary wearing of gloves may present a psychological barrier. This awareness also relates to carers, as previous experiences with professionals and particular assumptions or prejudices may colour attitudes necessitating sensitive handling.

13.4.2 Planning Care

The management of patients with MCS comprises supportive care, rehabilitation, and use of assistive devices. Whilst there is some evidence from other neurological disorders in support of the use of novel treatments, such as repetitive transcranial magnetic stimulation (rTMS), to date no benefit has been demonstrated for patients with MCS [30].

High-quality nursing care [27] is needed to minimise the risks of complications, as detailed throughout this book. In the short term, it is good medical practice to provide artificial nutrition and hydration to sustain any patient whose prognosis is uncertain. Medical treatments, including artificial nutrition and hydration, may be withdrawn later if they are considered futile [11]. Futility of treatment can be demonstrated based on establishment of clear goals prior to commencement of treatment. Case Study 13.1 illustrates selected aspects of patient care during the acute stage.

When planning care programmes, it is important to consider the balance of benefit versus burden from all treatments and interventions. Benefits of treatment might include:

- slowing the progress of disease;
- sustaining the patient's life;
- reducing disability and improving health; and
- relieving distress or discomfort [28].

Burdens of treatment include distress and suffering to the patient, their carers, and the wider community. Treatments may be considered overly burdensome if they are disproportionate to the likely benefits. Burden can derive from the risky, intrusive, destructive, exhausting, painful, or repugnant nature of a treatment, or from low benefit.

Management should include strategies to deal with:

- neurological status and general arousal levels [27];
- sensory stimuli and responses (touch, taste, smell, sound) [25];
- attempts to speak, eye contact, and visual tracking;

Case Study

Case 13.1	Harry

Harry, a 75-year-old retired man, lives with his wife. He suffers a subarachnoid haemorrhage (SAH) as the result of a ruptured aneurysm. Treatment by coiling is unsuccessful, so the neurosurgical team proceeds to clip the aneurysm. In the weeks following neurosurgery, Harry suffers complications, one of which is severe vasospasm, where the blood vessels in the brain spasm and constrict, resulting in ischaemia of the brain tissue. Harry also develops respiratory complications necessitating a 2 week stay in the neurointensive care unit (neuro-ICU), during which time he is sedated, intubated, and ventilated. When the sedation is withdrawn, the team notes that Harry is slow to wake, showing right sided hemiplegia and localising to the left only.

After discharge from the neuro-ICU, Harry's level of arousal improves. He demonstrates a defined sleep–wake pattern, but does not demonstrate any purposeful or intentional behaviours or any awareness of his environment. On one occasion, nursing staff report that Harry has spoken to them, saying 'Yes please' in response to the question, 'Would you like to be washed?' This is the only communication and indication that Harry has an awareness of his surroundings.

The MDT begins the Wessex Head Injury Matrix (WHIM) assessment [22]: a behavioural observation check list that allows for a systematic approach to the observation and recording of responses that can occur in disorders of consciousness. It can facilitate the prompt identification of any improvement or deterioration in a patient's level of consciousness. At the point of transfer to the rehabilitation unit, Harry is scoring 10 as the most advanced behaviour, which is defined as an 'expletive utterance'. This refers to the one occasion of spontaneous verbal communication he has demonstrated.

Due to Harry's low level of awareness, a swallow assessment has not been conducted. Nutrition and hydration are provided via a nasogastric tube, but given the limited progress in awareness, a percutaneous endoscopic gastrostomy (PEG) tube is inserted just before transfer to the rehabilitation unit.

- Management should include strategies to deal with;
- use of assistive technology [31, 32];
- sleep disturbances [33];
- following commands;
- social behaviours (dis-inhibition); and
- maintenance or regaining of movement of joints (e.g. splinting for contractures, postural tremor, clawed toes).

An intensive rehabilitation programme should be pursued for all patients with MCS, incorporating goal setting and regular reviews. This should involve all specialities and carers, since management and care cannot be provided in isolation. The MDT leader should plan and coordinate care tailored to the individual's needs. This might involve using evidence-based protocols with individualised modifications. Management should at all times utilise the best available evidence, including expert advice, to maximise prospects for recovery through MDT and carer goal setting. This does not prevent inclusion of other disciplines that might use their own assessments, as long as this occurs within a coordinated approach and with the full cooperation of the patient, their carers, and the MDT. Chapter 9 gives more detail on the goal-setting process.

Communication is the key to good planning, management, and care. The person with MCS may not be able to hold a conversation, but that should not stop MDT team members from informing them, seeking their consent for each procedure, or even obtaining their permission before entering their room. Withholding what may appear to be irrelevant information can lead to carer stress. For example, one patient's partner was observed becoming upset on finding that a change in management had been introduced since the last visit because they believed every change was for the worse. Education of carers as to the patient's condition, what to observe, and ways in which they can assist should enhance their understanding, lessen their fear and stress levels, and encourage them to provide information through their observations. Carers' observations reinforce or supplement staff observations and provide information on new areas of management and care for consideration. Good communication also creates a sense of trust between the carers and the MDT, especially the nurses.

13.4.3 Monitoring and Evaluating Care

Consciousness can only be inferred from behaviour, and this can be problematic for clinicians. Advances such as neuroimaging may prove to be more enlightening [34]. Most people with MCS are incapable of complex behaviours. If, when asked to obey simple commands like closing their eyes, a blink follows a few seconds later, it may be unclear as to whether this is a response to the command or whether the blink was a reflex action. Staff may miss or misinterpret changes in response which, despite increases in consistency, at first look random or coincidental. This occurs especially in staff new to the speciality, who lack knowledge and skills in assessment of this patient group, and in those who spend brief periods of time delivering care or who evaluate only during ward rounds. It may be necessary to be inventive and use props or markers to ensure a response is consistent and reliable. For example, marking tape placed a short distance in front of the foot of a person with MCS will show that they are making a positive response if they kick their toe beyond the tape. Since responses in people with MCS can be erratic, the MDT should not dismiss reports of changes observed by carers. Any reported change should be followed by careful observation for consistency and managed to facilitate improvement of the patient.

It is pointless asking people with MCS to follow commands which, because of limitations such as sensory, motor, or cognitive impairments (hearing, language processing, paralysis), they are unable to perform. Repeatedly asking someone to squeeze an assessor's hand, for example, may result in an intermittent random behaviour or a grasp reflex. Being able to follow a command is one of the important factors in distinguishing patients in VS from those with MCS, and misdiagnosis of VS has been reported [6, 7, 35]. Much is dependent on the nurse's assessment, implementation, monitoring, and evaluation of care.

Finally, because people may emerge from MCS, long-term effects should be borne in mind [12, 36]. Good nursing care, implemented, monitored, and evaluated in such a way as to avoid complications (e.g. bowel and bladder problems, pulmonary infections, electrolyte and liver function imbalance, seizures and dystonia), optimises quality of life, whatever degree of recovery and rehabilitation may be achieved [37, 38]. Case Study 13.2 continues to illustrate selected aspects of care of a patient with MCS in a rehabilitation unit.

Case Study

Case 13.2   Harry (Cont.)

Harry's wife is very anxious about the transfer from the acute hospital to the rehabilitation setting, as she has got to know many of the staff well. In the rehabilitation unit, she is encouraged to bring Harry's own clothes and personal items for his bed space. Over the next few days, the members of the MDT introduce themselves to Harry, his wife, and his children. Orientation to the hospital is given alongside the welcome booklet.

An initial part of Harry's rehabilitation involves asking the family to complete a communication and lifestyle questionnaire; this is done face to face with Harry's wife by the speech and language therapist (SLT), Harry's key worker. This personal information contributes to Harry's assessment and treatment planning. Assessment for appropriate seating and building up seating tolerance are priorities. Assessment of awareness can then begin.

The occupational therapist (OT) conducts a SMART assessment [25]. Alongside this, physiotherapy, music therapy, and speech and language therapy are carried out by specialist assessments and treatments. The MDT also continues using the WHIM.

Harry does not consistently show intentional communication. There is one more occasion where a spontaneous verbalisation occurs, but this is not repeated during his time in rehabilitation. A description of the specific speech and language therapy intervention follows.

The lifestyle and communication questionnaire reveals that Harry has been a passionate lover of food all his life, and amongst the activities that he and his wife particularly enjoy are cooking together and eating out. Despite only demonstrating very occasional evidence of awareness, it is decided to attempt a swallow assessment using oral trials. The rationale for this is to use oral intake and feeding – something that has been identified by Harry's family as very motivating for him – as a forum for assessing awareness and communicative intent. Determination of swallow function, safety, and prognosis for improvement are also important.

Ordinarily, prior to undertaking oral trials, an SLT would complete an oro–motor assessment of the key cranial nerves, to determine strength, speed, and range of movement of the bulbar muscles and begin to build a hypothesis around risk of swallow disorder and subsequent aspiration risk. This is done by asking patients to carry out specific movements with each bulbar muscle in turn. However, patients with disordered levels of consciousness present unique challenges when conducting a swallow assessment, as their ability to engage and participate is severely limited. Observation then becomes vital. From observing Harry performing spontaneous oral movements (yawning, grimacing, frowning), it is noted that he presents with a mild right upper motor neurone facial weakness, with normal tone throughout the rest of his facial muscles. Occasional spontaneous swallows are observed, approximately every 5 minutes at rest, after yawning and mouth care. There is no pooling or drooling of saliva.

A choice of yoghurts is presented to Harry at the start of each session, to determine if he is able to communicate a choice. The WHIM is conducted during these sessions. When Harry is sat out in his chair, a teaspoon of yoghurt is presented. In order to prepare him, the yoghurt pot is presented under Harry's nose in the hope of evoking a response via his sense of smell. The spoon and yoghurt are then placed on Harry's lips. Spontaneous mouth opening does not occur, but after four attempts, Harry does spontaneously lick his lips free of the yoghurt. Over the next 3 weeks, Harry is seen daily for short sessions repeating this activity; lip licking becomes more consistent, and nurses note an improvement in Harry's tolerance of mouth care. Hand over hand, facilitated self-feeding is then introduced with the aim of achieving spontaneous mouth opening when a spoon is presented. After three sessions, mouth opening is achieved sufficiently for a teaspoon-sized bolus of yoghurt to be placed in Harry's mouth. Spontaneous oral manipulation of the bolus occurs, and a swallow is triggered. This is then repeated with more teaspoons of yoghurt.

During a bedside swallow assessment, SLTs use the parameters of voice and cough after oral trials as indicators of overt aspiration. However, as Harry is non-verbal, it is not possible to use voice, and given the severity of his neurological presentation, it is difficult to know how reliable his airway response will be. Instrumental swallow assessment is discussed with Harry's family and the medical team. This is felt to be beneficial to determine swallow safety before increasing oral trials, as Harry is at high risk for aspiration pneumonia if an aspiration event occurs. Videofluoroscopy is deemed the most appropriate instrumental assessment, largely due to Harry's head position being rotated to the left due to his severe right neglect, making the view in fibre-optic endoscopic evaluation of swallow (FEES) challenging (see Chapter 5 for details of swallow investigations). Videofluoroscopy reveals that the pharyngeal phase is intact, but aspiration occurs on larger volumes of thin fluids because of lack of oral/tongue control of the bolus due to his low level of awareness, rather than any specific neurological weakness. Commencement of small amounts of thin fluids and pureed snacks is recommended.

Harry's wife is pleased with this progress and feels she can be directly involved, bringing in drinks and home-cooked food that she knows Harry will enjoy. Harry is supplied with a Provale cup (a specialist cup which delivers predetermined quantities of fluid) for his wife and staff to use for his drinks. He is upgraded to soft diet as his mouth opening in response to the spoon becomes consistent. His chest remains clear and his PEG feeds are reduced as his oral intake increases, with regular monitoring of his weight. The PEG remains in situ, however, as Harry is not able to meet all his nutritional and hydration needs orally.

Over time, Harry's wife takes over feeding him, which gives her a way of engaging and interacting with her husband even in the absence of communication. Harry is unable to indicate flavour preference, and at the end of his stay in rehabilitation his WHIM score is 14 for the highest level of behaviour ('mechanical vocalisation'), and the number of behaviours observed had increased to eight.

As with other patients living with the effects of stroke, assistive devices can be applied to support and enable patients with PDoC to make best use of their abilities. In Case Study 13.1, for example, Harry is able to drink using a specialised cup. Technology support for people with disabilities (including MCS) is a fast-growing field. New technologies such as gaze tracking are now well established for neurological disorders such as amyotrophic lateral sclerosis [39]. The potential of brain–computer interfaces (BCIs) for this patient group is beginning to be explored [40].

13.4.4 Long-Term Care

The prognosis for people with MCS is often uncertain, but may be many years. Long-term management and care may therefore need to be considered. Some may require ongoing rehabilitation because improvement may be slow but continue for years. Decisions will have to be made about the level of ongoing rehabilitation and care that is appropriate to the person's needs, as well as the setting in which this care will be delivered. Likely aspects of ongoing care include: nutrition and hydration; comprehensive social care, to maintain health and well-being and prevent pressure damage; physical therapy, to prevent contractures and maintain level of function; ongoing review, for early detection of any changes; and anticipation and treatment of infections or symptoms of distress.

Ongoing care may be delivered in various settings, and decisions about the long-term accommodation of the person with MCS can be difficult and stressful. Decisions about care at home are dependent both on community support and services available, as well asd the family's capacity to undertake home care. Modifications to the home may be required to accommodate necessary equipment such as hoist and tube feeding supplies. Health professionals need to consider the impact of such care; very high stress levels have been reported by families who care at home for a person with severe brain damage [41]. Respite care may also need to be considered as part of the package, if available. A trial period may be useful before committing to care at home, as well as consideration of what support carers may need for the situation to be sustainable. Conversely, if it is decided that care should not be provided at home then carers may need support to accept this decision.

Alternative accommodation options include a nursing home, specialist long-term rehabilitation hospital, and community group homes. The choice will depend on local availability, individuals' needs and preferences compared with details of service provision, and resourcing. Palliative care also has a role with people with severe and enduring illness, and referral should be considered if symptoms become burdensome or withdrawal of futile treatments is being considered.

Finally, decisions about continuance or withdrawal of treatments and resuscitation options should be considered through discussion between all involved, with clear plans made and instructions established. Decisions should be informed by consideration of the person's best interests, including what is known about their wishes, as well as the interests of their carers.

13.5 Locked-In Syndrome

The locked-in syndrome was first defined in 1966, and was redefined 20 years later as quadriplegia and anarthria with preservation of consciousness [10, 42]. It is rare, and caused by trauma or disease of the ventral pons, although extensive bilateral destruction of corticobulbar and corticospinal tracts in the cerebral peduncles may also be responsible (see Table 13.1).

Three categories are described [44]:

- *Classic.* Quadriplegia and anarthria, retained consciousness and vertical eye movement.
- *Incomplete.* The same as classic but with some additional voluntary movement.
- *Total.* Total immobility and inability to communicate, with full consciousness.

Typically, those affected have complete paralysis of voluntary muscles in all parts of the body except for the control of eye movement. Whilst horizontal gaze palsies are usual, patients usually retain upper eyelid control and vertical eye movement because of sparing of the mid-brain tectum. Associated problems can include blurred or double vision, impaired visual accommodation, vertigo,

TABLE 13.1	Causes and mechanisms of locked-in syndrome
Cause	**Mechanism**
Ischaemic	Basilar artery occlusion, stroke, hypotensive, hypoxic events
Haemorrhage	Haemorrhage within or into the pons
Traumatic	Direct brainstem contusion, vertebrobasilar axis dissection
Tumour	Primary or secondary metastasis
Metabolic	Central pontine myelinolysis
Demyelination	Multiple sclerosis
Infectious	Abscess, brainstem encephalitis

Source: Reproduced from Smith and Delargy [43], with permission from BMJ Publishing Group Ltd.

insomnia, and emotional lability. In one series, 6 of 44 recovering patients reported visual deficits, 39 said they cried or laughed more easily, 8 reported memory problems, and 6 had attentional deficits [45].

Most remain either in a chronic locked-in state or severely impaired, but early signs of recovery can be taken advantage of by multidisciplinary rehabilitation [43]. Early referral to specialist rehabilitation services is important. There is no cure for locked-in syndrome, but a wide range of therapies and assistive technologies may make significant improvements in quality of life, particularly in communication.

Initially, low-tech forms of alternative and augmentative communication such as AEIOU auditory and visual scanning (see Case Study 13.3) are used. However, a wide range of assistive computer interface technologies have been developed to exploit eye movements. These are used to drive a variety of communication devices, but also as a means for individuals to control their environment in relation to a variety of electrical and other appliances. For example, an eye-gaze system has been described based on the corneal–pupil reflection relationship technique. This is non-intrusive, and is calibrated by the user successively looking at nine points on the screen. Onscreen, the user has a main menu from which to select one of several controlling screens whereby they can type, place a telephone call, or turn appliances on or off [46]. Eye-gaze and eye tracking systems may be used to help patients communicate [46].

New direct brain interface mechanisms may provide future technological options. A BCI, also called a direct neural interface or brain–machine interface, is a direct communication pathway between the brain and an external device. Invasive BCI research has focused on replacing damaged sight and providing new avenues of function to paralysed people. Invasive BCIs are implanted directly into the grey matter of the brain. They provide the most effective communication of all BCI devices, but are prone to produce scar tissue, which can result in loss of signal. The first such implant was installed in a patient with locked-in syndrome in 1998, allowing them to learn to control a computer cursor. Partially invasive BCIs are devices implanted inside the skull but outside the brain. They produce better signals than non-invasive BCIs, where the bone of the skull deflects and deforms signals, and have a lower risk of scar tissue formation than invasive BCIs.

Case Study

Case 13.3 | Elizabeth

Elizabeth is 42 years old when she is admitted to a specialist rehabilitation centre following a haemorrhagic stroke in the brainstem region. Prior to her stroke, she worked as a full-time accountant, and she is mother to a 3-year-old daughter. She is referred with a provisional diagnosis of locked-in syndrome.

Elizabeth arrives with a cuffed tracheostomy tube in situ. The tracheostomy was performed 5 days after the brain haemorrhage, providing longer-term support for her airway. The majority of patients with locked-in syndrome require tracheostomy, at least initially, because:

- there is potential for damage to the respiratory control centre located in the medulla, resulting in physiological changes in breathing and subsequent need for ventilator support;
- bulbar muscles are weakened or paralysed, with resultant risk of airway obstruction from anatomical structures (e.g. low-toned base of tongue or vocal cord paralysis);
- paralysis of bulbar muscles is associated with risk of aspiration of food, fluid, or saliva into the airway, with the potential for development of aspiration pneumonia; and
- weakened respiratory musculature with resultant weak or absent cough reflex leads to an inability to clear chest secretions; a tracheostomy tube provides an entry point into the airway by which secretions can be removed via suctioning.

For 3 months prior to transfer, Elizabeth is free of chest infections and is receiving all nutrition and hydration via a PEG tube. First, the SLT assesses the effectiveness of Elizabeth's swallow function for saliva, in order to determine if it is appropriate to consider starting a tracheostomy tube weaning programme. The decision to commence a tracheostomy weaning programme is made by the MDT.

Speech pathology assessment of Elizabeth's bulbar muscles reveals low tone throughout her face, lips, and tongue. There is no observable swallow initiated either to command or reflexively. Reflexive bobbing and twitching movements are observed in the laryngeal area of the neck and in Elizabeth's facial muscles. No other reflexive or volitional movements are observed. Severe drooling of her saliva is observed due to the lack of movement of her lip, tongue, and throat muscles and the absent swallow reflex. Given the severity of deficits observed at the bedside, oral intake is not trialled.

Elizabeth's tracheostomy tube cuff is creating a barrier between her upper and lower airways, such that the flow of air occurs only through the tracheostomy tube to the lungs, bypassing the upper airway and larynx. This barrier (cuff) is helping prevent aspiration of oral secretions, but cuffs are not designed to prevent large-volume aspiration, and aspiration around them can occur [47]. The presence of a cuffed tracheostomy tube may impair swallowing, as there is loss of airflow in and around the larynx and laryngeal receptors, with reduced sensation [48]. Long-term, a cuffed tracheostomy tube may cause complications such as trachea-malachia, stenosis, and granulation [49], although these are reported less with newer cuff materials.

The MDT decides that given Elizabeth's clear chest status, short periods of cuff deflation should be trialled despite her high risk of aspiration of oral secretions. As cuffed tracheostomy tubes do not eliminate aspiration of secretions, it is likely that Elizabeth has been aspirating her oral secretions without detrimental impact on her respiratory health. Cuff deflation will expose Elizabeth to a more normal breathing and swallow experience and reduce risks of long-term complications associated with tracheostomy tubes.

Over 1 month, periods of cuff deflation are trialled and extended. By the end of the month, continuous cuff deflation is tolerated. Careful monitoring and documentation of Elizabeth's chest condition and respiratory status are essential. Detailed information about Elizabeth's swallow function and airway is required, so she is referred for a Fiberoptic Endoscopic Examination of Swallowing (FEES).

The FEES reveals severe dysphagia with copious amounts of saliva in the pharynx and severe subglottic stenosis, likely as a result of prolonged endotracheal intubation. This stenosis is occluding approximately 70% of her airway. Elizabeth also has myoclonus present throughout her pharynx, larynx, and base of tongue: rhythmical pulsing-type movements associated with lower motor neuron lesions, which, when severe, can compromise an individual's ability to breathe independently. Given these findings and the time since the initial brain haemorrhage, it is felt unlikely that Elizabeth will ever achieve full decannulation. Given her clear chest history, it is decided to continue with cuff deflation, and the tracheostomy tube is changed to a cuffless tube.

Elizabeth arrives at the rehabilitation centre with no established method of communication. As she has a medullary haemorrhage, it is not anticipated that she will have significant cognitive or linguistic impairments. A joint assessment between the SLT and OT reveals that Elizabeth has just two bodily movements under her control: she can raise her right thumb and she can reliably move her eyes up and down. Her thumb movement is inconsistent, due to muscle fatigue rather than impaired control, so eye movement is the chosen method of communication.

The level of linguistic understanding has to be determined. There are few assessments available for SLTs working with patients who have locked-in syndrome. Much of the assessment therefore comprises non-standardised material and informal observations of responses over time, allowing the clinician to build up a profile of her communicative strengths and weaknesses. The vertical eye movement is used as yes/no response, with Elizabeth rolling her eyes up for yes and lowering them for no. An assessment comprising paired yes/no questions is thus completed. For example, she might be asked, 'Is this a bell?' and then 'Is this money?', with a bell shown each time. In order to be scored correct, Elizabeth must answer both questions correctly (if non-paired questions were used, she would have a 50% chance for each of giving a correct answer by luck). Biographical questions are also employed; for example, 'Do you have a daughter?' (Yes), 'Do you have a son?' (No). A 60-question yes/no informal assessment is carried out, with Elizabeth scoring 60/60 correctly, indicating intact linguistic functioning.

The idea of AEIOU auditory/visual scanning is introduced as a broader means of communication (Figure 13.2). This is a low-tech form of alternative and augmentative communication involving the communication partner reading out letters from an alphabet board. The AEIOU row–column method of scanning was designed to speed up the system, because not all of the letters of the alphabet have to be read out each time. The communication partner starts by reading aloud the letters in the far left-hand column (AEIOU); the patient rolls their eyes up when they hear the letter at the beginning of the row containing the letter they want. For example, if Elizabeth wanted to spell the word GIRL, she would

A	B	C	D		
E	F	G	H		
I	J	K	L	M	N
O	P	Q	R	S	T
U	V	W	X	Y	Z

FIGURE 13.2 The AEIOU auditory/visual scanning device.

roll her eyes when the letter E was read out. The communication partner would then read aloud the letters contained in that row: EFGH. Elizabeth would roll her eyes up when the letter G was spoken, indicating the target letter was G. The communication partner would make a note of this and begin scanning again from A. This would then continue until Elizabeth had completed her message.

Although a time-consuming and laborious method (for both Elizabeth and the communication partner), this is an initial step. In the absence of any other method, it can literally 'unlock' an individual and enable a high level of communication. With practice, it can become fast and efficient, with short-cuts introduced. Eventually, it is common for both patient and communication partner not to require the board and for scanning to be done from memory.

A more high-tech aid is later introduced, aiming to support independent communication. However, after trialling the device, Elizabeth chooses to stay with the low-tech AEIOU method, describing it as quicker and easier for communication with people who know the system. Extensive education is provided to Elizabeth's key people on use of the technique, and a video demonstrating it is made in preparation for her discharge to a long-term care facility.

Elizabeth is re-referred to the specialist assistive communication service 1 year later for re-exploration of high-tech aids. On reassessment, Elizabeth is able to access an alphabet chart by direct eye gaze. The communication software is loaded on to a laptop and made accessible for wheelchair or bed usage. The software facilitates access to and writing of e-mails. Elizabeth still uses the low-tech AEIOU method at times.

Non-invasive BCIs have been trialled to power muscle implants and restore partial movement, but poor signal resolution makes the technology more difficult to control. All together, there is potential for such assistive technologies to radically enhance the lives of those living with locked-in syndrome [40].

Case Study 13.3 presents an account of the journey through rehabilitation of a patient with locked-in syndrome. Speech and language therapy rehabilitation is predominantly discussed, but her full rehabilitation programme was multidimensional and multidisciplinary, which is essential for an individual with significant impairments.

13.6 Conclusion

VS, MCS, and locked-in syndrome are rare outcomes of stroke, but when they occur, they are devastating for everyone. Nurses are central to care provision and make significant contributions at all stages of the patient journey. Through their round-the-clock presence on the ward, they assess and monitor change and maintain continuity. They are the cornerstone of communication, ensuring care management works in the best interest of the patient, their carers, and the MDT. Nurses are also the key link with carers, who are often invaluable in identifying and evaluating the needs and speeding the recovery of these patients. It is essential that nurses have a good understanding of the conditions; current evidence and best practice; areas where practice development, research, and technological innovation are revolutionising the patient experience; quality of life and survival; and carer and community contributions to management.

References

1. UK Stroke Forum Education & Training. Stroke-Specific Education Framework, United Kingdom: UK Stroke Forum 2010. Available from: http://www.stroke-education.org.uk/about. [30 November 2018]
2. Kitzinger, C. and Kitzinger, J. (2014). Grief, Anger and Despair in Relatives of Severely Brain Injured Patients: Responding without Pathologising. London: Sage.
3. Bauby, J.-D. (1997). The Diving Bell and the Butterfly: A Memoir of Life in Death. New York: Vintage.
4. Turner-Stokes, L. (2017). A matter of life and death: controversy at the interface between clinical and legal decision-making in prolonged disorders of consciousness. Journal of Medical Ethics 43 (7): 469–475.
5. Royal College of Physicians (2013). Prolonged Disorders of Consciousness. London: Royal College of Physicians.
6. Gill-Thwaites, H. (2006). Lotteries, loopholes and luck: misdiagnosis in the vegetative state patient. Brain Injury 20 (13–14): 1321–1328.
7. Schnakers, C., Vanhaudenhuyse, A., Giacino, J. et al. (2009). Diagnostic accuracy of the vegetative and minimally conscious state: clinical consensus versus standardized neurobehavioral assessment. British Medical Council Neurology 9 (1): 1–5.
8. Sannita, W.G. (2015). Responsiveness in DoC and individual variability. Frontiers in Human Neuroscience 9 (270): 1–2.
9. Parliamentary Office of Science and Technology (2015). Vegetative and Minimally Conscious States. London: Houses of Parliament.
10. Plum, F. and Posner, J.B. (1966). The Diagnosis of Stupor and Coma. Philadelphia: F.A. Davis Co.
11. British Medical Association (2007). Treatment of Patients in Persistent Vegetative State. London: British Medical Association: Medical Ethics Department.
12. Laureys, S., Boly, M., and Maquet, P. (2006). Tracking the recovery of consciousness from coma. Journal of Clinical Investigation 116 (7): 1823–1825.
13. Pignat, J.-M., Mauron, E., Jöhr, J. et al. (2016). Outcome prediction of consciousness disorders in the acute stage based on a complementary motor behavioural tool. PLoS One 11 (6): 1–16.
14. Varricchio, C.G. (2006). Measurement issues in quality-of-life assessments. Oncology Nursing Forum 33 (Suppl. 1): 13–21.
15. Pierce, E. and Braine, M. (2012). Nursing care of conditions related to the neurological system. In: Fundamentals of Medical-Surgical Nursing: A Systems Approach (ed. A.-M. Brady, C. McCabe and M. McCann), 326–363. Hoboken: Wiley-Blackwell.
16. Intercollegiate Stroke Working Party (2016). National Clinical Guidelines for Stroke. London: Royal College of Physicians.
17. Millwood, J., MacKenzie, S., Munday, R. et al. (2005). A report from an investigation of abnormal reflexes, lip trauma and awareness levels in patients with profound brain damage. Journal of Disability and Oral Health 6 (2): 72.
18. Scherb, C.A., Rapp, C.G., Johnson, M., and Maas, M. (1998). The nursing outcomes classification: validation by rehabilitation nurses. Rehabilitation Nursing 23 (4): 174–191.
19. Hiragami, F., Hiragami, S., and Suzuki, Y. (2016). A process of multidisciplinary team communication to individualize stroke rehabilitation of an 84-year-old stroke patient. Care Management Journals 17 (2): 97–104.
20. Cullen, N., Chundamala, J., Bayley, M., and Jutai, J. (2007). The efficacy of acquired brain injury rehabilitation. Brain Injury 21 (2): 113–132.

21. Magee, W.L. and Andrews, K. (2007). Multi-disciplinary perceptions of music therapy in complex neuro-rehabilitation. International Journal of Therapy and Rehabilitation 14 (2): 70–75.
22. Wilson, F.C., Elder, V., McCrudden, E., and Caldwell, S. (2009). Analysis of Wessex Head Injury Matrix (WHIM) scores in consecutive vegetative and minimally conscious state patients. Neuropsychological Rehabilitation 19 (5): 754–760.
23. Beaumont, J.G., Marjoribanks, J., Flury, S., and Lintern, T. (1999). Assessing auditory comprehension in the context of severe physical disability: the PACST. Brain Injury 13 (2): 99–112.
24. Magee, W.L. (2007). Development of a music therapy assessment tool for patients in low awareness states. NeuroRehabilitation 22 (4): 319–324.
25. Gill-Thwaites, H. and Munday, R. (2004). The Sensory Modality Assessment and Rehabilitation Technique (SMART): a valid and reliable assessment for vegetative state and minimally conscious state patients. Brain Injury 18 (12): 1255–1269.
26. MacKenzie, S., Gale, E., and Munday, R. (2006). Putney Auditory Single Word Yes/No Assessment (PASWORD). Development of a reliable test of yes/no at a single word level in patients unable to participate in assessments requiring a specific motor response: an exploratory study. International Journal of Language and Communication Disorders 41 (2): 225–234.
27. Pierce, E. and McLaren, S. (2014). Development of an assessment tool for the multi-disciplinary evaluation of neurological dependency (MEND). Scandinavian Journal of Caring Sciences 28 (1): 193–203.
28. National Health and Medical Research Council (2008). Ethical Guidelines for the Care of People in Post-Coma Unresponsiveness (Vegetative State) or a Minimally Responsive State. Melbourne: Australian Government.
29. Rodrigue, C., Riopelle, R.J., Bernat, J.L., and Racine, E. (2013). Perspectives and experience of healthcare professionals on diagnosis, prognosis, and end-of-life decision making in patients with disorders of consciousness. Neuroethics 6 (1): 25–36.
30. Lefaucheur, J.-P., André-Obadia, N., Antal, A. et al. (2014). Evidence-based guidelines on the therapeutic use of repetitive transcranial magnetic stimulation (rTMS). Clinical Neurophysiology 125 (11): 2150–2206.
31. Naudé, K. and Hughes, M. (2005). Considerations for the use of assistive technology in patients with impaired states of consciousness. Neuropsychological Rehabilitation 15 (3–4): 514–521.
32. Lancioni, G.E., Singh, N.N., O'Reilly, M.F. et al. (2015). Assistive technology to help persons in a minimally conscious state develop responding and stimulation control: performance assessment and social rating. NeuroRehabilitation 37 (3): 393–403.
33. Thaxton, L. and Myers, M.A. (2002). Sleep disturbances and their management in patients with brain injury. The Journal of Head Trauma Rehabilitation 17 (4): 335–348.
34. Laureys, S. and Schiff, N.D. (2012). Coma and consciousness: paradigms (re)framed by neuroimaging. NeuroImage 61 (2): 478–491.
35. Andrews, K., Murphy, L., Munday, R., and Littlewood, C. (1996). Misdiagnosis of the vegetative state: retrospective study in a rehabilitation unit. British Medical Journal 313 (7048): 13–16.
36. Taylor, C.M., Aird, V.H., Tate, R.L., and Lammi, M.H. (2007). Sequence of recovery during the course of emergence from the minimally conscious state. Archives of Physical Medicine and Rehabilitation 88 (4): 521–525.
37. Pierce, E., Cowan, P., and Stokes, M. (2001). Managing faecal retention and incontinence in neurodisability. British Journal of Nursing 10 (9): 592–601.
38. Chua, K.S., Ng, Y., Yap, S.G., and Bok, C. (2007). A brief review of traumatic brain injury rehabilitation. Annals Academy of Medicine, Singapore 36 (1): 31.
39. Hwang, C.-S., Weng, H.-H., Wang, L.-F. et al. (2014). An eye-tracking assistive device improves the quality of life for ALS patients and reduces the caregivers' burden. Journal of Motor Behavior 46 (4): 233–238.

40. Pasqualotto, E., Matuz, T., Federici, S. et al. (2015). Usability and workload of access technology for people with severe motor impairment: a comparison of brain-computer interfacing and eye tracking. Neurorehabilitation and Neural Repair 29 (10): 950–957.
41. Bastianelli, A., Gius, E., and Cipolletta, S. (2014). Changes over time in the quality of life, prolonged grief and family strain of family caregivers of patients in vegetative state: a pilot study. Journal of Health Psychology 21 (5): 844–852.
42. Haig, A.J., Katz, R.T., and Sahgal, V. (1987). Mortality and complications of the locked-in syndrome. Archives of Physical Medicine and Rehabilitation 68 (1): 24–27.
43. Smith, E. and Delargy, M. (2005). Locked-in syndrome. British Medical Journal 330 (7488): 406–409.
44. Bauer, G., Gerstenbrand, F., and Rumpl, E. (1979). Varieties of the locked-in syndrome. Journal of Neurology 221 (2): 77–91.
45. León-Carrión, J., Eeckhout, P., and Domínguez-Morales, M.D.R. (2002). Review of subject: the locked-in syndrome: a syndrome looking for a therapy. Brain Injury 16 (7): 555–569.
46. Wendt, O., Quist, R.W., and Lloyd, L.L. (2011). Assistive Technology: Principles and Applications for Communication Disorders and Special Education. Bingley: Emerald.
47. Ding, R. and Logemann, J.A. (2005). Swallow physiology in patients with trach cuff inflated or deflated: a retrospective study. Head & Neck 27 (9): 809–813.
48. Davis, D.G., Bears, S., Barone, J.E. et al. (2002). Swallowing with a tracheostomy tube in place: does cuff inflation matter? Journal of Intensive Care Medicine 17 (3): 132–135.
49. Epstein, S.K. (2005). Late complications of tracheostomy. Respiratory Care 50 (4): 542–549.

CHAPTER 14

Longer-Term Support for Survivors of Stroke and Their Carers

Judith Redfern[1], Clare Gordon[2], and Dominique Cadilhac[3,4]

[1]School of Nursing, University of Central Lancashire, Preston, UK

[2]Stroke Services, Royal Bournemouth and Christchurch Hospitals NHS Foundation Trust, Bournemouth, UK

[3]School of Clinical Sciences, Monash University, Clayton, VIC, Australia

[4]Stroke Division, Florey Institute of Neuroscience and Mental Health, Parkville, VIC, Australia

KEY POINTS

- Stroke survivors and carers should be assessed annually to ensure their needs are met.
- High-risk groups (e.g. under 65 years) may need additional assessment or follow-up.
- Health professionals should explore survivors' and carers' views about their concepts of recovery, since expectations vary.
- Recommended interventions should start as early as possible post-stroke, enabling a smooth transition from hospital to home and preparing survivors and carers for new circumstances and roles.
- Health professionals should consider pre-emptively discussing appropriate carer coping strategies and options for support.

This chapter maps to criteria within the following sections of the Stroke-Specific Education Framework (SSEF):

> *Looking back it was Sarah's determination [partner] that was so vital in these difficult weeks. Like many stroke sufferers I was so exhausted by the tiny details of everyday life – even the energy to get up and cross the room to answer the front door or the telephone – that stress of everyday life seemed so overly daunting and the idea of addressing a self-generated program of rehabilitation almost impossible. The more I sank into inky black inertia, the more Sarah battled on.*
> *(Extract from 'My Year Off' by Robert McCrum [2])*

14.1   Introduction

The preceding extract highlights one stroke survivor's experience of returning home and his perception of absolute emotional and physical dependence on his partner for support. In this chapter, we focus on the longer-term needs and support for people with stroke and their carers, such as Sarah. Traditionally, long-term support is referred to as the 'post-acute phase', incorporating hospital discharge and community rehabilitation (typically 3–6 months post-stroke). However, with the development of Early Supported Discharge services and other rehabilitation and community services (see Chapter 11), the average length of hospital stay in many countries has been reduced to just over 2 weeks, with half of survivors discharged from hospital within 7 days [3]. Now, longer-term support is more commonly defined as the phase after which most of the recovery of independence has occurred [4], and is focused on living with the condition in the future. Longer-term health service support for survivors of stroke and carers is underdeveloped [5]. Therefore, for survivors and their families, the process of living with stroke in the community involves a transition from dependence on health services to reliance on self-management and informal care [6].

To respond to the longer-term needs of survivors and carers, healthcare professionals should:

- understand the experience of living with stroke from a survivor and carer perspective;
- identify difficulties associated with self-management or caring in the longer-term; and
- be aware of the merits of different interventions for providing support to survivors and carers.

The following sections provide an outline of the context and need for support over the longer term, a summary of best-practice recommendations for management, and potential options for intervening with families and carers.

14.2 Longer-Term Consequences of Stroke, Informal Care and Costs

Approximately half of survivors have some form of lasting physical, cognitive, or psychological impairment. These survivors seek to regain a sense of normality, engage in meaningful activities or occupations, and accept changed capacities [7]. Following hospital discharge, many survivors remain dependent, with the majority cared for by an unpaid/informal carer, usually a family member or partner. It is to this group of carers that we refer in this chapter. An informal carer can be defined as:

> Someone who helps another person, usually a relative or friend, in their day-to-day life. This is not the same as someone who provides care professionally, or through a voluntary organisation. [8]

In the United Kingdom, more than 1 in 10 people are unpaid carers supporting people who are older, disabled, or seriously ill [9], saving public expenditure an estimated £119 billion per year in paid caregiving [10]. Carers of stroke survivors spend an average of 17–32 hours per week performing, for example, assistance with self-care, domestic duties, or community-based activities within 1 year post-stroke [11, 12]; this continues to hold true in the longer term [13]. To date, it is predominantly social services and voluntary organisations that provide support for carers in the United Kingdom and other countries, such as Australia. Funding services and support within healthcare have traditionally been focused on the stroke survivor, with less attention paid to the carer. However, the impact on carers may have important consequences for the health and well-being of both parties.

The costs of long-term care are substantial. The most important direct costs within 10 years of a first-ever stroke involve residential aged care facilities, informal care, and medications, with informal care making up between 20 and 27% of ongoing annual costs [13]. It is imperative that health professionals seek methods to provide a supportive healthcare model that actively seeks to regularly engage survivors and carers in accomplishing a two-way benefit: *enhancement of stroke survivors' recovery and minimisation of adverse carer outcomes* [7].

14.3 The Need for Support

14.3.1 Longer-Term Consequences for Survivors of Stroke

A large proportion of survivors are living with one or more physical, cognitive, and emotional problems up to 5 years post-stroke [5, 14], as indicated in the findings of two national surveys from the United Kingdom [5] and Australia [14] (Figure 14.1).

With ongoing problems, survivors often experience changes in social participation. For example, half of respondents in the UK Stroke Survivor Needs Survey reported lasting changes to their working conditions following stroke, two-thirds

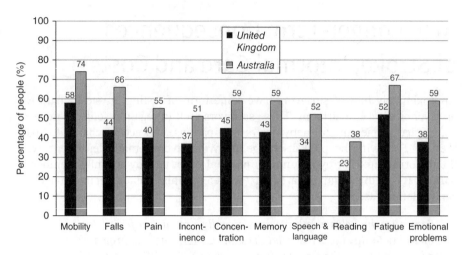

The long-term physical, cognitive and emotional problems reported in the UK and Australia

FIGURE 14.1 Proportion of people reporting longer-term physical, cognitive, and emotional problems post-stroke in the United Kingdom [5] and Australia [14].

reported negative changes to leisure activities, and 42% reported negative changes to their relationships [5]. These issues are described from the patient's experience in Case Study 14.1.

14.3.2 Long-Term Unmet Needs

I have difficulty coping with costs of incontinence pads, etc. required due to brother's incontinence ... In addition to other costs such as home help, district nursing service, medications etc., it is quite an effort to cope. [15]

Few national studies have examined unmet needs of stroke survivors beyond 1 year. In the UK Stroke Survivor Needs Survey, the majority of survivors felt they had unmet or partially met needs, particularly regarding emotional difficulties (39% with needs unmet), cognitive difficulties (59% with memory and 43% with cognition needs unmet), and fatigue (43% with needs unmet) [5]. These issues were consistent with Australian data, whereby 84% of survivors reported needs that were not fully met [14]. Unmet need was also associated with increased disability (physical disability, cognitive problems, fatigue) and sociocultural factors (ethnicity, younger age) [5, 14]. Notably, for every 1 year decrease in age, the number of needs reported as not fully met increased by 1% [14]. This highlights the particular needs of younger survivors.

Over half of survivors report unmet information needs [5]. In a systematic review of the educational needs of survivors and carers which included three studies of longer-term needs, both clinical and practical forms of information were requested [16]. More specifically, education was wanted on the psychological and social consequences of stroke; on recovery, the tasks of caring, and social activities; and on community support services and resources [16].

Case Study

Case 14.1 Brian

Brian is a 37-year-old coach driver. He lives independently in an annex to a house where his sister lives with her two primary school-age children. He has a long-term girlfriend, whom he tends to see at weekends. He enjoys gaming on his computer, spending time with his girlfriend, and going to the gym. Brian has a lacunar stroke that affects his right arm and leg. On leaving hospital, he has no functional movement in his arm, but he is beginning to weight-bear on his leg so he can transfer independently.

In the first year after returning home from his stroke, Brian is initially fiercely independent. His sister is involved in discharge planning and preparing him for home, but both emphasise that they have very separate lives, and his sister expresses that she does not want to be his carer. Initially, Brian receives assistance from community rehabilitation services, but once he is independent with his personal care needs, these services discharge him. This reflects the development of community services that primarily focus on physical rehabilitation needs. He continues to receive community occupational therapy (OT) and is followed up every 4–6 months by the hospital stroke service (consultant nurse clinic).

As Brian's mobility and arm function improve, he negotiates with his employer (with support from community OT) to return to work voluntarily, providing maintenance to the coaches that he used to drive. Brian is positive about this, and enjoys the social contact of being back at work. His participation in this is severely limited by his fatigue, and he can only manage 2 hours at work. He also relies on his sister to take him, so he is unable to go as often as he would like. He is still gaming at home in his spare time, but he breaks up with his girlfriend. After several months, he also acquires funding for a mobility scooter, and this enables him to access his gym. For a while, Brian loses weight and feels confident about his future, with a lifting in his low mood.

After 4 months, Brian has a post-stroke seizure whilst playing on his computer. This has a large impact on his confidence and he finds that he is even more fatigued. He is unable to use his mobility scooter due to the worry of having a seizure whilst driving, so he stops going to the gym. Soon after his seizure, Brian sees the stroke service follow-up clinic, which provides both him and his sister information and advice on post-stroke seizure and reviews his medication. The nurse facilitates a discussion between Brian and his sister about his needing support from her, and for a few months Brian moves into her home. Previously, he had helped significantly with his sister's childcare, but both feel that until his seizures are stable, this will not be possible, which results in his sister reducing her working hours. The follow-up clinic suggests his sister access carers' allowance, and provides support through the difficult discussions between the two on their roles and responsibilities.

Since Brian's seizure, he has given up his voluntary work on the coaches and stopped going to the gym. He spends a lot of time gaming. When reviewed 2 months later (6 months post-discharge), Brian is gaining weight and admits to being low in mood. The Greater Manchester Stroke Assessment Tool GM-SAT [18] is used to structure the 6-month assessment, and the results are communicated with Brian's local general practitioner (GP) and community stroke coordinator (with permission from Brian). The consultant nurse formally assesses Brian's mood and risk factors. She refers him to a counsellor through the Improving Access to Psychological Therapies programme [19]. She assesses that his body mass index (BMI) is near obese, and his blood pressure (BP) is also high. She asks the GP to monitor his risk factors, and suggests to Brian that once he feels his mood is more stable, they should discuss his weight gain. His BP control is monitored jointly between himself, the GP, and the stroke follow-up clinic, with the nurse encouraging Brian to take more responsibility for monitoring it himself. A written copy of the assessment is given to Brian, with key information on what was discussed to support retention of information.

Despite Brian requiring a large amount of support concerning his new post-stroke epilepsy, he is not entitled to follow-up through the epilepsy services because his epilepsy diagnosis has not been made by a neurologist. Therefore, the stroke follow-up service takes on this support. Once his epilepsy is stable at 18 months post-stroke, Brian is introduced to the idea that the stroke service cannot provide support indefinitely, and that this will need to be transferred over to primary care. Brian becomes anxious about this transition, with his main concerns being the relationships that he has formed with the consultant nurse over the last 2 years and the fact that he does not need to explain all the complexities of his condition at each consultation. Further, his experiences of primary care services have been of a general lack of knowledge around longer-term stroke needs. This reflects the lack of commissioning of longer-term stroke services amongst healthcare workers with the depth and breadth of knowledge required for post-stroke support.

Case Study

Case 14.2	**Eileen**

Eileen is 93 years old and lives with her husband, Derek (aged 90) in a bungalow on a large estate. Before Eileen's stroke, they both enjoyed long walks in the local countryside. Derek also enjoyed going to a photography group twice a week. Eileen did the vast majority of the shopping and all of the cooking. Whilst eating breakfast with Derek in the kitchen, Eileen suddenly loses the ability to speak and collapses on to the floor. She has a large left middle cerebral artery ischaemic stroke, resulting in severe expressive and receptive dysphasia and a severe right-sided weakness. On discharge from hospital, she is able to transfer with assistance of one, but remains incontinent of urine. She does not have any functional communication, and is increasingly frustrated by this.

At Eileen's 6-week review by the stroke service, she is no longer receiving any rehabilitation services. Derek appears anxious and negative, and although he brushes over any concerns initially, after more specific questioning he mentions that, at times, Eileen's frustration with her communication results in her hitting Derek – something very out of character. Due to Eileen's communication and physical disability, Derek is unable to leave her unattended. He relies on his neighbour to sit with Eileen for an hour each week whilst he goes shopping; otherwise, the furthest he ever goes is into the garden. Both Derek and Eileen are experiencing social isolation after her stroke, as neither is able to continue their previous roles or social activities. Derek is finding Eileen's aggressive behaviour and his new role as a carer difficult to cope with.

The stroke nurse formalises the assessment by completing an interview with Derek using the Caregiver Burden Index. She suggests some options available to Derek to help him cope with his additional responsibility as a carer, including the use of services such as home care, meals on wheels, and home sitting services. She suggests that Derek could speak to his GP about his anxiety.

Although difficult to assess, the stroke nurse recognises from Derek's responses that Eileen has changed since returning home and is displaying increased frustration and aggression linked to her severe communication disability. Derek feels able to manage Eileen's significant physical healthcare needs, but her complex personality changes and communication problems are a bigger concern and are having the greatest impact on him as a carer.

Carers also report inadequacies in social and financial support, with 21% receiving insufficient social support, 24% unable to access respite care, 28% reporting loss of income, and 50% experiencing increased personal expenses since the stroke [17]. Failing to meet the needs of survivors and provide carers with support has important implications for their health and well-being. In the Australian Stroke Survivor Needs Survey, it was found that there was a 14% increase in the odds of carers reporting moderate to extreme impacts on work, leisure, and relationships for every unmet need reported by the stroke survivor [17].

14.3.3 The Carer's Perspective

Seeking understanding of the caring experience from the carer's perspective, a review of qualitative literature identified 17 interview studies with carers of stroke survivors [20]. Interviews explored carers' perspectives of challenges experienced over time, positive aspects of caring, and coping strategies [21]. Carers reported feeling ill prepared for the caring role, particularly in relation to information and training, and having a negative emotional response (feeling distressed, uncomfortable, or unhappy) as a result of their changed role. These issues are exemplified in Case Study 14.1, and are further expanded on in Case Study 14.2. In contrast, strengthening relationships between couples or family members and giving the carer a sense of fulfilment and purpose were identified by some respondents as positive aspects of the caring role. In Case Study 14.1, Brian's sister was given support in how she could strengthen her relationship with her brother following his stroke and gradually take on and adapt to a carer role. This transition was made possible through having regular contact with a stroke follow-up clinic.

It is unclear why some carers view their new role more positively than others. The experience of caring has been described as a process of biographical disruption [22]; in other words, carers experience illness in a similar way to those who are ill, being confronted with dramatic changes in their understanding of life in relation to biography, self-identity, confidence, and social interaction [23]. The carer's experience of caring is defined by the degree of change and loss in their roles, responsibilities, and relationships and the way in which they are able to respond to this [23]. Various life adjustments accompany assumption of the caregiving role. For example, household and relationship roles for carers may change over the course of caregiving, including adopting duties previously attended to or shared with the survivor, such as managing finances, driving, cooking meals, and going grocery shopping [24]. In Case Study 14.1, the relationship between Brian and his sister – including the roles they both had in supporting each other – changed over time and was influenced by his varying needs and health conditions (e.g. his inability to help with childcare). The key to avoiding problems over the longer term appears to be both the quality of pre-existing stroke survivor–caregiver relationships and the coping strategies adopted in the post-stroke phase [25]. Therefore, health professionals should consider discussing with carers appropriate coping strategies.

Differences in the caring experience between those who are more used to caring responsibilities (typically older carers) and those who are new to the role (typically younger carers) have been reported [26]. This observation is supported by the theory of biographical disruption, since those already in a caring role may have less change and loss following the stroke. Traits and abilities that carers have identified as helpful in fostering a positive caring experience include asking for and receiving information and support (and, conversely, not suffering in silence), patience, humour, understanding the stroke survivor, and having one's own space to focus on self-care health and well-being [21, 27]. Concepts of 'returning to normality' for the stroke survivor and the 'tension of providing care' for informal carers may play an important role in adjustment [7]. In Case Study 14.2, the experience of an older couple is described, including the impacts on their life and relationship, and in particular the social isolation they experience.

14.3.4 Prevalence of Burden Amongst Carers

For caring, the term 'burden' can be defined as the 'emotional, physical and financial demands and responsibilities of an individual's illness that are placed on family members, friends or other individuals involved with the individual outside the healthcare system'. [28]. Burden may be objective (e.g. physical tasks performed as part of the caring role) or subjective (e.g. emotional adjustment required) [29]. The term 'burden' is often used interchangeably with the associated terms 'stress' or 'strain', although some hypothesise that burden is the result of stress creating negative emotional, social, environmental, and health-related consequences [30]. Pre-existing depressive symptoms may exacerbate the experience of burden [31].

Burden appears to be most prevalent pre-hospital discharge and may decrease over time as carers become more accustomed to their role [32]. It is estimated that between 25 and 54% of carers experience moderate to considerable burden as a consequence of caring for a stroke survivor [29]. Compared to age-matched non-carers, carers of stroke survivors also tend to have a poorer health-related quality of life [33]. An inverse relationship between the perceived burden and emotional health of carers means increased strain is often associated with poorer psychological outcomes, including anxiety and depression [34]. Estimates of the prevalence of mood disorders vary, with 30–35% reporting depressive symptoms [35] and 43–59% symptoms of anxiety [36–38]. Equally, the carer's ability to stay healthy and manage burden has an impact on survivor outcomes; for example, carer depressive symptoms have a significant negative impact on survivor quality of life, mood, and social participation [39]. However, it has been found that the amount of social support available to long-term carers may be an important factor in reducing psychological burden [40]. In Case Study 14.2, it was very important that the social isolation and its effect on the carer's mood (compounded by the complexity of the survivor's disabilities) were recognised by the stroke nurse and support was offered.

14.4 Responsibilities of Health and Social Care Professionals

In the case studies presented, long-term follow-up with stroke nurses or stroke clinics was critical in helping the survivors and their carer navigate a positive outcome through the dynamic process of adjustment. Where these services are unavailable, having consistent community services (e.g. through primary care) is essential. The importance of focusing on the longer-term needs of those with chronic conditions and their carers has been increasingly recognised in health and social care policies. In particular, the need to financially compensate carers is supported in many developed countries, including Canada, the United States, the United Kingdom, and Australia. However, service and financial support priorities are subject to change according to the political and economic climate. In Case Study 14.1, it was important that Brian and his sister were able to access financial support, since their ability to work changed following Brian's stroke.

Globally, guidelines on best clinical practice in stroke management include recommendations for longer-term support for survivors and address the role of carers [41–46]. However, in most cases, recommendations are brief and based on expert consensus rather than strong research evidence; such evidence is either inconclusive or lacking. Common factors across different guidelines include that:

- stroke survivors should be assessed for their rehabilitation and support needs, and reassessed if their health or social circumstances change (or annually, if not);
- carers should be assessed for their support needs, and reassessed if their health or social circumstances change (or annually, if not);
- tailored information and support should be provided for:
  - physical health needs;
  - psychological and emotional needs;
  - social needs, including financial benefits, leisure activities, driving, and return-to-work; and
- where the health professional is unable to provide support themselves, survivors and carers should be assisted to seek help from other statutory and voluntary sector organisations.

Most guidelines give no further detail on how to achieve these goals, how services should be integrated, who should take responsibility for different aspects of care, or when this should occur.

14.5 Identifying Those at Risk

My mother's stroke was mild and has not altered my life at all. I do have good support from my sister, husband, brother and sister-in-law. [15]

If the first recommendation given in any of the guidelines is to assess the needs of stroke survivors and carers then some form of assessment tool may be helpful. An array of tools exists to assess various aspects of health and well-being relating to the consequences of stroke, but most are not designed to assess stroke-specific problems or unmet needs from the survivor's or the carer's perspective.

Most tools use predefined categories to elicit responses; some were originally designed for research purposes, whilst others are clinical assessment tools. Specific clinical tools for assessing physical recovery, independence in activities of daily living, cognitive assessment, and emotional health can be found elsewhere. Here, we focus on assessments that can be used to identify carer burden and assess the unmet needs of carers and survivors.

14.5.1 Assessing Carer Burden

The Family Caregiver Alliance, a partially state-funded US not-for-profit organisation, has produced a comprehensive inventory of measures for use by health professionals in assessing aspects of the caregiver role and their consequences [47]. However, not all of these measures have been validated for use with carers of stroke survivors. The most commonly used assessments are summarised in two systematic reviews and presented in Table 14.1 [29, 57]. Not all of these measures were developed specifically for assessing burden post-stroke, or necessarily for use in practice; but all have been psychometrically tested with carers of stroke survivors. An example of application for practice is highlighted in Case Study 14.2, whereby the stroke nurse used a formal caregiver burden survey to guide a conversation on the carer's role in order to understand its potential impacts on Derek. Going through each of the domains of an assessment tool is important to ensure all areas of potential need are covered, and helps open dialogue between the carer and assessor on subjects that might otherwise not have been discussed. Carers should be assessed for their support needs and reassessed if their health or social circumstances change (or annually, if not) [60]. A number of studies provide evidence of specific stroke survivor and carer characteristics that increase the risk of poorer health and well-being in the longer term. Carer characteristics that predict greater burden include being younger, female, or in poor physical or mental health [20].

14.5.2 Assessing Needs of Survivors of Stroke

Several assessment tools have been developed to aid practitioners in assessing the ongoing needs of survivors, the latest of which was developed in conjunction with the World Stroke Organization (Table 14.2).

14.5.3 High-Risk Groups

Stroke survivors should be assessed for their rehabilitation and support needs, and reassessed if their health or social circumstances change (or annually, if not) [60].

Studies providing evidence of stroke survivor characteristics that predict greater burden include having severe physical, cognitive, behavioural, and emotional difficulties [20]. These characteristics also tend to result in greater proportions of unmet need (see earlier). Qualitative interviews with survivors reveal that those with more complex needs (e.g. those with communication difficulties and younger people) may fall through the net of services because they do not fit existing models of care or rigid policy criteria [61]. High-risk groups may require additional assessment or follow-up to ensure that their needs are met. Importantly, part of the risk assessment should explore individual recovery expectations and the amount of social support available to and utilised by survivors and carers [7, 40].

TABLE 14.1   **Commonly used tools for assessing burden in carers**

Name of assessment tool	Description	Author
Zarit Burden Interview	Originally developed to assess feelings of burden in carers of elderly people with dementia. Tool measures: (i) caregiver's health; (ii) psychological well-being; (iii) finances; (iv) social life; and (v) relationship between caregiver and care recipient	Zarit et al. [48]
Sense of Competence Questionnaire	Validated amongst carers at 6 and 17 mo post-stroke, 27 items on 3 subscales: (i) satisfaction with the impaired person as a recipient of care; (ii) satisfaction with one's own performance as a caregiver; (iii) consequences of involvement in care for the caregiver's personal life	Scholte op Reimer et al. [49]
Bakas Caregiving Outcome Scale	Validated amongst carers 4 mo post-stroke, 15 items covering: (i) caregiver and survivor characteristics; (ii) caregiver optimism; (iii) dependent-care tasks; (iv) appraisal; (v) depressive symptoms	Bakas and Champion [50], Bakas et al. [51]
Caregiver's Burden Scale	Validated in a mixed sample (83 carers of people with dementia, 76 carers of stroke survivors), 22 items covering: (i) general strain; (ii) isolation; (iii) disappointment; (iv) emotional involvement; (v) environment	Elmstahl et al. [52]
Preparedness for Caregiving Scale	Validated using data obtained at 6 wk and 9 mo after post-stroke hospital discharge, includes preparedness for: (i) providing physical care; (ii) providing emotional support; (iii) setting up in-home support services; (iv) stress of caregiving	Archbold et al. [53]
Caregiver Burden Inventory	Validated in 107 caregivers of confused older people, subscales cover a range of problems, including: (i) time dependence; (ii) developmental burden; (iii) physical burden; (iv) social burden; (v) emotional burden	Novak and Guest [54]
Caregiver Strain Index	Validated in 103 hospitalised hip fracture and heart disease patients, a brief 13-item, easily administered instrument with four domains: (i) patient characteristics; (ii) subjective perception of the caregiving relationship; (iii) caregiver emotional status; (iv) sociodemographics	Robinson [55]
Relatives Stress Scale	Developed with 38 carers of people with dementia, 15 items covering: (i) personal distress; (ii) degree of life upset; (iii) negative feelings towards care recipient	Greene et al. [56]

TABLE 14.2 **Assessment tools for assessing survivor and carer needs**

Name of assessment tool	Description	Author
Stroke Caregiver Unmet Needs Resource Scale	12-item scale for assessing carer unmet needs in relation to resources for managing the physical, emotional, and behavioural consequences of stroke; can be completed in person or by phone	Green and King [58]
Greater Manchester Stroke Assessment Tool (GM-SAT)	Assessment at 6 mo post-stroke, covers 34 topics relating to health, social, and emotional needs of stroke survivors and 1 topic relating to carer needs; available in a format designed for people with communication difficulties	Rothwell et al. [18]
Post Stroke Checklist (PSC)	11 items with dichotomous (yes/ no) answers relating to physical and emotional disability, life after stroke, and family relationships; designed to be used by clinicians at 3 mo, 6 mo, and annual reviews	Ward et al. [59]

14.6 Interventions to Support Stroke Survivors and Carers

National guidelines recommend providing information and support, but with little detail on what to provide or how it should be delivered. A meta-review of delivery of self-management support through routine rehabilitation therapy reported that delivery soon after the stroke event resulted in short-term (<1 year) improvements in basic and extended activities of daily living and reduced death and dependence [62]. It is therefore important that information and support interventions start as early as possible post-stroke, to assist in the transition from hospital to home and prepare survivors and carers for their new circumstances and roles.

In many countries, rehabilitation services such as those discussed in Chapters 8 and 9 are time-limited. The UK Intercollegiate Stroke Working Party reports that there is good-quality evidence that more therapy improves the rate of recovery and outcome within the first 6 months post-stroke, but there is little evidence to guide how much therapy should be provided. Therefore, continuation should take into account a survivor's willingness and capability to participate, and there should be measurable benefit from treatment [42]. Recommendations are limited by a lack of robust research on rehabilitation intensity in acute and longer-term settings [42]. Systematic reviews have investigated the effectiveness of specific interventions in improving the health and well-being of survivors and carers. Most include solely randomised controlled trials (RCTs), but whilst RCTs provide the strongest evidence for efficacy, complex interventions for longer-term support often do not lend themselves to evaluation with such a design. This is because it can be difficult to recruit and randomise participants, isolate the active ingredients of the intervention, implement the intervention in a trial context, and evaluate appropriate outcomes within a practical time frame [63, 64]. Complexity may explain the lack of strong evidence to support current guidance in this area. In addition, many studies have limited generalisability to other populations (e.g. studies of spouses may not be relevant to carers who are adult children) or settings where healthcare systems are different [65], and may lack consideration of ethnic/cultural minority groups, where caregiver/survivor expectations and experiences may vary [66].

Interventions can be categorised into the following groups: written information; education and practical training; psychoeducation, self-education, and psychological therapy; liaison work; respite care; peer support; and financial support (Table 14.3).

14.6.1   Written Information

Written information is a mechanism to encourage people to take more active roles in managing their health. Systematic reviews evaluating written information have consistently shown that without an active component, information alone does not lead to better health outcomes [64, 67, 68]. Even complex interventions with components targeting multiple stakeholders have been unsuccessful in influencing clinically relevant outcomes [84, 85]. However, there is evidence that passive educational interventions can improve patient and carer knowledge of stroke and aspects of patient satisfaction [67].

14.6.2   Education and Practical Training

The evidence for more active educational intervention is mixed. One in-hospital hands-on training programme delivering procedural education to survivors and carers stood out in all reviews as the only intervention to demonstrate a positive effect on survivor well-being in the first year [86]. However, an attempt to replicate the effects in a multi-centre study failed [87]. In-hospital written proformas were given to staff to promote hands-on training with families, but staff uptake was poor [88]. Practical training may improve the transition to home and subjective health outcomes, but successful implementation requires that complex processes such as motivating staff and influencing professional behaviour are addressed. Research on community-based training, as opposed to delivery in hospital or pre-discharge, is lacking.

14.6.3   Psychoeducation, Self-Management, and Psychological Therapy

Despite multiple reviews of interventions in this area, the evidence for psychoeducational interventions is limited, with only two RCTs of interventions to enhance survivor self-efficacy (self-confidence) [74]. Neither intervention had an impact on psychological outcomes (including self-efficacy), although Johnston's workbook

TABLE 14.3 Interventions to support survivors and carers in the longer term

Intervention	Description and examples	References for further information
Written information	Passive written information without active instruction includes generic information leaflets or booklets; personally tailored information; patient-held health records; and complex interventions targeting multiple stakeholders (patients, carers, and primary care professionals) using generic and tailored information updated at multiple time points	Redfern et al. [64], Forster et al. [67], Legg et al. [68]
Education and practical training	These have an active educational component, including lectures, hands-on procedural training, and case reviews conducted either in person, by phone, or via the Web	Redfern et al. [64], Bakas et al. [65], Forster et al. [67], Legg et al. [68], Brereton et al. [69]
Psychoeducation, self-management, and psychological therapy	These interventions can be distinguished from generic education by their psychological component, aiming to reinforce personal strengths, resources, and coping skills to help participants manage their own health in the longer term. Interventions tend to be delivered by individuals from psychological or psychiatric disciplines or health professionals with specific training and supervision. Self-management interventions, rooted in self-efficacy theory, are one type of psychoeducation. Psychological therapies include cognitive behavioural therapy (CBT), motivational interviewing, problem solving, and goal setting	Redfern et al. [64], Legg et al. [68], Hackett et al. [70], Lui et al. [71], Hackett et al. [72], Foster et al. [73], Jones and Riazi [74]
Liaison work	Liaison work is not a discipline in itself. The role may entail utilising components discussed elsewhere in this table, but also focuses on linking with social services, benefits agencies, and the voluntary sector	Ellis et al. [75]
Respite care	Respite (formal or informal) is a means for carers to take a short-term break from responsibilities and activities. Traditional locations for services include day centres, hospitals, and home-based services	Hanson et al. [76], Shaw et al. [77]
Peer support	Peer support entails provision of emotional, appraisal, and informational assistance by a person of similar characteristics and with experiential knowledge of stroke. It can be delivered in acute care settings, during home visits, via telephone follow-up calls, through Web-based support, and via leisure-focused activities	Stroke Foundation [46], Dennis [78], Kessler et al. [79], Morris and Morris [80], Stewart et al. [81], Smith et al. [82], Tamplin et al. [83]
Financial support	Financial support may include payment for loss of income for carers or assistance in covering out-of-pocket costs, including home adaptations and equipment	Addo et al. [96], Department of Health and Social Care [97]

intervention resulted in improved functional recovery for the self-management group, as compared to controls [89]. A more recent RCT of an intervention to improve memory self-efficacy demonstrated a significant improvement in the intervention arm during the first year, and improved quality of life in younger participants compared to controls, but with no impact on mood or social participation [90, 91]. Several small trials of self-management programmes for long-term stroke recovery have also been inconclusive [92].

Reviews of psychological therapy for the prevention and treatment of depression in survivors have demonstrated small but significant effects on mood in prevention, but not in treatment of those diagnosed with depression at the outset [70, 72]. The evidence for the ability of psychological therapy to prevent or treat post-stroke fatigue remains insufficient [93]. Group educational support, counselling, and home-based problem-solving sessions show no effect on carer burden [68].

14.6.4 Liaison Work

A systematic review of liaison work concluded that it benefited specific groups of stroke survivors and carers, including reducing death and disability and improving satisfaction with service provision in survivors with mild to moderate disability [75].

14.6.5 Respite Care

Little research has examined the benefits of respite care for carers of stroke survivors. A recent cross-sectional study of the association between satisfaction with respite care and carer burden amongst people with acquired brain injury (70% stroke) found that survivors and carers were highly satisfied with the respite centre. However, high levels of burden remained, as did low levels of overall life satisfaction [94]. Evidence of increased institutionalisation amongst survivors following respite care suggests it is used more as a form of crisis management than as a routine part of the caring process [77]. Proactive intervention to prevent crises is imperative.

14.6.6 Peer Support

Peer support is not routinely recommended in clinical guidelines, as there is no conclusive evidence to support it. Nonetheless, stroke voluntary sector services and peer-support groups can play an important role in helping community integration [42]. Therefore, consensus-based recommendations in the Australian guidelines include that carers should be provided with information about the availability and potential benefits of local stroke support groups and services, at or before the patient's return to the community [46]. Recent case examples of peer-support programmes entail: visits in the acute care setting by experienced stroke survivors and carers [79, 80]; home visits [81]; telephone follow-up calls [79]; Web-based support [82]; and leisure-focused activities in the form of a choir for people with aphasia [83]. One RCT provided evidence of a positive influence on mood for carers, but not survivors [82]. Observational and qualitative findings suggest that informational and psychological benefits for recipients are likely to be linked to personal preference [79]. Guidance on peer-support groups, including advice on setting up a group and useful contacts, is available through the US Stroke Association Web site (www.strokeassociation.org). Other peer support resources can be found via the UK Stroke Association and the Australian Stroke Foundation enableme Web site (www.enableme.org.au [95]).

14.6.7   Financial Support

Socioeconomic factors play a role in most aspects of stroke recovery and care, but no studies have examined the impact of financial support on stroke survivors and carers [96]. In many high-income countries (HICs) with strong social support policies, they may be eligible for financial support. The UK 2014 Care Act focuses on financial support for carers, and provides factsheets on the subject [97]. Local authority support is often means-tested, so not all survivors and carers are eligible.

14.6.8   Other Potential Interventions for Long-Term Support

More recently, and with increasing access to technology, the benefits of e-health in promoting well-being and long-term support post-stroke are being explored. Importantly, use of technology may improve access to health professionals or online support groups, reducing inequity. Technological support includes telestroke programmes and use of apps and Web-based programmes to encourage self-management, promote behaviour change, and ultimately improve health outcomes [98–100]. In the era of computer-literate stroke survivors and carers, such interventions may prove worthwhile, and health professionals should keep up with developments in this field.

14.7   Supporting Working-Age Survivors of Stroke

One in four strokes occurs in working-age people, and the proportion experiencing first stroke at a younger age is increasing [101, 102]. Younger survivors and carers may have additional age-related needs, for example in relation to employment and family relationships (including raising young children) [14, 103].

Return-to-work is important for psychological, social, and financial reasons. However, one-quarter of working -age stroke survivors do not return to paid or unpaid work [104]. A systematic review of the social consequences of stroke in working-age people identified factors enabling return-to-work, including:

vocational rehabilitation; flexibility and support in the workplace; social benefits; and family support [105]. An RCT of a tailored workplace intervention for stroke survivors showed significant increase in return-to-work amongst the intervention group compared to controls [106].

Generic rehabilitation is mostly insufficient to meet the needs of younger people [105, 107], and long-term care options are often inadequate or inappropriate. The UK-based national charity Different Strokes offers information and support for younger people [108]. Little is known about the needs of younger carers, despite the increased burden in this group [109]. The World Stroke Organization and most national charity Web sites cover issues related to living with stroke at a younger age, but much remains to be done. Independence in activities of daily living is the strongest predictor of return to paid work within 12 months post-stroke [104]. However, as highlighted in Case Study 14.1, whilst efforts to return to work by Brian were important in increasing his social participation, he could only work up to 2 hours per day due to his fatigue. Therefore, conversations with employers on realistic work participation are needed to ensure a successful outcome for all parties. Nurses, in conjunction with their multidisciplinary colleagues, have an important role in educating patients about setting realistic and achievable goals for their recovery, including return-to-work.

14.8 Conclusion

This chapter presents an overview of the unmet long-term needs of survivors of stroke and their carers, as well as potential interventions to meet these needs and improve well-being. The area lacks a strong research base to support policy and practice decisions related to effective long-term support. Novel approaches using e-health solutions may reduce inequity of access to support. Health professionals should discuss options for support and appropriate carer coping strategies pre-emptively to enhance well-being for both survivor and carer.

Dedication

This chapter is dedicated in memory of Judith Redfern, who lost her battle with cancer in February 2018, prior to the publication of this book. Judith started her research career in 1993 as a student working at the Home Office on the British Crime Survey. After graduating in Mathematics and Psychology, she moved into health services research. Her first research post was at University College London, working with Ann Bowling on a study into the appropriateness of outpatient care in the North Thames region. Judith has made an important contribution to the field of stroke since 1999, including a national study into the longer-term needs of stroke survivors. Jude joined the University of Central Lancashire in 2013 and was a Senior Research Fellow until her death in February 2018. During this time, she contributed to various research outputs, including the development of the Stroke Patient Concerns Inventory.

References

1. UK Stroke Forum Education & Training. About the SSEF. Available from: http://www.stroke-education.org.uk/about [30 November 2018].
2. McCrum, R. (2015). My Year Off: Rediscovering Life After Stroke. London: Pan Macmillan.
3. Campbell, J., Tyrrell, P., Bray, B., and Kavanagh, K. (2014). How Good is Stroke Care? First SSNAP Annual Report. London: Royal College of Physicians.
4. Intercollegiate Stroke Working Party (2012). National Clinical Guidelines for Stroke. London: Royal College of Physicians.
5. McKevitt, C., Fudge, N., Redfern, J. et al. (2011). Self-reported long-term needs after stroke. Stroke 42 (5): 1398–1403.
6. Jones, F., Riazi, A., and Norris, M. (2013). Self-management after stroke: time for some more questions? Disability and Rehabilitation 35 (3): 257–264.
7. Graven, C., Sansonetti, D., Moloczij, N. et al. (2013). Stroke survivor and carer perspectives of the concept of recovery: a qualitative study. Disability and Rehabilitation 35 (7): 578–585.
8. Department of Health (2007). National Stroke Strategy. London: Department of Health.
9. Office of National Statistics. 2011 Census Analysis: Unpaid Care in England and Wales, 2011 and Comparison with 2001. London: Office of National Statistics; 2013.
10. Buckner, L. and Yeandle, S. (2011). Valuing Carers 2011. London: Carers UK.
11. Dewey, H.M., Thrift, A.G., Mihalopoulos, C. et al. (2002). Informal care for stroke survivors: results from the North East Melbourne Stroke Incidence Study (NEMESIS). Stroke 33 (4): 1028–1033.
12. Tooth, L., McKenna, K., Barnett, A. et al. (2005). Caregiver burden, time spent caring and health status in the first 12 months following stroke. Brain Injury 19 (12): 963–974.
13. Gloede, T.D., Halbach, S.M., Thrift, A.G. et al. (2014). Long-term costs of stroke using 10-year longitudinal data from the North East Melbourne Stroke Incidence Study. Stroke 45 (11): 3389–3394.
14. Andrew, N.E., Kilkenny, M., Naylor, R. et al. (2014). Understanding long-term unmet needs in Australian survivors of stroke. International Journal of Stroke 9 (SA100): 106–112.
15. National Stroke Foundation (2002). Stroke Care Outcomes: Providing Effective Services: SCOPES Report. An Evaluation of Victorian Stroke Services. Melbourne: National Stroke Foundation.
16. Hafsteinsdottir, T.B., Vergunst, M., Lindeman, E., and Schuurmans, M. (2011). Educational needs of patients with a stroke and their caregivers: a systematic review of the literature. Patient Education and Counseling 85 (1): 14–25.
17. Andrew, N.E., Kilkenny, M.F., Naylor, R. et al. (2015). The relationship between caregiver impacts and the unmet needs of survivors of stroke. Patient Preference and Adherence 9: 1065–1073.
18. Rothwell, K., Boaden, R., Bamford, D., and Tyrrell, P.J. (2013). Feasibility of assessing the needs of stroke patients after six months using the GM-SAT. Clinical Rehabilitation 27 (3): 264–271.
19. Clark, D.M. (2012). The English Improving Access to Psychological Therapies (IAPT) Program. In: Dissemination and Implementation of Evidence-Based Psychological Interventions (ed. R.K. McHugh and H. Barlow), 61–77. Oxford: Oxford University Press.
20. Greenwood, N., Mackenzie, A., Cloud, G.C., and Wilson, N. (2008). Informal carers of stroke survivors – factors influencing carers: a systematic review of quantitative studies. Disability and Rehabilitation 30 (18): 1329–1349.

21. Greenwood, N., Mackenzie, A., Cloud, G.C., and Wilson, N. (2009). Informal primary carers of stroke survivors living at home-challenges, satisfactions and coping: a systematic review of qualitative studies. Disability and Rehabilitation 31 (5): 337–351.
22. Bury, M. (1984). Chronic illness as biographical disruption. Sociology of Health and Illness 6: 1122–1133.
23. Greenwood, N. and Mackenzie, A. (2010). Informal caring for stroke survivors: meta-ethnographic review of qualitative literature. Maturitas 66 (3): 268–276.
24. Masry, Y.E. (2010). Understanding the Experiences of Caring for Someone After Stroke: A Qualitative Study of Caregivers and Stroke Survivors. Sydney: University of Sydney.
25. El Masry, Y., Mullan, B., and Hackett, M. (2013). Psychosocial experiences and needs of Australian caregivers of people with stroke: prognosis messages, caregiver resilience, and relationships. Topics in Stroke Rehabilitation 20 (4): 356–368.
26. Mackenzie, A. and Greenwood, N. (2012). Positive experiences of caregiving in stroke: a systematic review. Disability and Rehabilitation 34 (17): 1413–1422.
27. Quinn, K., Murray, C., and Malone, C. (2014). Spousal experiences of coping with and adapting to caregiving for a partner who has a stroke: a meta-synthesis of qualitative research. Disability and Rehabilitation 36 (3): 185–198.
28. World Health Organisation. A Glossary of Terms for Community Health Care and Services for Older Persons. Available from: http://apps.who.int/iris/handle/10665/68896 [30 November 2018].
29. Rigby, H., Gubitz, G., and Phillips, S. (2009). A systematic review of caregiver burden following stroke. International Journal of Stroke 4 (4): 285–292.
30. Camak, D.J. (2015). Addressing the burden of stroke caregivers: a literature review. Journal of Clinical Nursing 24 (17–18): 2376–2382.
31. Tang, W.K., Lau, C.G., Mok, V. et al. (2011). Burden of Chinese stroke family caregivers: the Hong Kong experience. Archives of Physical Medicine and Rehabilitation 92 (9): 1462–1467.
32. Visser-Meily, J.M., van den Bos, G.A., and Kappelle, L.J. (2009). Better acute treatment induces more investments in chronic care for stroke patients. International Journal of Stroke 4 (5): 352–353.
33. Parag, V., Hackett, M.L., Yapa, C.M. et al. (2008). The impact of stroke on unpaid caregivers: results from the Auckland Regional Community Stroke study, 2002–2003. Cerebrovascular Diseases 25 (6): 548–554.
34. Denno, M.S., Gillard, P.J., Graham, G.D. et al. (2013). Anxiety and depression associated with caregiver burden in caregivers of stroke survivors with spasticity. Archives of Physical Medicine and Rehabilitation 94 (9): 1731–1736.
35. Berg, A., Palomaki, H., Lonnqvist, J. et al. (2005). Depression among caregivers of stroke survivors. Stroke 36 (3): 639–643.
36. Atteih, S., Mellon, L., Hall, P. et al. (2015). Implications of stroke for caregiver outcomes: findings from the ASPIRE-S study. International Journal of Stroke 10 (6): 918–923.
37. Smith, L.N., Norrie, J., Kerr, S.M. et al. (2004). Impact and influences on caregiver outcomes at one year post-stroke. Cerebrovascular Diseases 18 (2): 145–153.
38. Anderson, C.S., Linto, J., and Stewart-Wynne, E.G. (1995). A population-based assessment of the impact and burden of caregiving for long-term stroke survivors. Stroke 26 (5): 843–849.
39. Klinedinst, N.J., Gebhardt, M.C., Aycock, D.M. et al. (2009). Caregiver characteristics predict stroke survivor quality of life at 4 months and 1 year. Research in Nursing and Health 32 (6): 592–605.
40. Cumming, T.B., Cadilhac, D.A., Rubin, G. et al. (2008). Psychological distress and social support in informal caregivers of stroke survivors. Brain Impairment 9: 152–160.
41. National Institute for Health and Care Excellence (2015). Stroke Rehabilitation. London: National Institute for Health and Care Excellence.

42. Intercollegiate Stroke Working Party (2016). National Clinical Guidelines for Stroke. London: Royal College of Physicians.
43. Lindsay, P., Bayley, M., McDonald, A. et al. (2008). Toward a more effective approach to stroke: Canadian best practice recommendations for stroke care. Canadian Medical Association Journal 178 (11): 1418–1425.
44. Miller, E.L., Murray, L., Richards, L. et al. (2010). Comprehensive overview of nursing and interdisciplinary rehabilitation care of the stroke patient: a scientific statement from the American Heart Association. Stroke 41 (10): 2402–2448.
45. National Institute for Health and Care Excellence (2013). Long Term Rehabilitation After Stroke. London: National Clinical Guideline Centre.
46. Stroke Foundation (2017). Clinical Guidelines for Stroke Management. Melbourne: Melbourne Stroke Foundation.
47. Family Caregiver Alliance (2012). Selective Caregiver Assessment Scales: A Resource Inventory for Practitioners. San Francisco: Family Caregiver Alliance.
48. Zarit, S.H., Reever, K.E., and Bach-Peterson, J. (1980). Relatives of the impaired elderly: correlates of feelings of burden. The Gerontologist 20 (6): 649–655.
49. Scholte op Reimer, W.J., de Haan, R.J., Pijnenborg, J.M. et al. (1998). Assessment of burden in partners of stroke patients with the sense of competence questionnaire. Stroke 29 (2): 373–379.
50. Bakas, T. and Champion, V. (1999). Development and psychometric testing of the bakas caregiving outcomes scale. Nursing Research 48 (5): 250–259.
51. Bakas, T., Champion, V., Perkins, S.M. et al. (2006). Psychometric testing of the revised 15-item bakas caregiving outcomes scale. Nursing Research 55 (5): 346–355.
52. Elmstahl, S., Malmberg, B., and Annerstedt, L. (1996). Caregiver's burden of patients 3 years after stroke assessed by a novel caregiver burden scale. Archives of Physical Medicine and Rehabilitation 77 (2): 177–182.
53. Archbold, P.G., Stewart, B.J., Greenlick, M.R., and Harvath, T. (1990). Mutuality and preparedness as predictors of caregiver role strain. Research in Nursing and Health 13 (6): 375–384.
54. Novak, M. and Guest, C. (1989). Application of a multidimensional caregiver burden inventory. The Gerontologist 29 (6): 798–803.
55. Robinson, B.C. (1983). Validation of a caregiver strain index. Journal of Gerontology 38 (3): 344–348.
56. Greene, J.G., Smith, R., Gardiner, M., and Timbury, G.C. (1982). Measuring behavioural disturbance of elderly demented patients in the community and its effects on relatives: a factor analytic study. Age and Ageing 11 (2): 121–126.
57. Visser-Meily, J.M., Post, M.W., Riphagen, I.I., and Lindeman, E. (2004). Measures used to assess burden among caregivers of stroke patients: a review. Clinical Rehabilitation 18 (6): 601–623.
58. Green, T.L. and King, K.M. (2011). Relationships between biophysical and psychosocial outcomes following minor stroke. Canadian Journal of Neuroscience Nursing 33 (2): 15–23.
59. Ward, A.B., Chen, C., Norrving, B. et al. (2014). Evaluation of the post stroke checklist: a pilot study in the United Kingdom and Singapore. International Journal of Stroke 9 (Suppl. A100): 76–84.
60. National Institute for Health and Care Excellence (NICE). Stroke Rehabilitation in Adults. Clinical guidelines C162. National Institute for Health and Clinical Excellence; 2013.
61. Mold, F., Wolfe, C., and McKevitt, C. (2006). Falling through the net of stroke care. Health and Social Care in the Community 14 (4): 349–356.
62. Parke, H.L., Epiphaniou, E., Pearce, G. et al. (2015). Self-management support interventions for stroke survivors: a systematic meta-review. PLoS One 10 (7): e0131448.

63. Redfern J. Methods for Developing and Evaluating Randomised Controlled Trials of Complex Interventions: Case Study of Stroke Secondary Prevention. London: University of London; 2007.

64. Redfern, J., McKevitt, C., and Wolfe, C.D. (2006). Development of complex interventions in stroke care: a systematic review. Stroke 37 (9): 2410–2419.

65. Bakas, T., Clark, P.C., Kelly-Hayes, M. et al. (2014). Evidence for stroke family caregiver and dyad interventions: a statement for healthcare professionals from the American Heart Association and American Stroke Association. Stroke 45 (9): 2836–2852.

66. American Psychological Association. Cultural diversity and caregiving. Available from: http://www.apa.org/pi/about/publications/caregivers/faq/cultural-diversity. aspx [30 November 2018].

67. Forster, A., Brown, L., Smith, J. et al. (2012). Information provision for stroke patients and their caregivers. Cochrane Database of Systematic Reviews 11 (Art. No.: CD001919). https://doi.org/10.1002/14651858.CD001919.

68. Legg, L.A., Quinn, T.J., Mahmood, F. et al. (2011). Non-pharmacological interventions for caregivers of stroke survivors. Cochrane Database of Systematic Reviews 10 (Art. No.: CD008179). https://doi.org/10.1002/14651858.CD008179.

69. Brereton, L., Carroll, C., and Barnston, S. (2007). Interventions for adult family carers of people who have had a stroke: a systematic review. Clinical Rehabilitation 21 (10): 867–884.

70. Hackett, M.L., Anderson, C.S., House, A., and Halteh, C. (2008). Interventions for preventing depression after stroke. Cochrane Database of Systematic Reviews 3 (Art. No.: CD003689). https://doi.org/10.1002/14651858.

71. Lui, M.H., Ross, F.M., and Thompson, D.R. (2005). Supporting family caregivers in stroke care: a review of the evidence for problem solving. Stroke 36 (11): 2514–2522.

72. Hackett, M.L., Anderson, C.S., House, A., and Xia, J. (2008). Interventions for treating depression after stroke. Cochrane Database of Systematic Reviews 4 (Art. No.: CD003437). https://doi.org/10.1002/14651858.CD003437.

73. Foster, G., Taylor, S.J., Eldridge, S.E. et al. (2007). Self-management education programmes by lay leaders for people with chronic conditions. Cochrane Database of Systematic Reviews 4 (Art. No.: CD005108). https://doi.org/10.1002/14651858. CD005108.

74. Jones, F. and Riazi, A. (2011). Self-efficacy and self-management after stroke: a systematic review. Disability and Rehabilitation 33 (10): 797–810.

75. Ellis, G., Mant, J., Langhorne, P. et al. (2010). Stroke liaison workers for stroke patients and carers: an individual patient data meta-analysis. Cochrane Database of Systematic Reviews 5 (Art. No.: CD005066). https://doi.org/10.1002/14651858.CD005066.

76. Hanson, E.J., Tetley, J., and Clarke, A. (1999). Respite care for frail older people and their family carers: concept analysis and user focus group findings of a pan-European nursing research project. Journal of Advanced Nursing 30 (6): 1396–1407.

77. Shaw, C., McNamara, R., Abrams, K. et al. (2009). Systematic review of respite care in the frail elderly. Health Technology Assessment 13 (20): 1–224, iii.

78. Dennis, C.L. (2003). Peer support within a health care context: a concept analysis. International Journal of Nursing Studies 40 (3): 321–332.

79. Kessler, D., Egan, M., and Kubina, L.-A. (2014). Peer support for stroke survivors: a case study. BMC Health Services Research 14 (1): 256.

80. Morris, R. and Morris, P. (2012). Participants' experiences of hospital-based peer support groups for stroke patients and carers. Disability and Rehabilitation 34 (4): 347–354.

81. Stewart, M.J., Doble, S., Hart, G. et al. (1998). Peer visitor support for family caregivers of seniors with stroke. Canadian Journal of Nursing Research 30 (2): 87–117.

82. Smith, G.C., Egbert, N., Dellman-Jenkins, M. et al. (2012). Reducing depression in stroke survivors and their informal caregivers: a randomized clinical trial of a Web-based intervention. Rehabilitation Psychology 57 (3): 196–206.

83. Tamplin, J., Baker, F.A., Jones, B. et al. (2013). 'Stroke a Chord': the effect of singing in a community choir on mood and social engagement for people living with aphasia following a stroke. NeuroRehabilitation 32 (4): 929–941.

84. Redfern, J., Rudd, A.D., Wolfe, C.D., and McKevitt, C. (2008). Stop Stroke: development of an innovative intervention to improve risk factor management after stroke. Patient Education and Counseling 72 (2): 201–209.

85. Wolfe, C.D., Redfern, J., Rudd, A.G. et al. (2010). Cluster randomized controlled trial of a patient and general practitioner intervention to improve the management of multiple risk factors after stroke: stop stroke. Stroke 41 (11): 2470–2476.

86. Kalra, L., Evans, A., Perez, I. et al. (2004). Training carers of stroke patients: randomised controlled trial. British Medical Journal 328 (7448): 1099.

87. Forster, A., Young, J., Nixon, J. et al. (2012). A cluster randomized controlled trial of a structured training programme for caregivers of inpatients after stroke (TRACS). International Journal of Stroke 7 (1): 94–99.

88. Clarke, D.J., Hawkins, R., Sadler, E. et al. (2014). Introducing structured caregiver training in stroke care: findings from the TRACS process evaluation study. BMJ Open 4 (4): 1–10.

89. Johnston, M., Bonetti, D., Joice, S. et al. (2007). Recovery from disability after stroke as a target for a behavioural intervention: results of a randomized controlled trial. Disability and Rehabilitation 29 (14): 1117–1127.

90. Aben, L., Heijenbrok-Kal, M.H., Ponds, R.W. et al. (2014). Long-lasting effects of a new memory self-efficacy training for stroke patients: a randomized controlled trial. Neurorehabilitation and Neural Repair 28 (3): 199–206.

91. Aben, L., Heijenbrok-Kal, M.H., van Loon, E.M. et al. (2013). Training memory self-efficacy in the chronic stage after stroke: a randomized controlled trial. Neurorehabilitation and Neural Repair 27 (2): 110–117.

92. Cadilhac, D.A., Hoffmann, S., Kilkenny, M. et al. (2011). A phase II multicentered, single-blind, randomized, controlled trial of the stroke self-management program. Stroke 42 (6): 1673–1679.

93. Wu, S., Kutlubaev, M.A., Chun, H.Y. et al. (2015). Interventions for post-stroke fatigue. Cochrane Database of Systematic Reviews 7 (Art. No.: CD007030). https://doi.org/10.1002/14651858.

94. Smeets, S.M., van Heugten, C.M., Geboers, J.F. et al. (2012). Respite care after acquired brain injury: the well-being of caregivers and patients. Archives of Physical Medicine and Rehabilitation 93 (5): 834–841.

95. Stroke Foundation. Enable me Melbourne: helping you with your own stroke recovery. Available from: https://enableme.org.au [30 November 2018].

96. Addo, J., Ayerbe, L., Mohan, K.M. et al. (2012). Socioeconomic status and stroke. An Updated Review 43 (4): 1186–1191.

97. Department of Health and Social Care. Care Act 2014 part 1: factsheets. Available from: http://www.gov.uk/government/publications/care-act-2014-part-1-factsheets [30 November 2018].

98. Mc Kinstry, B., Hanley, J., and Lewis, S. (2015). Telemonitoring in the management of high blood pressure. Current Pharmaceutical Design 21 (6): 823–827.

99. Vloothuis, J., Mulder, M., Nijland, R.H. et al. (2015). Caregiver-mediated exercises with e-health support for early supported discharge after stroke (CARE4STROKE): study protocol for a randomized controlled trial. British Medcial Council Neurology 15: 193.

100. Jones, K.M., Bhattacharjee, R., Krishnamurthi, R. et al. (2015). Methodology of the Stroke Self-Management Rehabilitation Trial: an international, multisite pilot trial. Journal of Stroke and Cerebrovascular Diseases 24 (2): 297–303.

101. Busch, M.A., Coshall, C., Heuschmann, P.U. et al. (2009). Sociodemographic differences in return to work after stroke: the South London Stroke Register (SLSR). Journal of Neurology, Neurosurgery, and Psychiatry 80 (8): 888–893.
102. Rothwell, P.M., Coull, A.J., Giles, M.F. et al. (2004). Change in stroke incidence, mortality, case-fatality, severity, and risk factors in Oxfordshire, UK from 1981 to 2004 (Oxford Vascular Study). The Lancet 363 (9425): 1925–1933.
103. Kersten, P., Low, J.T., Ashburn, A. et al. (2002). The unmet needs of young people who have had a stroke: results of a national UK survey. Disability and Rehabilitation 24 (16): 860–866.
104. Hackett, M.L., Glozier, N., Jan, S., and Lindley, R. (2012). Returning to paid employment after stroke: the Psychosocial Outcomes in Stroke (POISE) Cohort Study. PLoS One 7 (7): e41795.
105. Daniel, K., Wolfe, C.D., Busch, M.A., and McKevitt, C. (2009). What are the social consequences of stroke for working-aged adults? A systematic review. Stroke 40 (6): e431–e440.
106. Ntsiea, M.V., Van Aswegen, H., Lord, S., and Olorunju, S.S. (2015). The effect of a workplace intervention programme on return to work after stroke: a randomised controlled trial. Clinical Rehabilitation 29 (7): 663–673.
107. Medin, J., Barajas, J., and Ekberg, K. (2006). Stroke patients' experiences of return to work. Disability and Rehabilitation 28 (17): 1051–1060.
108. Different Strokes. About Different Strokes. Available from: https://differentstrokes.co.uk/about-us [30 November 2018].
109. van den Heuvel, E.T., de Witte, L.P., Schure, L.M. et al. (2001). Risk factors for burn-out in caregivers of stroke patients, and possibilities for intervention. Clinical Rehabilitation 15 (6): 669–677.

APPENDIX A

The Stroke-Specific Education Framework (SSEF)

The SSEF consists of 16 Elements of Care, based on the quality markers in the UK National Stroke Strategy and related to the stroke strategies in all four UK countries.

Within each Element of Care there are various numbers of key competences that reflect the 'knowledge and understanding' and 'skills and abilities' a member of staff should possess if they work in that area of stroke care delivery. Icons at the start of each chapter indicate content in that chapter linking to that element. The SSEF is a freely available resource for anyone interested in stroke care to use. Each of the 16 elements is comprised of variable numbers of knowledge and skills components. At the beginning of each chapter there are icons to reflect the SSEF element fully or partially covered.

http://www.stroke-education.org.uk/framework

The SSEF 16 Elements of Care

E1: Awareness raising

Members of the public and health and care staff are able to recognise and identify the main symptoms of stroke and know to treat it as an emergency.

E2: Managing risk

Those at risk of stroke and those who have had a stroke are assessed for and given information about risk factors and lifestyle management issues so that action can be taken to reduce overall vascular risk.

E3: Information

Those affected by stroke have access to practical advice, emotional support, advocacy, and information throughout the care pathway and lifelong.

E4: User involvement

Those affected by stroke are meaningfully involved in the planning, development, delivery, and monitoring of services.

Stroke Nursing, Second Edition. Edited by Jane Williams, Lin Perry, and Caroline Watkins.
© 2020 John Wiley & Sons Ltd. Published 2020 by John Wiley & Sons Ltd.

E5: Assessment (TIA)

Immediate referral for appropriately urgent specialist assessment and investigation is considered in all patients presenting with a TIA or minor stroke.

E6: Treatment (TIA)

All people with TIA or minor stroke are followed up 1 month after the event, in either primary or secondary care.

E7: Urgent response

All people with suspected acute stroke are immediately transferred by ambulance to a receiving hospital providing hyper-acute stroke services.

E8: Assessment (stroke)

People with suspected acute stroke receive an immediate structured clinical assessment from the right people.

E9: Treatment (stroke)

People who have had a stroke have prompt access to an acute stroke unit and spend the majority of their time at hospital in a stroke unit with high-quality stroke specialist care.

E10: Specialist rehabilitation

People who have had a stroke access high-quality rehabilitation and, with their carer, receive support from stroke-skilled services as soon as possible, in hospital, immediately after transfer, and for as long as needed.

E11: End-of-life care

People who are not likely to recover from their stroke receive care at the end of their lives, which takes account of their needs and choices.

E12: Seamless transfer of care

A workable, clear discharge plan that has fully involved the individual (and their family where appropriate) is developed by health and social care services, together with other services such as transport and housing.

E13: Long-term care

A range of services are in place and easily accessible to support the individual long-term needs of those affected by stroke.

E14: Review

Those affected by stroke are offered a review of their health and social care status and secondary prevention needs from primary care services, typically within around 6 weeks and 6 months of leaving hospital.

E15: Participation in community

Those affected by stroke are enabled to live a full life in the community.

E16: Return to work

Those affected by stroke are enabled to participate in paid, supported, and voluntary employment.

Index

Note: Page numbers in *italics* refer to figures, those in **bold** refer to tables.

Stroke Nursing, Second Edition. Edited by Jane Williams, Lin Perry, and Caroline Watkins.
© 2020 John Wiley & Sons Ltd. Published 2020 by John Wiley & Sons Ltd.